Atlas of Diseases of the Breast

Atlas of Diseases of the Breast

Synopsis of Clinical, Morphological, and Radiological Findings. With a Consideration of Special Investigation Methods

By Volker Barth
With the Technical Assistance of Manfred Hesse

Translated by Leo G. Rigler and Richard A. Steidl

294 Figures, Mostly in Color

1979
Year Book Medical Publishers Chicago and London

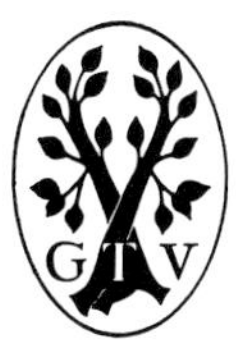

Georg Thieme Publishers Stuttgart

Privatdozent Dr. med. VOLKER BARTH,
Röntgeninstitut, Katharinenhospital,
D-7000 Stuttgart, FRG

Ing. MANFRED HESSE,
Photoabteilung, Katharinenhospital,
D-7000 Stuttgart, FRG

Prof. LEO G. RIGLER, M.D.,
Department of Radiological Sciences,
The Center of the Health Sciences,
University of California,
Los Angeles, CA 90024, USA

RICHARD A. STEIDL, M.D.
Chief, Department of Radiology,
Kaiser Permanente Medical Center,
Fontana, California, 92335, U.S.A.
Assistant Clinical Professor of Radiology
Loma Linda University Medical Center,
Department of Radiation Sciences,
Loma Linda, California, 92350, U.S.A.

Library of Congress Cataloging in Publication Data

Barth, Volker.
Atlas of diseases of the breast.

Translation of Atlas der Brustdrusenerkrankungen.
Bibliography: p.
Includes index.
1. Breast—Diseases—Atlases. I. Title. [DNLM:
1. Breast diseases—Atlases. WP17 B284a]
RG491.B3713 618.1'9 78-23552
ISBN 0-8151-0418-9

Distributed in continental North, South and Central America, Hawaii, Puerto Rico, the Philippines, the United Kingdom and Eire by YEAR BOOK MEDICAL PUBLISHERS, INC.

Typesetting: Stauffer+Cie., Basel, System TXT
Printed in Germany by W. Kohlhammer GmbH, Stuttgart
ISBN 3 13 542401 4 (Thieme)
ISBN 0-8151-0418-9 (Year Book)

This book is dedicated to my wife Christa
and my children Stephan, Christina, Andrea
and Corinna

Preface

"Thorough knowledge of breast anatomy and pathology is a *conditio sine qua non* for the interpretation of mammograms."

This statement by H. Ingleby—made years ago—is still of greatest importance today.

Only a few specialists master both the anatomic pathology of the breast and the interpretation of mammograms. The pathologist considers the breast solely from the viewpoint of the morphologist. Often he is unaware of the methods, goals and problems of radiology. The definitive finding in the histologic interpretation of the breast is the presence of epithelial proliferation, and the role of microcalcifications is secondary. The clinical radiologist, on the other hand, relies on the x-ray film and palpation. Epithelial proliferations cannot be differentiated in the mammogram. Microcalcifications (less important to the pathologist) become in radiological diagnosis a "guiding track" on which the diagnosis of a pathological process can be based. This book is not only meant to facilitate the interpretation of the mammogram through comparison of radiograph and substrate by the radiologist; it is also meant to advance the necessary understanding between radiologists and pathologists and concomitantly to help further the results of the work in related of morphology in medicine.

In radiological work and particularly in the development of mammography, I was greatly aided by the knowledge of pathology and anatomy acquired over many years of study under Dr Friedrich Leicher of the Institute of Pathology at Ludwigsburg. Very early I was allowed to familiarize myself with the problems of the histology of the breast and to learn the interpretation of cytological specimens. After further developing my knowledge of cell morphology at the Cytological Institute of the Karolinska Hospital in Stockholm under Prof Dr Josef Zajicek, I was able to undertake the interpretation of aspiration material from the breast myself.

With the help of my teacher Prof Dr Friedrich Heuck I started in 1969 to develop a plan for the comprehensive diagnosis of the breast. Together with a thorough clinical examination, such diagnostic tools as mammography, galactography, electronic thermography, plate thermography and cytology of aspirates and secretions were used, depending on the individual case. This more comprehensive diagnosis was made possible in great part through the help of the Grimminger Foundation, which gave the hospital the use of their AGA thermovision camera. President Eugen Grimminger deserves particular thanks.

Approximately 13,000 patients have been examined so far by our group. Thanks to excellent cooperation with the surgical clinic, the radiation therapy clinic and the Institute of Pathology, I was able to photograph and present radiologically many surgical specimens and correlate them with the histologic results. For this reason it was possible, together with the pathologists Dr Brigitte Kraus and Dr Friedrich Leicher, to present to the 52nd German Congress of Radiology in Stuttgart in 1972 the results of comparative radiological and anatomical findings which serve as the basis of this book, completed after five years of preparation.

The completion of such a book is not possible without help. I am particularly thankful to my teachers in radiology—Prof Dr Friedrich Heuck—and in pathology—Dr Friedrich Leicher—who through advice and action have pushed me to complete this atlas and through their many proposals for improvement have largely contributed to its final form—concrete and to the point. I also sincerely thank the director Prof Dr Hans Cain of the Institue of Pathology of the Katharinenhospital and his co-worker, Dr Brigitte Kraus, who have given me access to numerous histological specimens and the material for histological drawings.

I received valuable ideas for the format of the present synopsis from Dr Gerhild Schumann who together with Prof Dr Wilhelm Doerr published an excellent atlas on pathological anatomy. She also provided the histological macrosections in this atlas. Dr Gerhard Heller (Institute of Pathology, Ludwigsburg) helped me with the gathering and preparation of autopsy material. In particular he provided me with the pictures of the normal breast. Ms Brigitte Bast gave me valuable help in preparation of microradiographs.

For friendly and professional cooperation with the surgical clinic of Katharinenhospital I wish to thank its director, Prof Dr Walter Behrends, and his assistants, Drs Heinz Fürnrohr, Ursula Gerhard, Gerd Deiml, Hubertus Ey and Eckard Walter, who provided me with surgical specimens, specimen radiographs and unusual medical observations.

I am indebted to everyone who helped me with material collection and preliminary work for this book—to my colleagues Drs Dietrich Bach, Peter Jochman, Hans Peter Maurer and Levente Mitrovics, and last but not least to the remaining associates and technical assistants, in particular Wolfgang Bernhard, Regine Haug, Gila Müller, Brigitte Katz (Institute of Pathology, Ludwigsburg), Irene Kuhn and Anette Robinson; without their help this work would not have been conceivable.

The publication of an atlas with many color plates creates problems not only for the author but the publisher as well, and these cannot always be solved without help. I therefore would like to thank the following companies for their material support: Tropon-Werke Köln-Müllheim, Kodak-AG Stuttgart, Agfa-Gevaert Leverkusen, C.H.F. Röntgen-Müller Hamburg, Siemens Erlangen and Dupont Frankfurt.

Dr med hc Günther Hauff not only sponsored the publication of this atlas but also through personal initiative provided its excellent makeup. Mr Achim Menge assisted me with much effort and patience.

Stuttgart, April 1979 VOLKER BARTH

Foreword

The great expansion of mammography for the detection and diagnosis of breast lesions in recent years, especially its use as a screening procedure for the early detection of clinically unsuspected tumors, has made it imperative that knowledge in this field be as wide-spread and deep as possible. There are a large number of volumes in English or translations which are dedicated to this enterprise. None, however, in the American literature adequately correlate the mammographic findings with the gross anatomy, the histology, and the cytology of breast lesions. This atlas, already a popular, highly-prized recent addition to the German literature on diseases of the breast, contains also extensive demonstrations of both electronic and plate thermography and of specimen radiography and an unusual emphasis on galactography. Superb illustrations with the brief but excellent discussions by Privatdozent Volker Barth will permit the reader to improve his understanding of the significance of the normal and abnormal findings in the mammogram. The book presents a synthesis of the information gained by the application of these various methods of breast examination. For these reasons, the translation of this atlas was undertaken to bring this extensive knowledge to the American physician, especially to radiologists and pathologists and all others concerned with breast diseases.

There are minor differences in the designation of the various forms of carcinoma of the breast. The author, for example, uses the term "simple solid carcinoma" in a more specific fashion than is usually the case in the American literature. The reader will find a few footnotes explaining certain designations which do not conform to the common American terminology, but such differences are uncommon. I am confident that a study of this volume will be most rewarding.

Los Angeles, April 1979

LEO G. RIGLER

Foreword to the German Edition

Technical and methodological developments have improved the radiographic demonstration of the breast to such an extent that mammography is now one of the most valuable special diagnostic examinations in clinical radiology. Based on growing knowledge of the radiologically demonstrable structures, the radiographic analysis of the healthy and diseased breast developed to amazing accuracy. While there are remarkable and widely accepted textbooks by leading experts, an organized short comparative radiographic-morphological atlas of the breast demonstrating macroscopically the anatomical and pathological appearances, the histologic and microradiographic findings and the cytology and thermography either concomitantly or synoptically has been a need. Volker Barth presents this monograph of the breast with this goal in mind.

Comparison of the morphological findings in the radiograph with the anatomic specimen and subsequent examination of the tissues and cells can only be done by who is also knowledgeable in pathological anatomy and cytology. My co-worker and chief physician, Volker Barth, is well experienced in pathology after working several years at the Pathologic Institute of Ludwigsburg under Friedrich Leicher. In addition, he aquired an early knowledge in cytology, which was furthered by his work with Joseph Zajicek in Stockholm. An understanding of cytology was the basis for the development of mammography and supplementary methods (galactography, electronic thermovision and plate thermography, the cytological examination of thin-needle biopsies or secretions) and allowed critical evaluation of the results of these various studies. Excellent interdepartmental cooperation with the Surgical Clinic under Walter Behrends and the Pathologic Institute under Hans Cain of Katharinenhospital in Stuttgart facilitated the tedious work of comparing the preoperative radiologic-morphologic findings with the anatomic specimen and the histological-microradiographic findings. The illustrations in this atlas represent a selection of examples from more than 13,000 patients. The spectrum of morphological findings of the breast ranging from in vivo images to the macroscopic and microscopic analysis of structures may also be considered the basis of the early recognition of disease, particularly malignant tumors. On this basis each imaging system, be it a radiograph, xeroradiograph, thermogram or histological image, is given its place in clinical diagnosis.

Volker Barth's atlas is not only the result of extensive comparison studies but also the evidence of the value of morphologic findings in the demonstration of disease. The atlas not only should close a gap as a reference book, but also will bring radiology and pathology even closer to clinical medicine and will further serve as a valuable aid for the practicing radiologist in the interpretation of mammograms.

I am convinced that this book will stimulate the further development of long-wave x-ray examination. Almost every physician who has already written a book knows something about the fascination of the scientist who, irrespective of the demands on his time, makes personal sacrifices to contribute toward the improvement of medical practice. This atlas will be a success and will reward the hard work of both author and publisher if it becomes a contribution toward early recognition and cure of human suffering.

Stuttgart, Autumn 1976 FRIEDRICH HEUCK

Contents

Introduction

The basis for mammographic diagnosis was developed through comparative studies by anatomists, pathologists and radiologists (SALOMON 1913, KLEINSCHMIDT 1927, DOMINGUEZ 1929, RIES 1930, WARREN 1930, GERSHON-COHEN et al 1937, LEBORGNE 1953, INGLEBY and GERSHON-COHEN 1960, BUTTENBERG and WERNER 1962, EGAN 1963 and 1969, GROS 1963, BÖHMIG 1964, GERSHON-COHEN 1966 and 1970, DOBRESTSBERGER 1967, WOLFE 1967, HAMPERL 1968, BÄSSLER 1970 and 1971 and 1975, OZZELLO 1970, HÜPPE 1970, PRECHTEL 1971 and 1974, HOEFFKEN 1977, PICARD 1974, ANASTASSIADES 1974 and many others).

Radiographs of surgical specimens were made and analyzed. Microcalcifications were of greatest interest (BLACK 1965, GALLAGER 1969, KOEHL 1970, SNYDER 1971, BAUERMEISTER 1973, MENGES 1974). SCHWARZ (1969) and DAVIES (1974) used histological macroscopic slides which were compared with the radiographs.

LEVITAN et al (1964) studied the different types of microcalcifications histologically confirming the presence of calcium by radiography.

HASSLER (1969) reported on "microradiographic" examinations done with 4-mm thick tissue sections of the breast. Of particular interest was the pattern of calcifications of benign and malignant breast tumors. Important information was found concerning the relationship between the tumor and its surrounding structures.

Thermographic examinations were introduced into routine breast diagnosis by GERSHON-COHEN (1965), HABERMANN (1968), JONES (1969), TRICOIRE (1970), VAILLANT (1970) and GROS and co-workers (1972).

The cytological examination of aspirated material from breast tumors was developed by ZAJDELA (1975) of the Fondation Curie-Institut du Radium in Paris and FRANZEN and ZAJICEK (1968) of the Karolinska-Institut in Stockholm.

The high degree of diagnostic accuracy (over 90%) of carcinoma of the breast using inspection and palpation, radiography and cytology applies primarily to larger carcinomas. The preinvasive carcinomas represent only a small portion of the total number of breast carcinomas that are identified. The known typical mammographic signs are rarely found at this early stage. Pathomorphologic examinations revealed that it is possible to recognize certain carcinomas of the breast in their *preinvasive phase*—in other words, to make the diagnosis prior to full development of malignancy (BÄSSLER 1975). *Lobular* and *ductal* carcinoma in situ are considered to be the preinvasive stages of a tumor. Both cause typical morphological changes in the lobules and lactiferous ducts. Under certain conditions these changes may be recognizable radiographically.

In order to diagnose preinvasive carcinoma radiographically, structural changes occurring prior to the known changes of an invasive carcinoma must be identified. This will only be possible if the radiologist has a basic knowledge of pathological anatomy of the breast and is able to correlate it with the radiograph. (INGLEBY is quoted by GERSHON-COHEN, 1970, as follows: "thorough knowledge of breast pathology is a sine qua non for interpretation of breast films.")

Particularly important findings of the morphological-radiological analyses of the breast were reported by INGLEBY and GERSHON-COHEN in their monograph "Comparative Anatomy, Pathology and Roentgenology of the Breast."

The present book is a further contribution to the morphological-radiographic analysis of the abnormal breast. Microradiographs are presented only when necessary to bridge histological and radiographical anatomy.

The normal breast, benign changes of the breast and mastopathy with its extensive radiographic-anatomical variations are discussed most extensively. Such benign changes of the breast represent most of the daily, diagnostic, routine work of the practitioner and surgeon. Our findings are based on studies of 13,000 patients. The cooperation between our colleagues in the surgical and radiation-therapy clinics, the pathology department and the central radiology department was an absolute prerequisite for our examinations. Without the cooperation of the different specialities, it would also not be possible to properly and intelligently treat the abnormalities of the breast detected radiographically.

Examination of the Breast—Methods and Results

The breast may be examined in many ways which may be combined as *extended diagnosis of the breast*. In addition to inspection and palpation, radiographic examination (mammography), measurement of skin temperature (thermography), aspiration of cells with a thin needle (thin-needle biopsy) and open biopsy to determine microscopic structure (histology) are also used. The radiographic examination of biopsy specimens (specimen radiography) is used to localize pathological changes, particularly microcalcifications and enlarged lobules.
Comparison of the radiographic-anatomical image of sections of the breast with the histological image is done by microradiography. Complementary examinations are the filling of the lactiferous ducts of the secreting breast (galactography), aspiration of cysts followed by cytological examination of the aspirate and radiographic examination of the "empty cyst" following filling with air (pneumocystography).

Clinical examination

Inspection and palpation are an integral part of any breast examination. Inspection helps to determine whether both breasts are of equal size, whether there is retraction of the nipple or the skin and whether there are pathological changes in the skin. Nipple retraction may often be seen only when the arms are raised. Retraction of the skin is, in many cases, only noticeable when the thorax is stretched or with a marked forward-bending maneuver to demonstrate the "forward-falling breast." Tumors of the skin (hyperkeratosis and other benign changes) may simulate tumors in the parenchyma of the breast on the mammogram, leading to unnecessary surgical intervention.
Palpation of the breast allows detection and localization of areas of induration and nodules. Palpation is correlated with the radiographs. Generally, a nodule which cannot be confirmed radiographically is aspirated since up to 10% of all breast carcinomas are occult radiographically (Barth and co-workers, 1974).
Cysts, particularly if incompletely filled, may be overlooked during palpation. They are best found by palpating the breast with the hand flat upon the chest muscles. The cyst will slide along the palpating fingers when the hand is tilted.
Palpation of the axilla, infraclavicular and supraclavicular fossae and soft tissues of the neck will detect enlarged lymph nodes. Nodules up to the size of a bean may be found in both axillae in almost every woman. In 80% of the cases, there are lipomas. Lipomas and enlarged lymph nodes can be differentiated cytologically. *Changes in the inframammary fold* are commonly overlooked during inspection and palpation. Malignancies in this region are not rare (Figs **162**, **163**). The area is best examined with the breasts elevated or the patient supine.
Pressure upon the retroareolar lactiferous sinuses produces secretion from the nipple in *secreting breasts*. Five percent of 10,500 women examined by us showed spontaneous or provoked increased secretions (Barth and co-workers, 1975).

Radiographic examination

Mammography

In our own facility radiographs are done with a special, low-kV x-ray unit (Mammomat, Siemens). Depending on the size of the breast, between 25 and 32 kV are used. The maximum wave length in this kV range is from 0.6 to 0.75 Å (Seifert, 1975). This allows identification of the different soft tissues (fat and connective tissue, breast parenchyma, blood vessels).
A special mammographic film is used (Definix Medical, Kodak AG). Developing time is 8 minutes, temperature of the developer is 26 °C (79 °F).

The following diagnoses are made:
a) juvenile, dense, minimally radiolucent,
b) normally arranged excretory glands,
c) involuted with focal opacities,
d) atrophic with marked substitution of parenchyma by fat,
e) benign changes (cyst, fibroadenomas and others),
f) fibrous or fibrocystic mastopathy,
g) malignant tumor.

Typical signs of malignancy in the mammogram are:
a) stellate opacities which are spiculated with retraction of the surrounding tissue,
b) typical localized carcinomatous microcalcifications,
c) non-homogeneous ribbon-like and reticulated densities,
d) circumscribed thickening or retraction of the skin and/or nipple,
e) either increased radiolucency or opacity with thickened pathological vessels surrounding an atypical density,

Routine mammography as part of the routine examination of the breast permits the following:

a) diagnosis and differential diagnosis of palpable tumors,
b) early recognition of preinvasive or invasive occult tumors,
c) recognition and localization of the microcalcifications of benign and malignant epithelial proliferations,
d) diagnosis of mastopathy—recording as well as follow-up of increased-risk patients.

The accuracy of the method is shown in Table 1.

In our own studies the accuracy of mammography, when used alone, is 90% in the diagnosis of carcinoma. Combined with inspection, palpation, thermography and thin-needle biopsy, its accuracy is 95% (Barth and co-workers, 1974).
The number of open biopsies could be reduced significantly with the routine application of extended breast diagnosis (particularly percutaneous thin-needle biopsy). If preceded by various well established methods of diagnosis, such biopsies could be made more accurate. From the original findings the ratio of benign to malignant processes in the biopsy material shifted in favor of the malignancies. According to de Luca (1974) the ratio of malignant to benign lesions changes from the figure of 1:7 to 1:4 following 10 years of the utilization of radiographic methods in routine diagnosis. In our own material the ratio changed to 1:3. For the past two years, however, the rate of benign diagnoses in the biopsy material has again increased relative to carcinoma. This is explained by the selective removal of microcalcifications of which histologically 70% are benign proliferations of the epithelium (for example, with mastopathy). It should, however, not be overlooked that removal of microcalcifications from the breast also eliminates a number of pre-neoplastic changes which, at the time of removal, cannot histologically be classified as carcinomas.

Specimen radiography

Biopsy material from the breast or sections of tissue 0.5 to 1 cm in thickness from breasts which have been surgically removed are examined with an x-ray beam of 15 kV and 800 MAS using mammography film. The specimen radiography is done routinely when circumscribed non-palpable lesions (microcalcifications, enlarged lobules, occult carcinomas) have to be removed. Specimen radiography should prove that the suspicious structures noted on mammography have been completely removed. Using the specimen radiograph the pathologist is able to process the suspicious areas optimally. It seems practical and unavoidable that small x-ray generators producing soft x-ray beams will be installed in the pathology department to make histological examination more accurate.

Microradiography

Microradiography of soft tissues was developed by Goby (1913), Dauvillier (1930) and particularly by Lamarque (1936) and Sievert (1936). The method consists of radiography of a thin object with very soft x-ray radiation using a film with the finest grain emul-

Table 1. The accuracy of the various groups of examiners using this method (from W. Hoeffken und M. Lanyi: *Roentgen Examination of the Breast,* Thieme, Stuttgart, 1973)

Author	Total Number	Number of Histological Examinations			Accuracy of Mammographic Diagnosis (in Percentage)		
		Total	Malignant	Benign	Total	Malignant	Benign
Asch (1963)	500	259	84	175	90.0	86.0	84.0
Buttenberg and Werner (1962)	860	158	–	–	96.1	91.9	99.8
Clark and co-workers (1965)	1580	1580	475	1105	87.1	79.0	90.0
Dorman and Labusch (1958)	157	157	–	–	86.6	88.9	80.0
Egan (1964)	3818	1217	728	489	94.6	97.1	91.0
Friedman and co-workers (1966)	2022	776	233	543	72.8	68.0	75.0
Gershon-Cohen and co-workers (1954)	210	210	47	163	94.7	85.0	97.0
(1960)	1500	536	–	–	98.0	–	–
Hessler and Gershon-Cohen (1965)	213	215	58	157	88.8	91.4	98.1
Kaufmann (1969)	–	619	259	360	56.5	61.0	53.3
Kremens (1958)	1000	372	124	248	62.6	98.8	97.9
Lanyi and co-workers (1966)	440	140	–	–	77.0	–	–
Lohbeck and Frischbier (1966)	–	525	194	331	–	88.0	79.0
De Luca and Wentworth (1966)	5000	700	175	525	–	85.2	–
Martinelli and co-workers (1969)	300	186	23	163	87.1	86.3	–
Muntean (1961)	488	168	79	89	90.9	92.4	92.1
Phillip and co-workers (1964)	50	50	20	30	48.0	50.0	46.0
Picard and Desprez-Curely (1959)	2500	569	430	139	82.2	86.4	67.6
Rogers and co-workers (1966)	3379	1270	441	859	80–88	70–88	76–96
Samuel and Young (1964)	450	245	–	–	82.4	–	–
Skinner (1963)	294	174	53	121	90.0	92.5	90.0
Warren (1930)	–	–	–	–	85.0	–	–
Weinstein and Endlich (1966)	13	13	–	13	92.0	–	92.0
Wolfe (1964)	2000	749	161	598	89.0	92.0	88.0

sion. The radiograph is further enlarged under the light microscope. The following factors play a role in microradiography:

a) object to be examined,
b) quality of radiation using low kV,
c) characteristics of the film or the plate using a fine grain emulsion and the microscopic examination of the microradiograph.

The object
Images of 50-micron-thick cuts of biopsy material are microradiographically produced and compared with the microscopic section. The cuts must be smooth and of equal thickness. Differences in thickness cause variations in absorption of the x-ray beam and may lead to wrong conclusions about the density of the tissues.
The value of microradiography lies in the additional information obtained about the physical density of the different areas (fat and connective tissue, lobules, lactiferous ducts) (BARTH, 1979). The anatomic relationships of the different structures are easier to demonstrate topographically in the microradiograph (because of the increased thickness of the section) than in histological section (Figs **8**a, b, **9**a, b).

X-rays for the microradiographic examination
The special generator Micro 81 (Philips-Müller GmbH Hamburg) is used to expose the sections with a beam of 15–18 kV, 10 mA for 3 to 5 minutes. The maximum wave length of this soft radiation is 0.77 Å. Film focal length with this special unit is 30 cm. At this distance there is no geometric unsharpness in the microradiograph.

Characteristics of photoemulsion for microradiography
Finest grain emulsions (high-resolution plates, Kodak) are used. These are laid down upon glass plates so that it is possible to examine the developed and fixed microradiographs microscopically without additional preparation. The radiographs can be enlarged 400 times microscopically without sacrificing quality because of the fine grain of the emulsion.
Histological sections, 8 microns thick, are prepared for comparison with the microradiograph. It is important to make these cuts as close as possible to the tissues used for microradiography to allow the most accurate micro-radiographic-histological comparison of the structures shown.
Extensive description of the microradiographic method of examining the tissues of the breast is found in BARTH (1979).

Demonstration of lactiferous ducts with contrast media (galactography)

When there is spontaneous or provoked secretion from the breast the duct is filled with contrast medium. First, it is necessary to dilate the opening of the lactiferous duct with a lymphangiography needle. Via a tear duct cannula attached to a tuberculin syringe, 0.5 to 1 cc of water soluble contrast medium (Endografin 50 FL) is injected into the duct. The filling is terminated when the patient complains about increasing pain in the breast which may be evidence of extravasation of the contrast material from the lactiferous ducts into the periductal stroma. Following removal of the cannula from the duct and occlusion of the duct with a collodium film (Collodium liquid) radiographs of the breast (galactographs) are made by the technique described on page 68.
The filling of the ducts with contrast medium permits evaluation of their lumen and proof or disproof of intraductal epithelial proliferation (see page 68).
Galactography is a very valuable method and the only one permitting proof of circumscribed proliferation of the epithelium of the lactiferous ducts in vivo. It is technically simple.
Occasionally, a localized or generalized mastitis will occur as a complication which usually can be well controlled with anti-inflammatory medication (oxyphenbutazone), (BARTH et al., 1975).

Thermography

The heat emission of the breast is determined by its deep and superficial vessels. The heat emission varies individually and may change secondary to inflammation and malignancy of the breast. The thermographic examinations are done following cooling of the breast. The skin temperature can be measured by two methods:
a) electronic thermovision,
b) TRICOIRE's plate thermography.

Electronic thermovision

The examinations are done with a thermovision camera (AGA Sweden). A semiconductor crystal of indium antimonid serves as an infrared detector; it changes its electrical resistance with infrared exposure. To achieve necessary sensitivity, the crystal is cooled with liquid nitrogen. The detector checks the surface of a body in point-by-point fashion with a rotating mirror and converts the infrared into electrical signals to be exhibited on an oscilloscope screen. The result is a heat pattern in black and white; the hottest areas are white, the coldest black. The heat pattern may be photographed with a polaroid film.
Both breasts are shown *en face* and laterally. It is possible to get an isothermal image using a color filter permitting registration of differences in temperature of different areas.
Temperature differences of less than 1 °C are insignificant; those between 1.0 and 1.5 °C are questionable. Differences over 2 °C suggest carcinoma. Also considered symptomatic of malignancy is a hot spot and increased nipple temperature following cooling. The warm nipple occurs with retroareolar intraductal epithelial proliferations and is an important diagnostic sign when electronic thermovision or plate thermography is used.

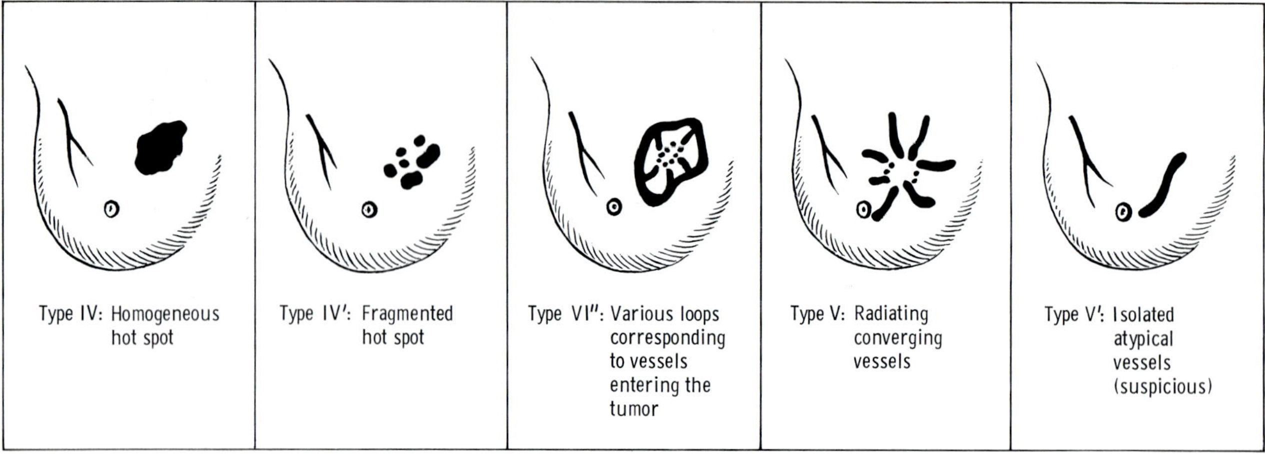

1 *Plate thermography.* Atypical heat distribution and vascular pattern with malignant tumors.

Plate thermography (thermographie en plaque)

In 1964, F.J. Fergason discovered that certain cholesterol crystals have the same ability as liquid crystals to change color following a change in temperature. Selawry and Holland started experiments in 1966 using liquid crystal thermography in medicine. Crystals are painted on the skin of the patient and the resulting colors photographed.
In 1970, Tricoire used liquid crystals on heat conductive foil. Temperature differences of 0.3 °C can thus be made visible as color differences. The different colors range from black-brown to maroon, reddish, orange-yellow-green, green, green- to marine-blue and violet. Interestingly enough, so-called "warm" colors like red or brown correspond to the lowest temperature while the deep blue reflects the highest skin temperature. The color changes occur in seconds. Atypical vascular supplies are recorded. The following diagnoses are made (Tricoire et al, 1970) (Fig **1**):

- I) no hormonal activity (pre-puberty, senescence),
- II) normal vascularization,
- II') hypervascularization (pregnancy, mastodynia, premenstrual syndrome) (Fig **266**),
- III) thermographically indifferent benign tumor (palpable),
- III') cold spot in parenchyma (benign palpable tumor),
- IV) homogeneous hot spot (malignant tumor),
- IV') fragmented hot spot (malignant tumor),
- IV") various loops corresponding to vessels entering the tumor (malignant),
- V) radiating converging vessels (malignant) (Fig **258**),
- V') isolated atypical vessels (suspicious).

The results of these methods for identifying malignant tumors with electronic thermovision and with plate thermography are identical according to our own experience with 5700 patients. The accuracy of the procedures varies widely. Our own experience in all examinations resulted in 20% false negative and 30% false positive findings.

Thermographic examination is a valuable *supplement* to clinical, radiographic and cytological examination. Because of the large number of false negative results, it cannot be used as a mass screening procedure.
Temperature measurement with the thermovision camera is done at the beginning of extended breast diagnosis and followed by mammography. Clinical examination and plate thermography are done at the end. Compression of the breast during mammography and by palpation did not produce a corresponding change in either thermovision image or plate thermography.

Cytology

Thin-needle biopsy of solid nodules

Palpable nodules in the breast are aspirated with a very thin needle (0.17 mm). Non-palpable densities can be aspirated only if it is certain that they can be reached with the tip of the needle. Aspiration of groups of microcalcifications without palpable findings are not recommended because they are usually missed with the needle. Suspected microcalcifications are removed operatively, localized with specimen radiography and examined histologically after embedding in paraffin in serial sections.
After sterilization of the skin, the suspicious lesion is aspirated *without local anesthesia* (edema of the tissue makes palpation more difficult). With a special instrument (Cameco–Sweden) a vacuum is produced in a disposable 20-cc syringe. The needle is placed into the nodule and is moved back and forth several times. Cell material is thereby aspirated into the lumen of the needle. After elimination of the vacuum, the needle is removed from the nodule and the content is ejected onto a glass slide. The specimen is spread out carefully with a cover-slip, and a Pappenheim stain is done. The puncture site is to be compressed for two minutes to avoid a hematoma.
The cytological findings of thin-needle biopsy at our clinic are evaluated as follows:

Table 2. Value of aspiration cytology in diagnosis of benign breast masses (from Zajdela, Ghossein, Pilleron and Ennuyer, *Cancer* 35: 499, 1975).

Histologic diagnosis	No.	Cytologic diagnosis Concord.		Prob. malig.		False pos.		Inadequate smear	
Adenoma and fibrocystic disease	568	491/568	86.4%	31/568	5.4%	3*/568	0.5%	43/568	7.5%
Benign cystic tumors	371	355/371	95.6%	11/371	2.9%	–		5/371	1.3%
Lipoma	31	22/31	71%	–		–		9/41	29%
Inflammation	53	46/53	86.7%	–		–		7/53	13.2%
Tuberculosis	2	1/2		–		–		1/2	
Actinomycosis	1	0/1		–		–		1/0	
Granular cell myoblastoma	1	1/1							
Total	1027	916/1027	89.2%	42/1027	4%	3/1027	0.3%	66/1027	6.4%

* Two cases proved to be fibroadenoma and one fibrocystic disease.

a) no cell material—fat and/or connective tissue,
b) no suspicious epithelium from lobules or lactiferous ducts,
c) inflammatory cells (leukocytes, lymphocytes, histiocytes),
d) proliferating epithelium—not indicative of malignancy (mastopathy),
e) proliferating epithelium with atypical cells and nuclei—suspicious of malignancy,
f) definite malignant epithelium.

The accuracy of cytological examination and the quantity of diagnostic cells depend on the experience of the cytologist and of the physician performing the aspiration.
Tables 2 and 3 by Zajdela and co-workers (1975) show accuracy of diagnosis of benign and malignant changes in a large number of patients.
Despite the great accuracy of thin-needle biopsy, *only a positive smear* establishes the diagnosis of carcinoma. *A negative smear does not exclude malignancy.* This applies particularly when an attempt is made to aspirate a non-palpable lesion.

Cyst puncture

Cysts are aspirated and their contents completely removed. The cyst cavity is filled with a volume of air half that of the fluid removed, and radiographs in two planes are made (pneumocystogram). Changes in the wall of the cyst are thereby proved or disproved (Fig **160**).
The liquid content of the cyst is centrifuged and the sediment examined cytologically. Cytological findings are grouped as stated above (thin-needle biopsy).

Cytological examination of secretions from the breast

Cells found in breast secretion are always examined. The underlying reason for the secretion may thus be determined. Cell-free smears are found in hormonal- or drug-induced galactorrheas.
The smear may also be cell-free with papillomas and carcinomas. *Negative cytological examination therefore does not exclude an intraductal carcinoma.*
Foam cells are degenerated epithelial cells which may form in cysts. If they are found, cystic change of the acini is assumed to be present. Foam cells are found alone or with epithelium from the lactiferous ducts.
Portions of intraductal papillomas are found in small compact epithelial groups with retroareolar location of the tumor. The cells have a basophilic cytoplasm. The nuclei are half-moon shaped and lie eccentrically in the cell (Fig **92** b). Irregular epithelium (with plump cells, often with naked nuclei) and cell groups with hyperchromatic nuclei may be found in cases with atypical epithelial proliferation of the lactiferous ducts, carcinoma in situ and infiltrating male- or female-breast carcinoma (Figs **113** b, **270** a).
Of 319 smears from the secreting breast, 20.6% were free of cells. Normal duct epithelium and/or foam cells were

Table 3. Value of aspiration cytology in diagnosis of carcinoma of the breast (from Zajdela, Ghossein, Pilleron and Ennuyer, *Cancer* 35: 499, 1975).

Histological diagnosis	No.	Cytologic diagnosis Concord.		Prob. malig.		False neg.		Inadequate smear	
Carcinoma	1731*	1526*/1731	88%	53/1731	3%	63/1731	3.6%	89/1731	5%
Melanoma	2	2/2		–		–		–	
Malignant lymphoma	9	9/9		–		–		–	
Fibrosarcoma	3	2/3		1/3		–		–	
Total	1745	1539/1745	88%	54/1745	3%	63/1745	3.6%	89/1745	5%

* Including 36 cases of colloid carcinoma, 3 of adenoid cystic carcinoma and 2 of carcinoma with squamous metaplasia. All diagnosed by aspiration cytology.

found in 64.4% and portions of a papilloma in 5.7%. Proliferating and atypical epithelium was present in 5.7% of the examinations (BARTH, et al, 1975).
The cytological diagnosis of intraductal carcinoma is unreliable. The cytological findings in seven intraductal carcinomas were as follows: no cells in two cases, degenerating ductal epithelium with foam cells in two additional cases and proliferating and atypical epithelium found on the smear only in the remaining three cases (BARTH and co-workers, 1975).
In ten cases with a normal mammogram, diagnosis of intraductal papilloma was made by cytology with only a few drops of secretion. The diagnosis was confirmed by galactography. In two patients the exact origin of the atypical cells in the smear could not be localized by galactography. Repeated cytological examinations of the secretions and repeated galactography are necessary in such cases. Blind biopsy is useless.

In our experience the diagnosis of carcinoma can be made in 95% when inspection, palpation, radiographic examinations, thermography and thin-needle biopsy are combined. These results apply predominantly for the larger carcinomas. Carcinomas in the preinvasive or preclinical stage make up only a small portion of the total number of malignancies. Typical signs of cancer are not present in the mammogram in such cases. VON FOURNIER and associates (1975) detected 3% of 301 carcinomas in the preinvasive phase. Out of 259 carcinomas we examined, 10 carcinomas in situ were found.
The *value of the different examinations mentioned* in detecting cases of carcinoma in situ and clinically occult invasive carcinoma can, according to our experience with 13,000 patients and 259 histologically proved carcinomas, be classified in the order of their utility as follows:

a) mammography supplemented by galactography, pneumocystography and specimen radiography;
b) thin-needle biopsy with cytological examination of aspirated cell material; cytological examination of smears from the secreting breast and of aspirated material from cysts;
c) history, inspection and palpation;
d) thermography.

The Normal Breast

Anatomy

The breast consists of 15 to 20 lobes with a corresponding number of ducts ending at the nipple. They dilate beneath the areola to form the lactiferous sinuses. The lobes are of different size and each consists of 30 to 80 lobules. The lobules are most prominent in the middle and peripheral (near the thoracic wall) portions of the breast (Figs **5–7**, **15–19**).

Mastion

The lobules consist of *terminal lactiferous ducts* and *acini*. A loosely covering intralobular connective tissue* lies between acini and terminal lactiferous ducts and around the lobules and smaller lactiferous ducts. The intralobular tissue is induced hormonally and develops from supporting fibrous tissue lying between the lobules and surrounding the larger lactiferous ducts.

RAHN (1972) coined the term *mastion*** corresponding to physiological-pathological units in the liver (hepaton), kidney (nephron) and bone (osteon). The mastion is the functional unit composed of glandular epithelium, intralobular connective tissue and the perilobular connective tissue*** of the lobule (Figs **8**a, b). Between the epithelium and the intralobular connective tissue there are close functional relationships governed predominantly by hormonal influences (BÄSSLER, 1970; NIZZE, 1972).

RAHN (1972) proved that within the breast there is a flow of secretions not only into the lumen of the acinus but also from the glandular epithelium into surrounding connective tissue. It is therefore believed that there is a fluid exchange between intralobular connective tissue and the glandular epithelium.

In the child-bearing age the mastion consists of glandular epithelium, supporting interlobular (perilobular) and covering intralobular connective tissue (Fig **12**b). Physiological *involution* of the mastion characterizes premature and partial aging of breasts. It begins with hyalinization of peri- or interlobular connective tissue and leads to complete disappearance of intralobular tissue. Atrophy of the glandular epithelium follows with complete replacement of the lobules by connective tissue and fat. The changing from epithelial proliferation to regression dominates breast development not only from birth to child-bearing age to senescence but also during each menstrual cycle and pregnancy. With *proliferative changes* of the epithelium of the breast loose intralobular connective tissue can be found. The premenstrual phase is a typical example for this type of proliferation. Histologically this phase can be recognized by marked proliferation of capillaries in the acini, enlargement of tubules and formation of secretion-filled additional acini. The loose interlobular tissue contains an increased amount of secretions and also exhibits delicate fibers difficult to stain. INGLEBY and GERSHON-COHEN (1960) demonstrated these changes in macrosections of the breast. Such changes also were observed in histological macrosections of our own material.

The postmenstrual cycle of the breast may be used as an example of epithelial regression with consecutive changes in intralobular connective tissue. In this stage there are only a few capillaries in the lobules. The edema is gone; the condensed intralobular tissue consists of thickened, deeply stained collagen fibers. The acini are collapsed; some deteriorate. The residual lumen is filled with desquamated epithelium and debris. There is round-cell infiltration of intralobular tissue.

Interlobular tissue surrounding the lobules coalesces with interlobular connective tissue of adjoining mastions which may lead to extensive fibrosis. If so, it will no longer be possible to distinguish individual lobules by mammography (Fig **15**). Mastion interlobular tissue is denser in the *microradiograph* than lobules with their tissue (Figs **8**a, b). The lobule is radiolucent and divided by mesh-like intralobular connective tissue. If interlobular connective tissue is missing in a mastion, the lobules are surrounded by fat and appear denser. Vessels supplying lobules are easily recognizable (Figs **9**, **10**).

* The term "Mantelbindegewebe" is used by the author to designate the covering connective tissue within the lobule and has been translated as the intralobular connective tissue. It is responsive to hormonal changes much as are the terminal ducts and acini of the lobule. This connective tissue is an intrinsic part of the lobule and of course of the mastion as well.

** The term "Mastion" is not used in the English language literature in the descriptions of the anatomy or pathology of the breast. The term coined by Rahn is, however, fully explained in the translation of the author's description of this functional unit.

*** The term "Stützbindegewebe" is used by the author to designate the supportive connective tissue which is outside the lobule and is translated as interlobular or perilobular connective tissue. While it is a part of the mastion and participates in some of its changes, it is not affected by hormonal changes as is the intralobular connective tissue. The interlobular tissue is a part of the stroma.

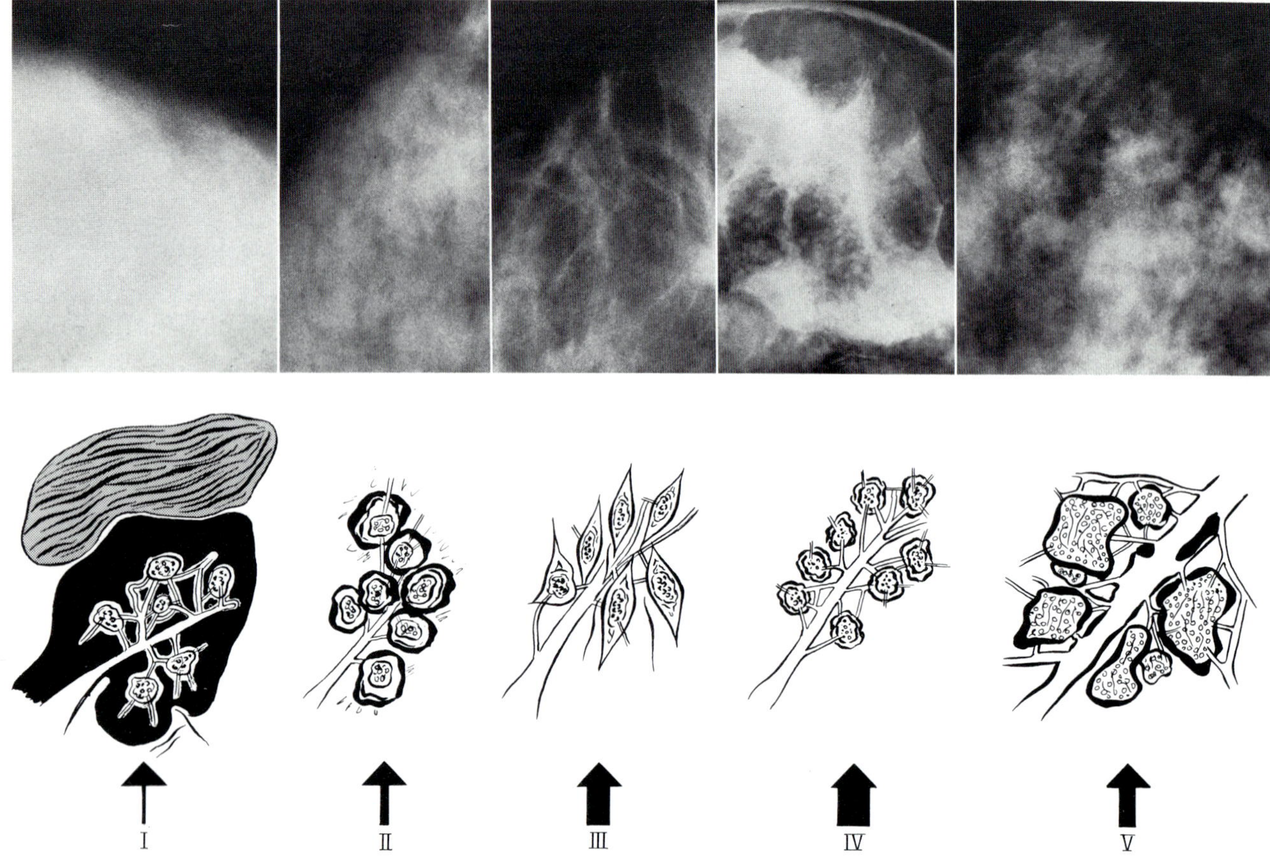

2 Lactiferous duct with multiple lobules surrounded by interlobular tissue of different thicknesses. Ease of recognition of lobules in each mammogram corresponds to arrow thickness. The mastion in IV is the easiest to identify.

I) Mastion with extensive interlobular tissue confluent with the interlobular tissue of the surrounding mastions. Radiographically: homogeneous density (Figs 11–14).

II) Involution of interlobular connective tissue. Radiographically: mastion identifiable as spotty shadow (Fig 31b).

III) Interlobular tissue arranged in form of stroma septa. Lobules lie between septa. Radiographically: opacities with stripe and band shapes (Fig 54).

IV) Absence of interlobular connective tissue. Lobules are surrounded by fat. Radiographically: very fine nodular opacities (Figs 15–19).

V) Irregularly enlarged lobules with little interlobular connective tissue (pregnancy, adenosis, epitheliosis). Radiographically: large irregular opacities (Figs 77–86a, 194, 196).

Mammographic appearance of the mastion is as follows:

a) The individual mastion cannot be identified if its interlobular connective tissue is prominently developed. It is confluent with the adjoining mastions and forms a homogeneous shadow (Fig **2** I).
b) With relatively little interlobular tissue in the mastion, it appears as a spotty, partially oval, unsharp opacity with sawtooth-like contours. The acini lie within these opacities (Fig **2** II).
c) Regression of interlobular tissue to thin septa leads to delicate linear lines in the mammogram. The acini lie between these thin lines. This type of mastion occurs in the involuted breast (Fig **2** III).
d) In the absence of interlobular connective tissue, the lobule appears as a very fine nodular density in portions near the chest wall and in midportions of the mammogram. Its radiographic diameter is rarely greater than 2 mm (Fig **2** IV).

The size of the mastion in the mammogram depends on:

a) number and width of acini,
b) amount and arrangement of intralobular areolar tissue,
c) extent of perilobular stroma.

Lobule changes dependent on perilobular tissue are shown in Fig **2**. Arrow thickness corresponds to distinctness of respective mastion in mammogram.

The studies of Ingleby and Gershon-Cohen (1960) of macrosections showed that with anovulatory menstrual cycles there is no proliferation of the lobules. Lobules may be absent also in fibrous mastopathy, so one cannot expect to find lobules in every mammogram with reduced interlobular connective tissue.

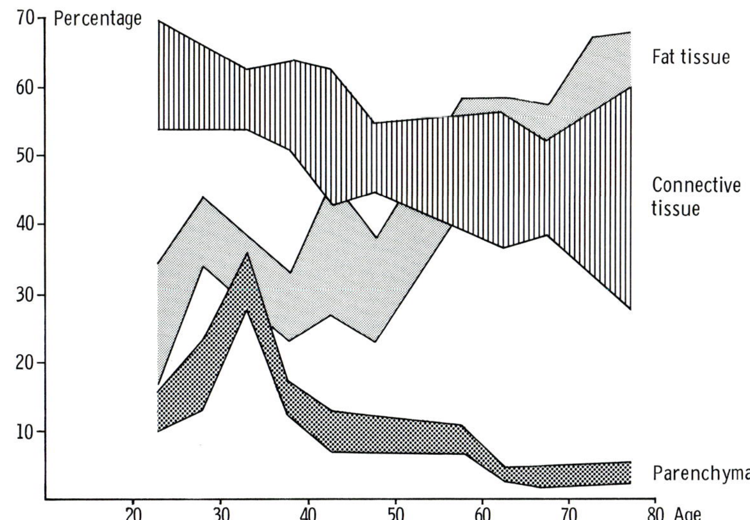

3 Age-dependent progression and regression of fat, connective and glandular tissue. Area determination by macrosections. (From: Prechtel, K.: Fortschr. Med. 89: 1312, 1971)

Development—Maturation—Atrophy

There is significant growth of the breast at the end of intrauterine life. Subsequently the breast grows longitudinally with branching of the ductal system and formation of lobules. These changes are most pronounced at puberty. The formation of lobules begins one to two years following menarche with continuous growth up to age 30, until 15 to 20 lobes with a corresponding number of lobules are formed. Involution of the lobules in the female begins at age 35. Walchshofer (1930) differentiates three stages of physiological involution:
In the *early stage* there is regression of glandular epithelium with associated regression of intralobular connective tissue.
In the *second stage* (ages 40 to 80) there is only a minimal amount of the glandular parenchyma. Interlobular connective tissue is very coarse; intralobular is absent.
In the *third stage* all glandular remnants have disappeared and been replaced by fat.
Progression and regression of glandular parenchyma, fat and connective tissue and their age-dependent changes are shown in Fig **3** by Prechtel (1971).
Regression of glandular tissue and its replacement by connective tissue is rarely detectable mammographically.
There are no significant changes in the mammogram within the first short period after menopause. Patients followed over a period of six years show no structural changes that would suggest substitution of glandular structures by fat. Further experience over a longer period of time is obviously necessary to evaluate regression of glandular tissue radiographically.

Hormonally induced changes of the breast

Morphogenesis of the breast is regulated by multiple hormones. *Essential hormones* are estrogen and progesterone as well as the hormones of the anterior pituitary gland (somatotropic hormone [STH], adrenocorticotropic hormone [ACTH], prolactin). Indirectly effective *hormones* are thyroxin, insulin and the glucocorticoids. Interaction of these hormone complexes regulates breast development. Estrogen, STH and the adrenocorticotropic hormones control proliferation of the *ductal system*. Ovarian hormones, STH, steroids and prolactin regulate *development of lobules*. Experiments on rats and mice demonstrate that irregular and excessive doses of estrogen lead to enlargement and cystic dilatation of lobules and to an increase in perilobular connective tissue. Prolonged administration causes cystic fibrosis of the breast (Lang and co-workers, 1972).
Preparations with a large content of gestagenic hormones can cause changes similar to chronic cystic mastopathy. Duct ectasias with cysts in the acini and accumulation of secretions occur. Large densities, irregular structures and cysts are identifiable radiographically.
Increased density of breast structures in the child-bearing age may be found radiographically following a single administration of estrogen in low dosage. There is a general increase in density detectable only by mammographic comparison over a longer period of time.

Anatomy, physiology, growth, aging and hormonal regulation have been discussed.
The three stages of development as demonstrated radiographically are as follows:
a) juvenile,
b) child-bearing age,
c) involuted.

The juvenile breast

Two to three years prior to the first menstrual period, there is very rapid breast enlargement. Displacing fat, the lactiferous ducts divide and grow into surrounding tissue. Before the first menstrual period, the breast consists of multiple lactiferous ducts and connective tissue with a minimal amount of fat.

Lobules develop after the first menstrual period and are not present before the first ovulation. *Intra*lobular and *inter*lobular connective tissues are differentiated (Figs **11–14**). At the beginning of the third decade, lobules become less dense. During the menstrual cycle they are influenced hormonally and become irregular. Incomplete development of the terminal portions of the gland are common, so cysts may develop early (Figs **44**, **45**). Increased proliferation of intralobular tissue may in young girls frequently cause fibroadenomas (Figs **53**a, **54**) which may regress spontaneously.

The *mammogram* is characterized by well-developed dense interlobular tissue. Up to age 20 the breast is very dense and homogeneous with a relatively high degree of x-ray density. Hence, its structures cannot be differentiated radiographically. A small rim of fat is located between breast and skin (Figs **13**, **14**a). In these dense breasts fibroadenomas can be seen radiographically only if located at the edge of the breast, if palpable or if they cause generalized enlargement of the breast. Such nodules should be checked clinically and cytologically in girls of age 10 to 18. The unnecessary removal of juvenile breast parenchyma may lead in later years to underdevelopment and deformity. The younger the patient at the time of surgery, the greater the risk (Fig **25**). Because of the increased stroma, juvenile breasts are difficult to interpret radiographically, so inspection, palpation, thin-needle biopsy and thermography should be preferred to radiographic examination of juvenile nodular changes.

The breast during child-bearing age

Interlobular connective tissue regresses and is replaced by fat. The breast becomes more radiolucent. At the beginning and in the middle of the third decade, more lobules become differentiated. Their greatest development is during lactation following pregnancy. The outline of the lobules is more irregular in multiparous than in nulliparous women. Ectasia of major and terminal lactiferous ducts also is more common in multiparous than in nulliparous women. All types of the mastion (Fig **2**) are identifiable in mammograms from child-bearing age. There are areas rich in stroma alternating with low-stroma areas in which lobules also are identifiable if present (Fig **15**). In two thirds of all women, the greatest development is in the upper outer quadrant. The remaining third shows equal distribution over the four quadrants. The lactiferous sinuses appear as band-like densities behind the nipple.

After marked regression of interlobular connective tissue, the lobules become located within septa of the stroma (trabeculi). Fine band-like opacities can be seen mammographically, in which is located epithelium with potential for growth. For this reason cancer is as likely in breasts with a large amount of fat and very little stroma (erroneously called "empty breasts" by radiologists) as in those rich in stroma and quite radiopaque.

Toward the middle of the fourth decade along with hormonal imbalance, there is regular growth of parenchyma and regression of lobules and lactiferous ducts. Duct ectasia and small cysts may be seen in the galactogram. This is physiological in this age group.

The involuted breast

The lobules atrophy beginning at age 40 and are replaced by fat and connective tissue. Two forms are differentiated radiographically:

a) Rich in fat with multiple *fine septae*. Mammograms of this type of breast are relatively easy to interpret. Carcinomas measuring 2 to 3 mm may be diagnosed (Fig **119**). Potentially malignant, markedly atrophic, lobular parenchyma may be present in the delicate septae. Serial survey mammography therefore is indicated in the atrophic breast.
b) Replacement of parenchyma of the lobules by connective tissue may lead to a *homogeneous fibrosis* of the breast. Focal or diffuse densities are noted radiographically. There is dilatation of lactiferous ducts and formation of small cysts within the atrophic lobules which, if there is secretion, can be demonstrated on the galactogram (Figs **20**, **21**). The conversion of "small-cystic breast fibrosis" to fibrocystic mastopathy is continuous and often can only be differentiated histologically.

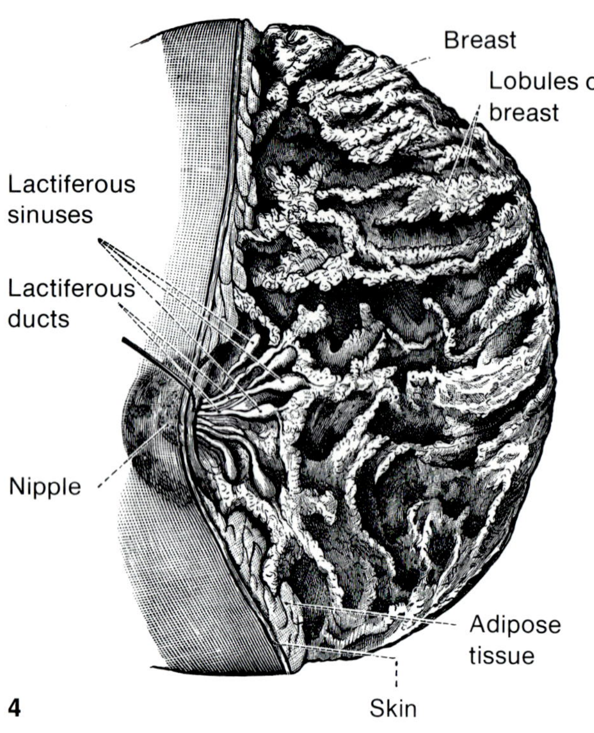

4

4 Breast during lactation. Half of the skin and subcutaneous fat has been removed. Lactiferous ducts with sinuses (ampullae) and lobes are exposed. (From Toldt and Hochstetter: Anatomischer Atlas, Band II, Urban und Schwarzenberg, München 1961).

5 *Galactogram* of lactiferous duct and two lobes. Lobules appear within the lobes as multiple small nonhomogeneous, unsharp densities of marked contrast. Interlobular supporting connective tissue lies between lobules (nonopacified areas).

6 a, b. *Histology*, magnif 40×.

a) Lobules with branching ducts and tubulo-alveolar end portions. Many small myoepithelial cells lie between perilobular fat.

b) Large lactiferous duct with some secretions. Periductal (interlobular) loose connective tissue.

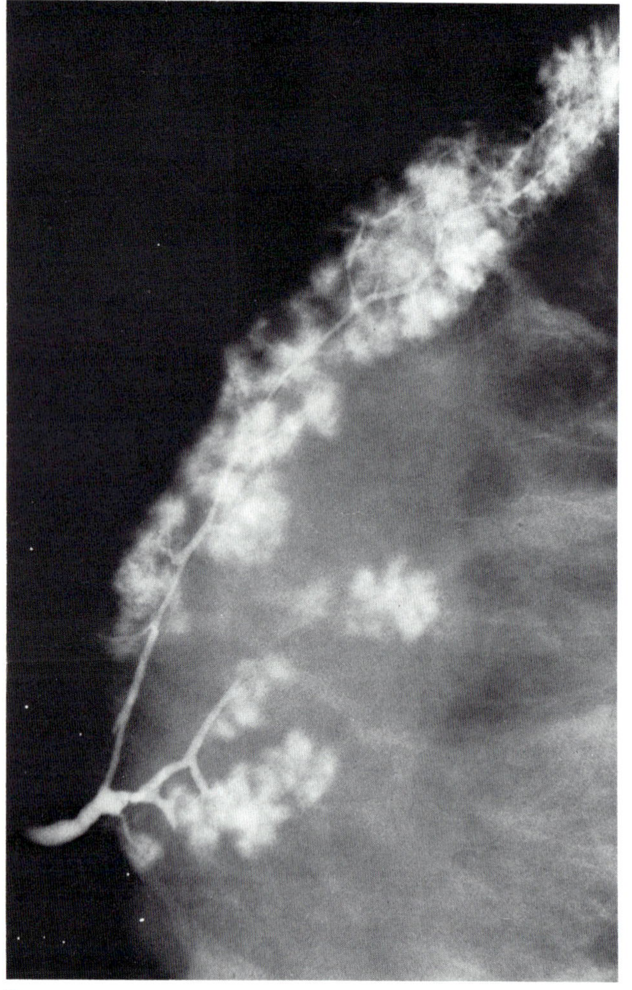

5

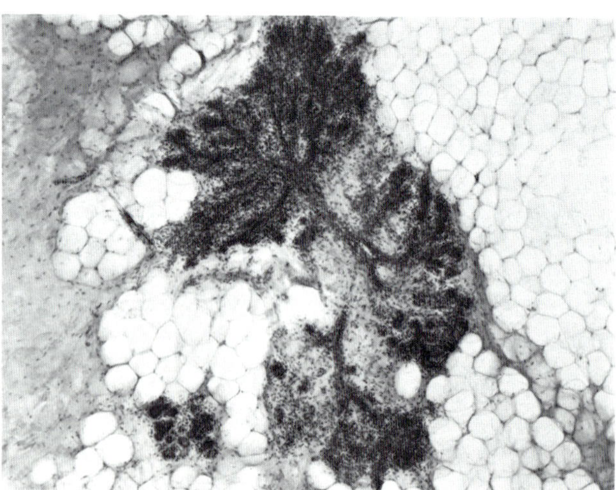

6a

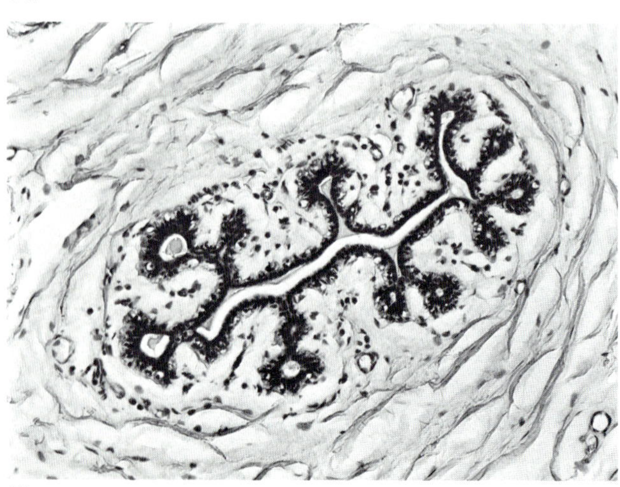

6b

7 36-year-old female, two pregnancies. *Galactogram,* magnif 2×.
Multiple, contrast-filled lactiferous ducts surrounded by small, less radiopaque lobules. Perilobular connective tissue lies between.

8 a, b. Terminal lactiferous ducts and lobules.
Microradiographic-histological comparison, magnif 80×.
a) Lobules (3—dark areas) consisting of acini, terminal lactiferous ducts and intralobular tissue (mesh-like densities). Perilobular connective tissue (1—clear), with lactiferous ducts (2) passing through. Terminal lactiferous ducts lie in a mesh-like fashion in the lobules (upper edge).
b) Histology. Lactiferous ducts with several partially atrophic and microcystically changed lobules. Little *intra*lobular connective tissue. Sclerosing and partially hyalinized *inter*lobular connective tissue.

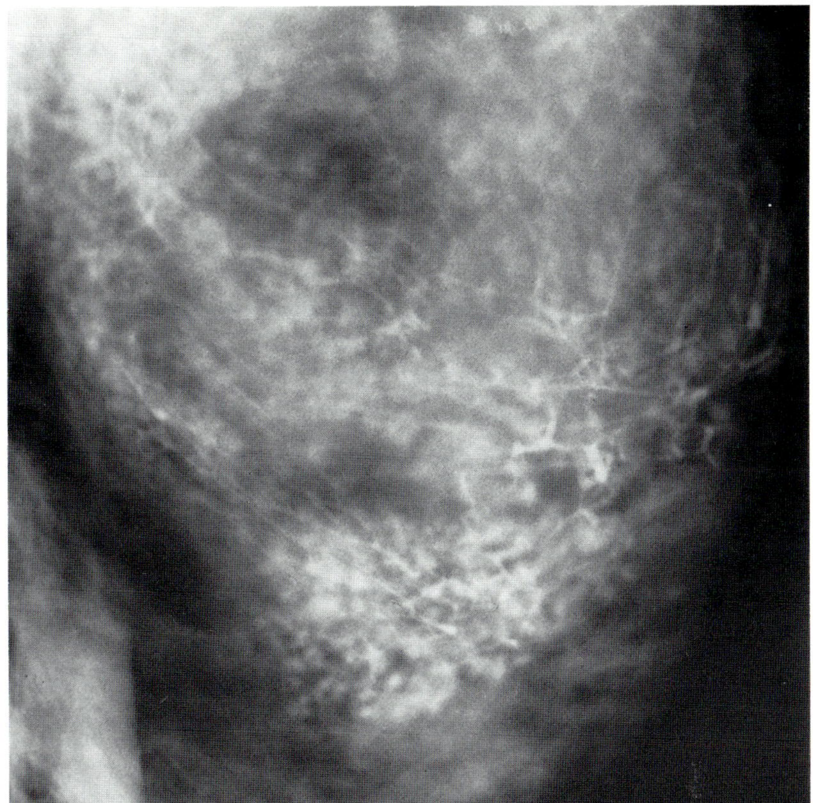
7

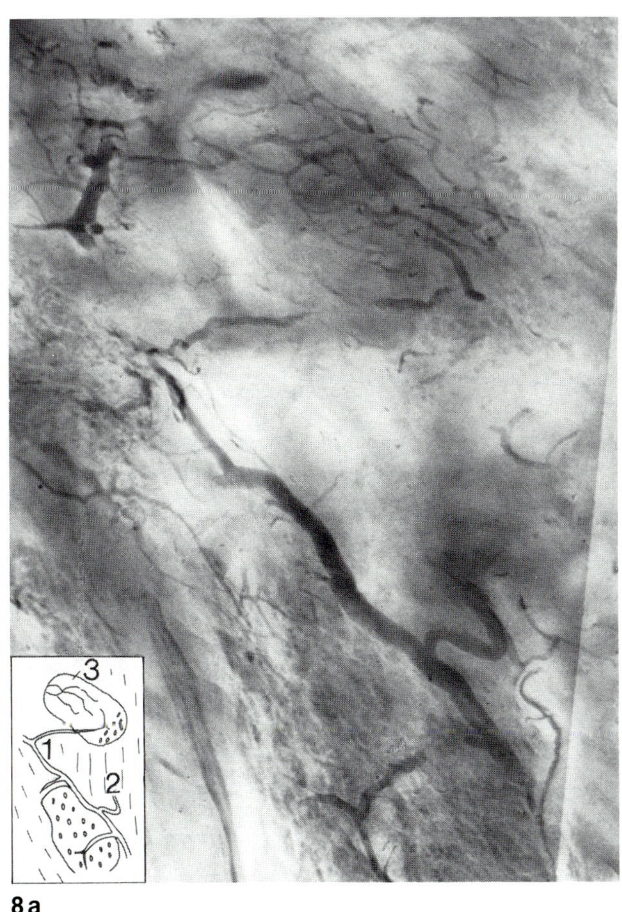

8a

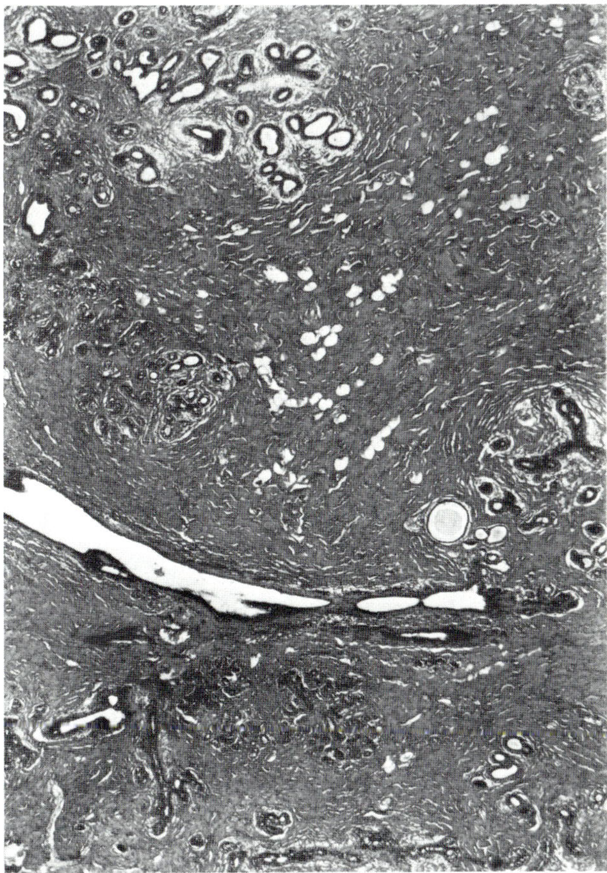
8b

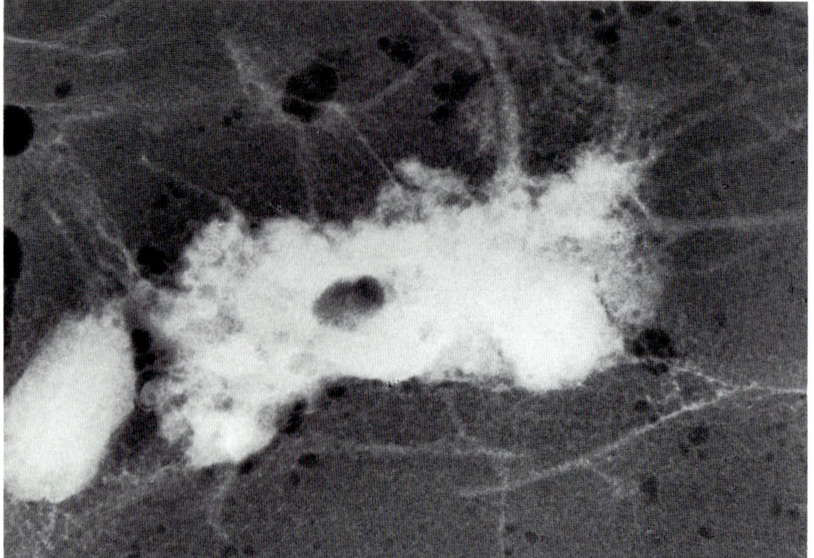

9a

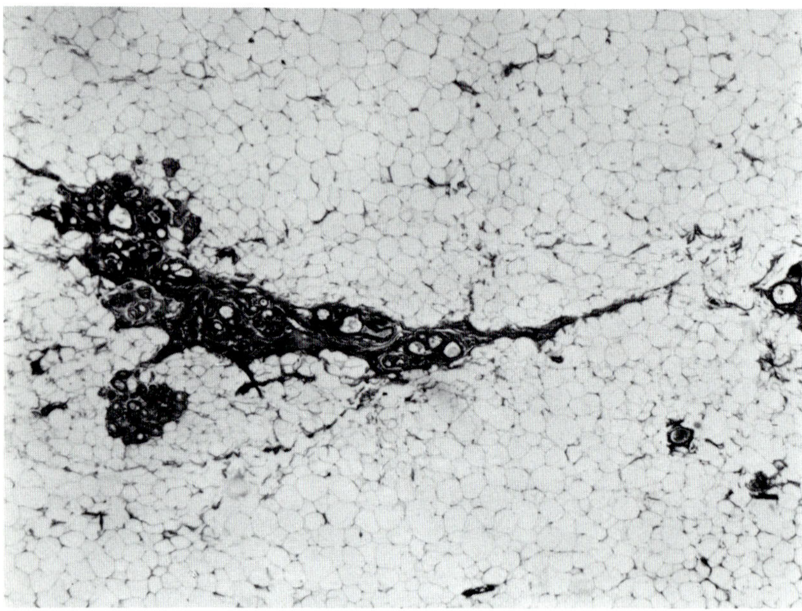

9b

9 a, b. Mastion with diminished perilobular tissue.
Microradiographic-histologic comparison, magnif 80×.

a) Nonhomogeneous, irregular, well-defined opacity with central lucency due to dilated lactiferous duct. Next to it fat with supplying blood vessels.

b) Island of stroma with many small, partially microcystic lobules. Perilobular adipose tissue.

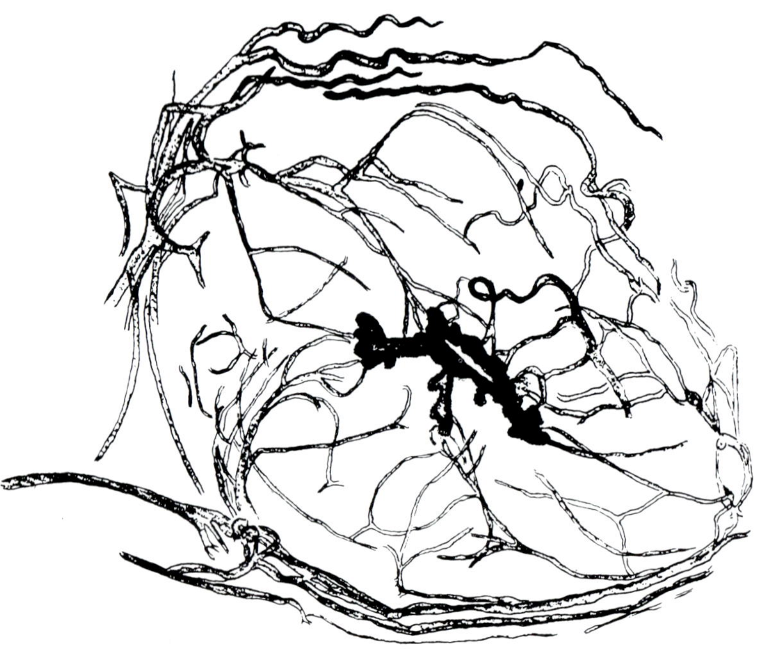

10 Vascular supply of a lobule (center) by extensive capillaries (From Ingleby and Gershon-Cohen, 1960).

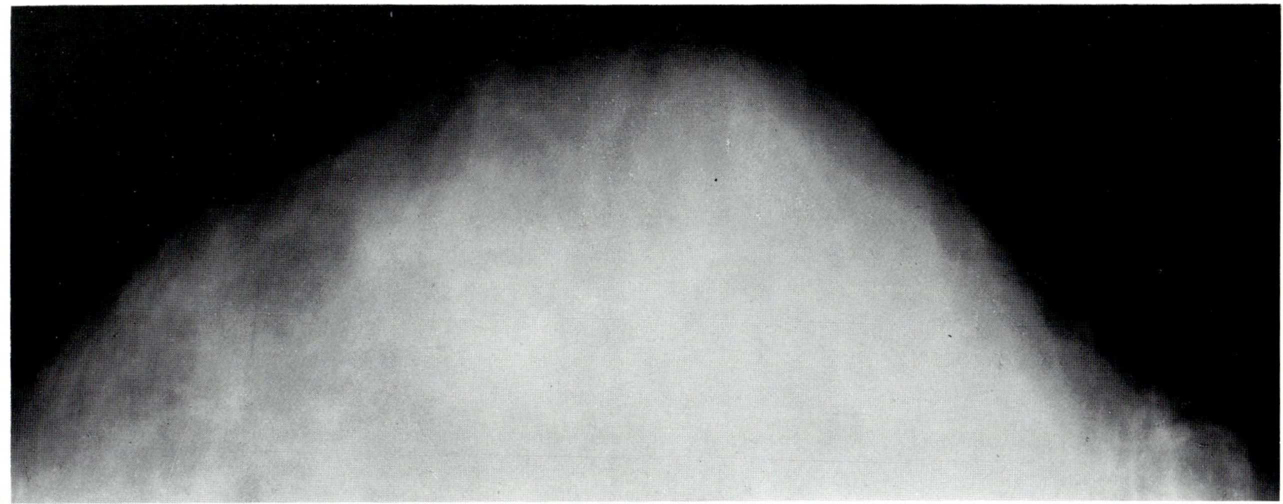
11

18-year-old female, right breast. Bilateral mastectomy because of marked carcinophobia (Figs 11–14).

11 *Mammogram* (cranio-caudal). Homogeneous, dense, slightly radiolucent breast with increased fat deposition in the inner quadrant (left).

12 a, b. *Cytology and histology.*
a) Specimen of thin-needle biopsy consisting of compact epithelial lining from a lobule. Nuclei of different sizes. Delicate rim of cytoplasm. A large fat cell lies above the epithelium.
b) Histology, magnif 40×. Markedly developed loose interlobular connective tissue, a lactiferous duct (near top), 4 lobules. Within the lobules extensive intralobular tissue with terminal lactiferous ducts. Acini are not yet present.

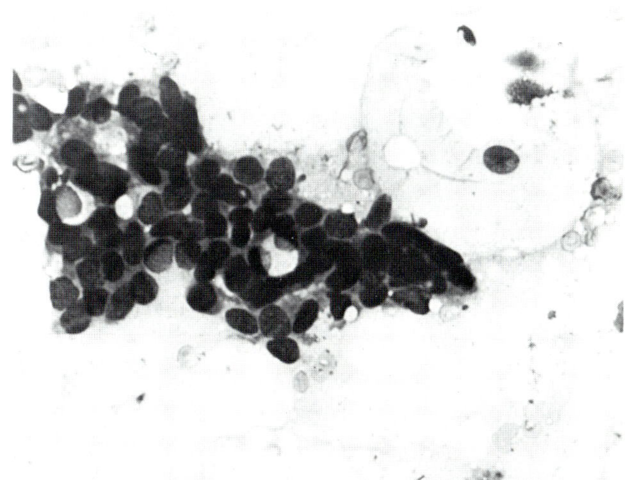
12 a

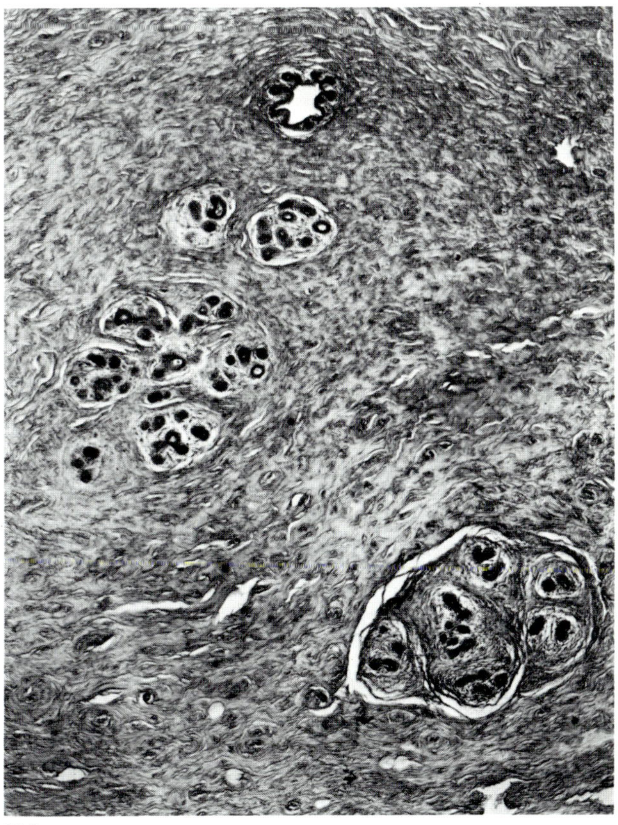
12 b

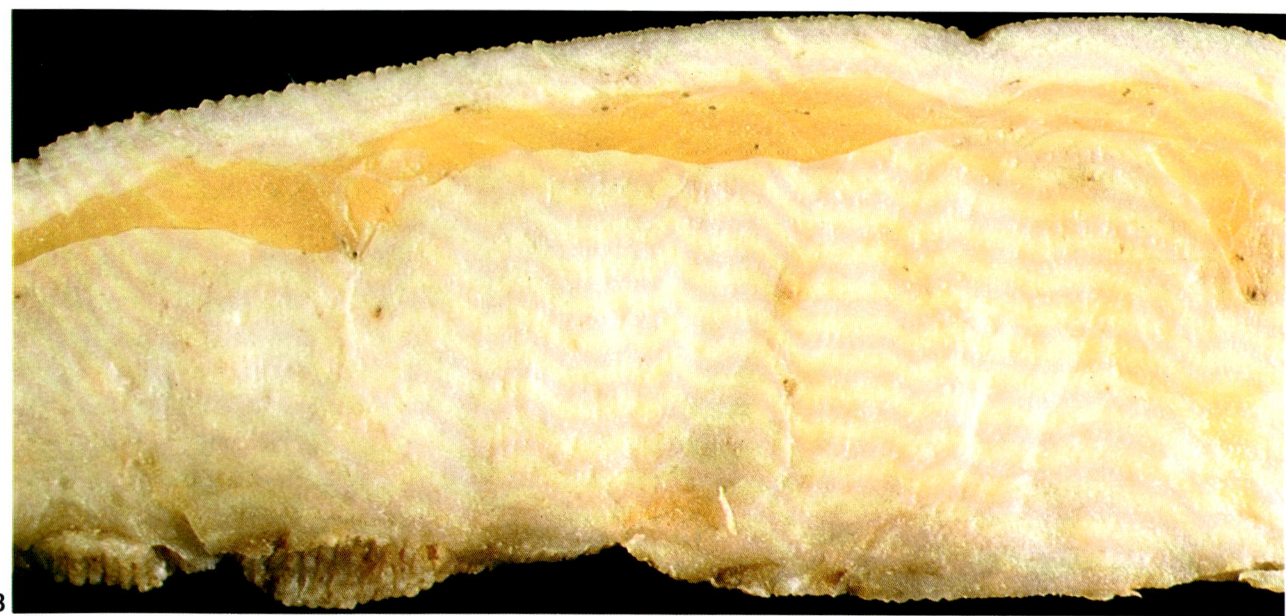
13

13 *Macroscopic view* of the cut surface. Skin, subcutaneous rim of fat, gray-white breast. Individual lactiferous ducts and blood vessels in cross section.

14 a, b. *Histological-radiological comparison.*
a) Histological macrosection. Markedly developed interlobular connective tissue with lobules varying in size. Beginning infiltration of fat on right side and center.
b) Specimen radiograph. Subcutaneous fat, radiolucent. Breast homogeneously radiopaque. Areas with an increased amount of fat are more radiolucent.

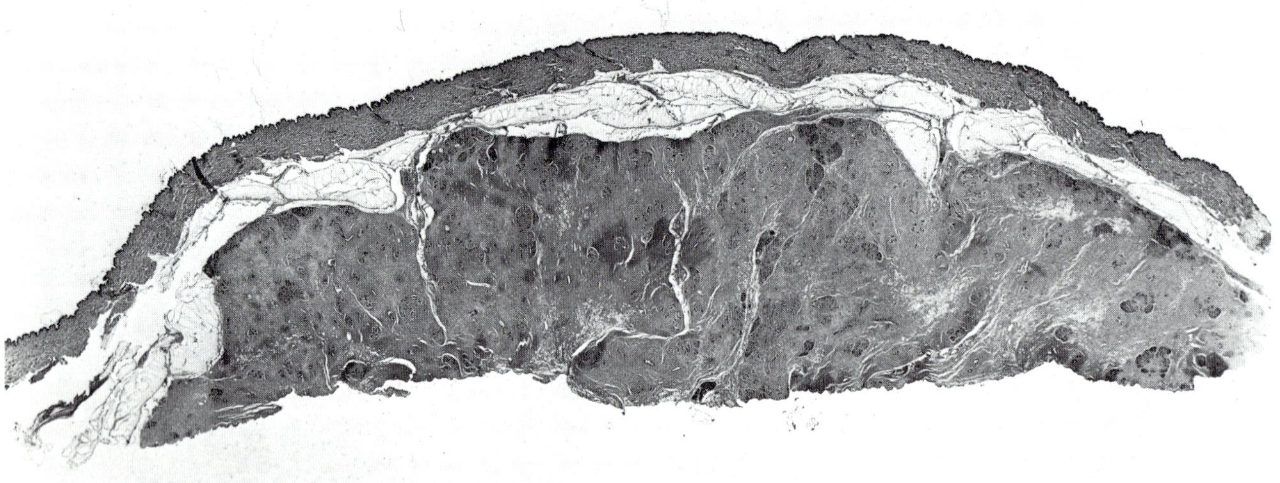
14 a

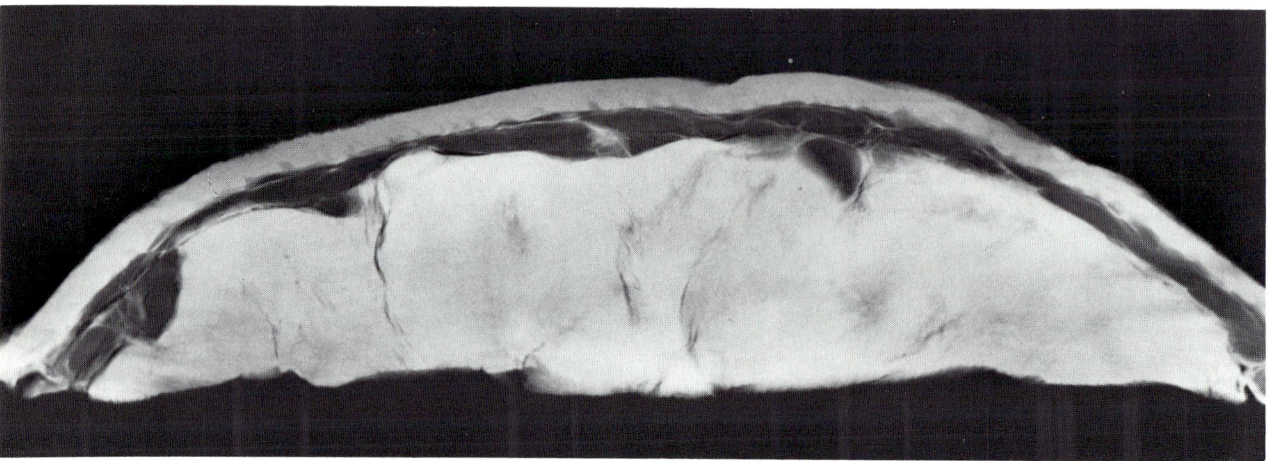
14 b

28-year-old female, two pregnancies, right breast (Figs 15–19).

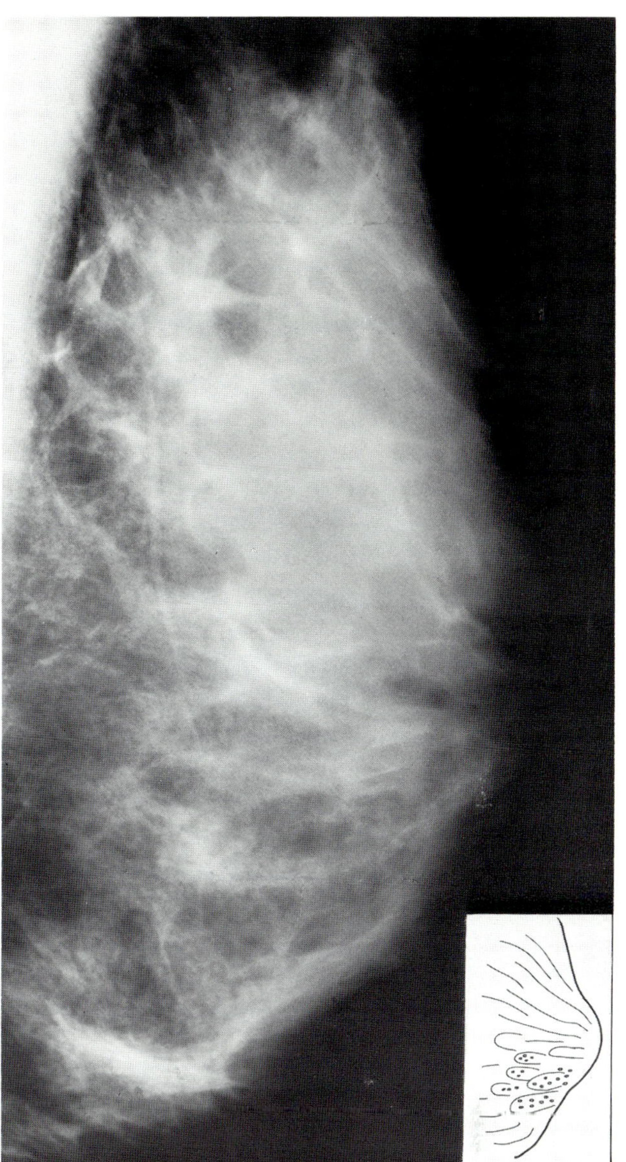

15 *Mammogram.* Lateral view, medio-lateral projection. Upper quadrants are radiopaque because of a large amount of interlobular tissue. Much less interlobular tissue in the lower quadrants. Lobules appear as very fine nodular opacities.

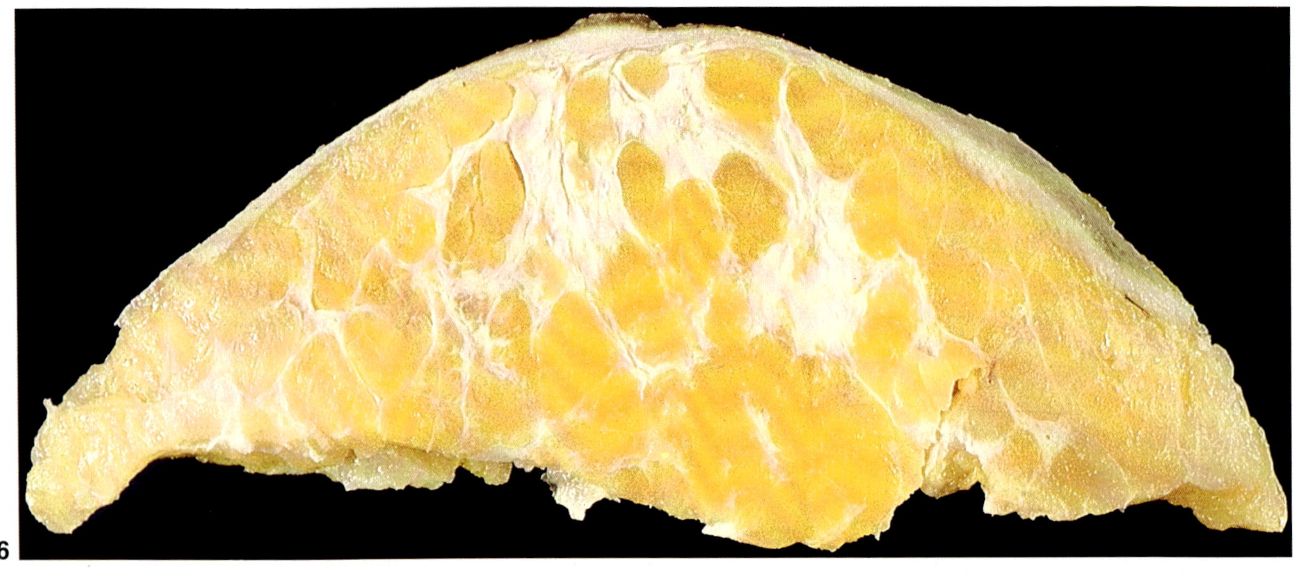

16

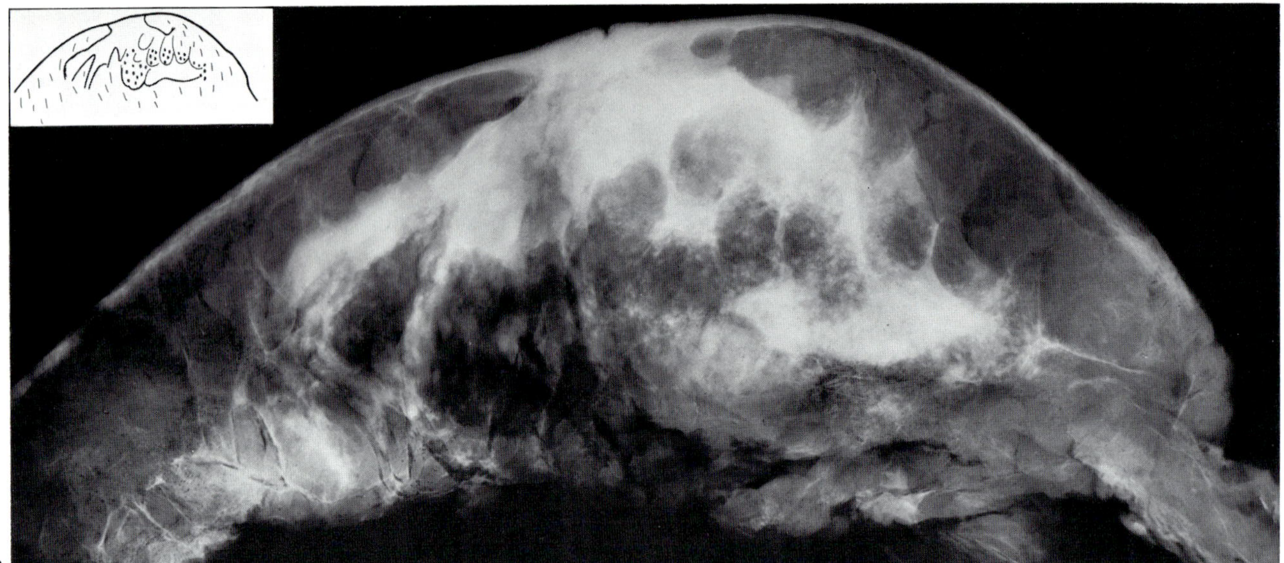

17a

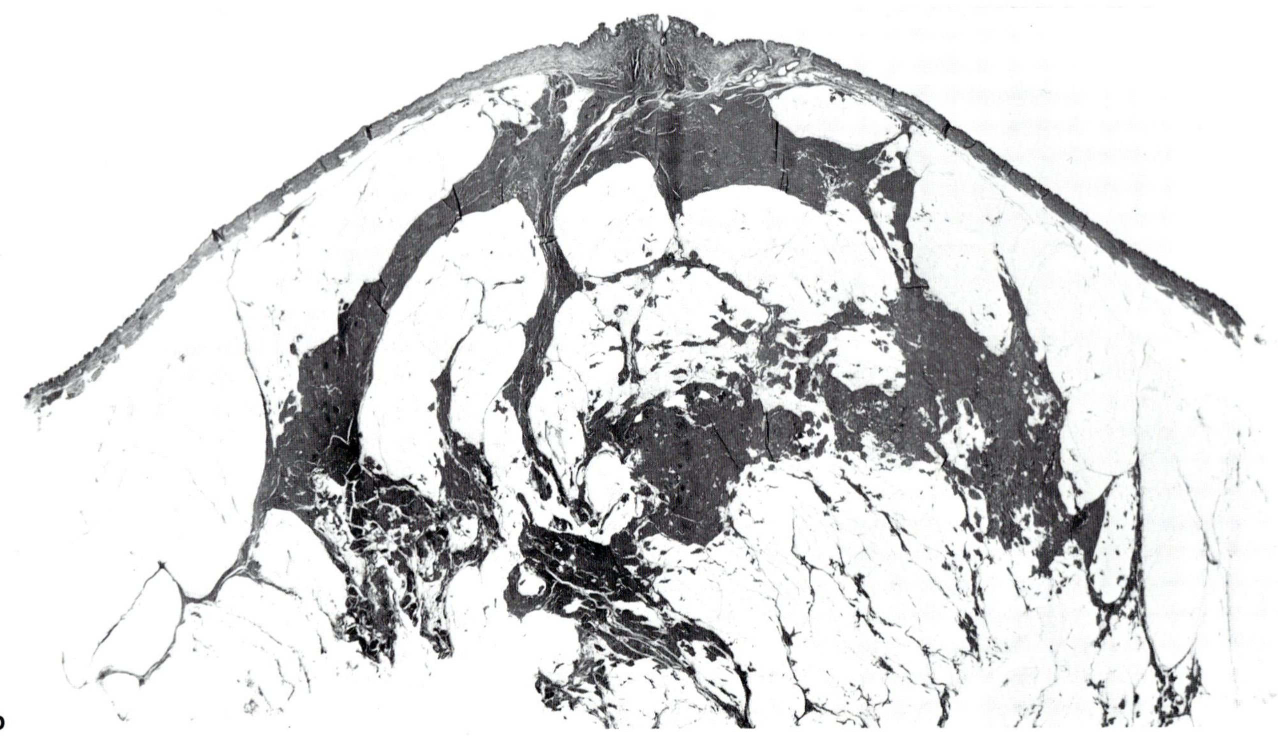

17b

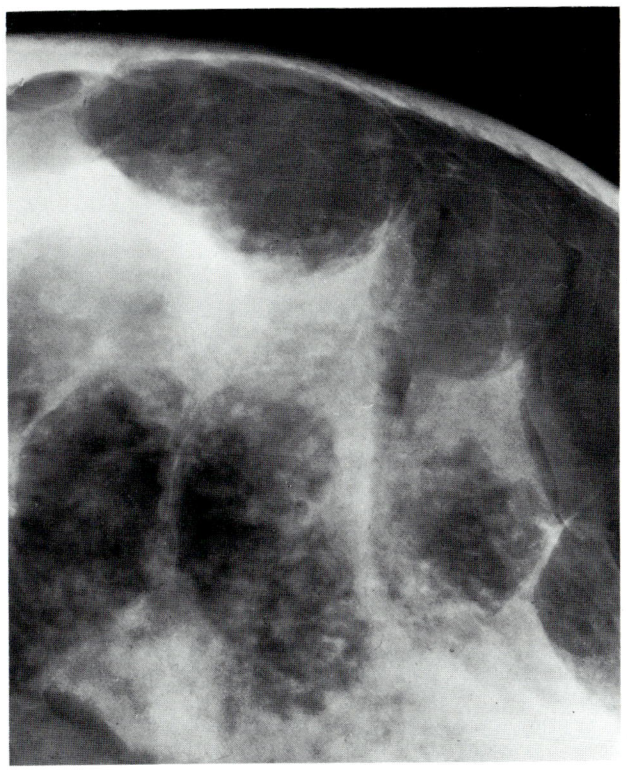

18a

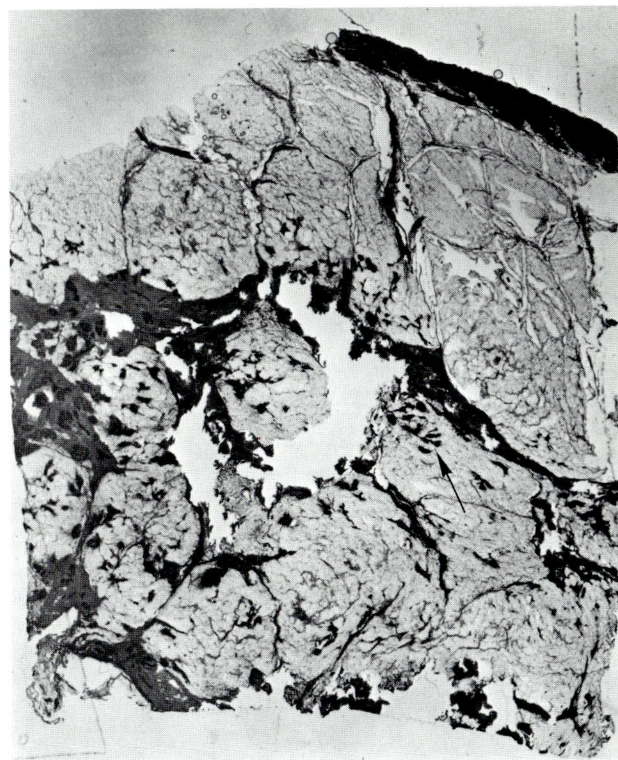

18b

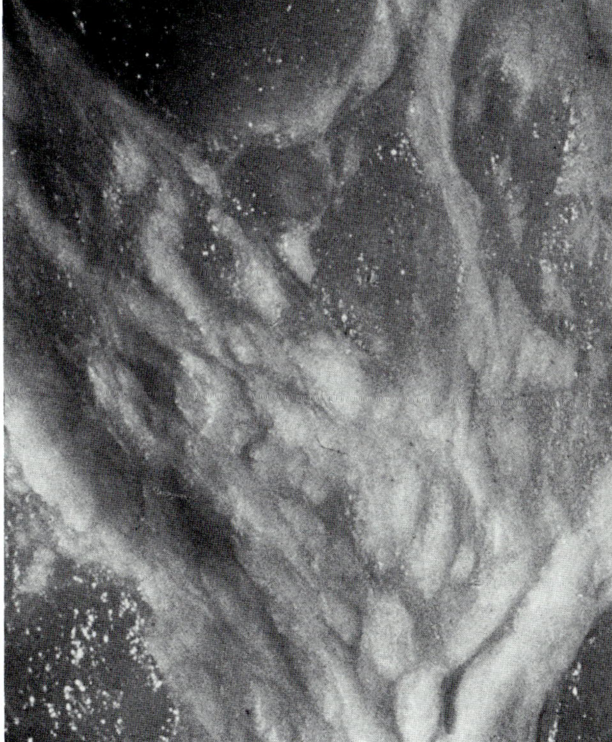

18c

19

◁ **16** *Cut surface of the surgical specimen.* Several lobes are surrounded by fat. Lobules appear as gray-white spots within the lobes (compare with Fig 18c).

◁ **17** a, b. *Radiological-anatomic comparison.*
a) Specimen radiograph. Lobes are demonstrated as non-homogeneous, band-like opacities. Fine, fleck-like opacities represent lobules (compare with Fig 18a).
b) Histological macrosection, magnif 2×. Broad bands and opacities representing stroma, lactiferous ducts and blood vessels. Minute lobules surrounded by fat in periphery and center (compare with Fig 18b).

18 a-c. Lobe and lobules. Enlargement of sections of Figs 16 and 17.
a) *Specimen radiograph.* Band-shaped opacities (interlobular tissue) surrounded by very fine nodular densities (lobules), magnif 5×.
b) *Histological macrosection.* Connective tissue trabeculi connected with the skin by Cooper's ligaments. Lactiferous ducts and lobules are located in the trabeculi as well as surrounding fat (compare with Fig 19) (magnif 5×).
c) *Anatomy of cut surface.* Lobules (oval) next to band-like septa of stroma surrounded by fat (magnif 10×).

19 *Histological section* of Fig 18b, magnif 60×. Lobule surrounded by fat without perilobular connective tissue. Sclerotic intralobular connective tissue with lactiferous ducts and acini.

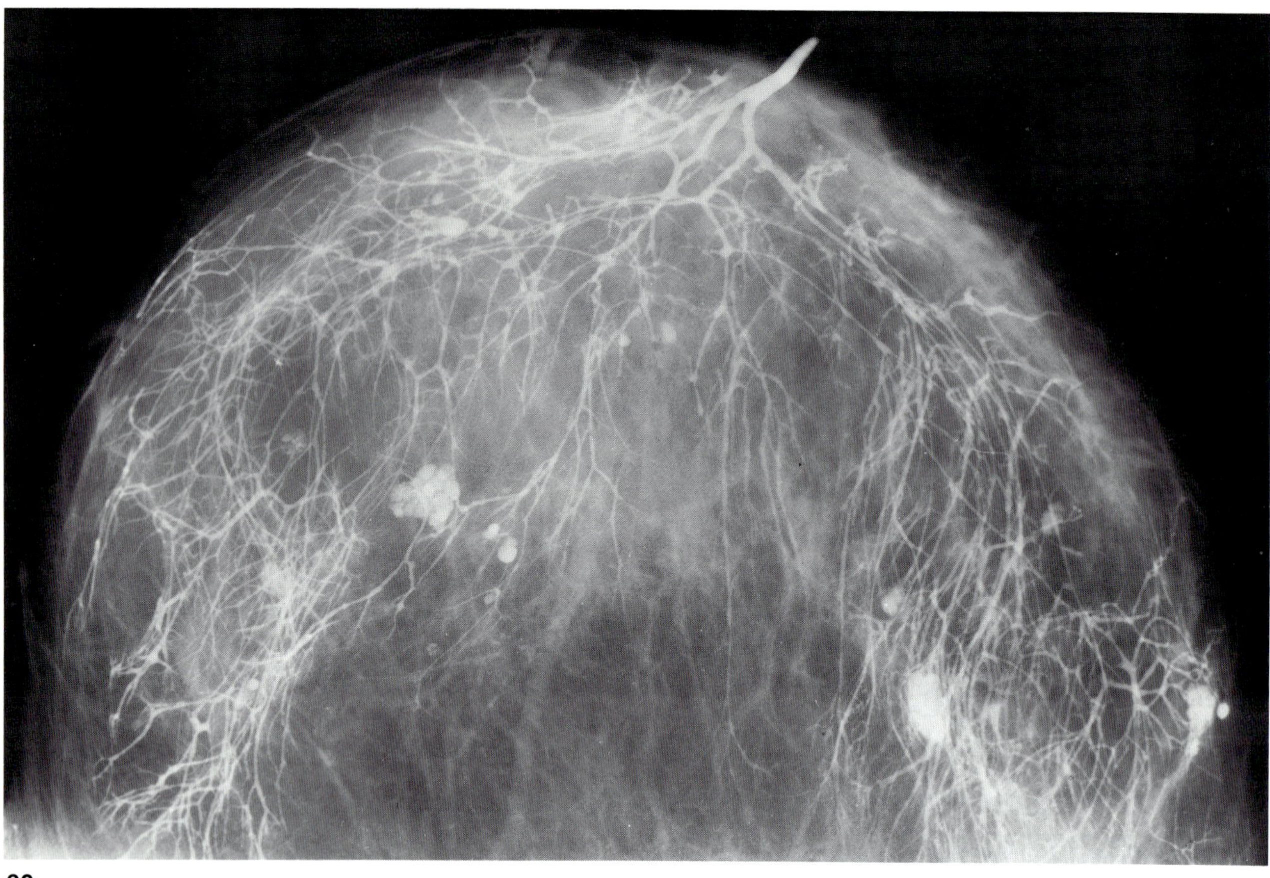

20

58-year-old female, right breast. Minimal serous secretion (Figs 20–22).

20 *Galactography.* Multiple delicate lactiferous ducts with circumscribed dilatations and conglomerations of cysts in the periphery (area of involuted lobules).

21 *Anatomic specimen,* magnif 5×. Dilated lactiferous ducts with cystic changes. Below are ducts of normal width.

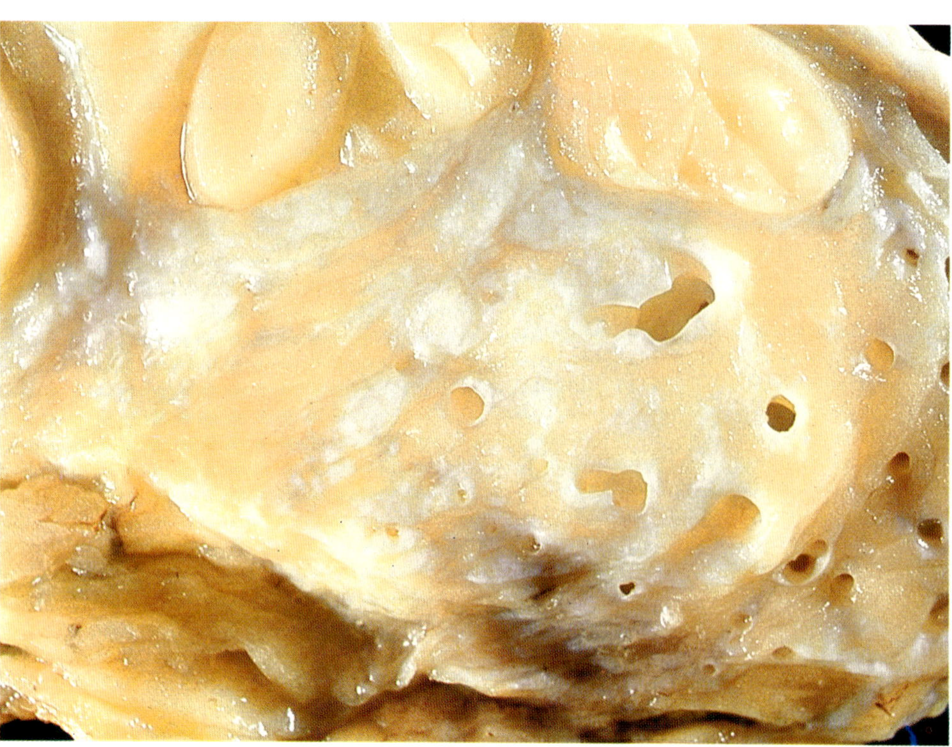

21

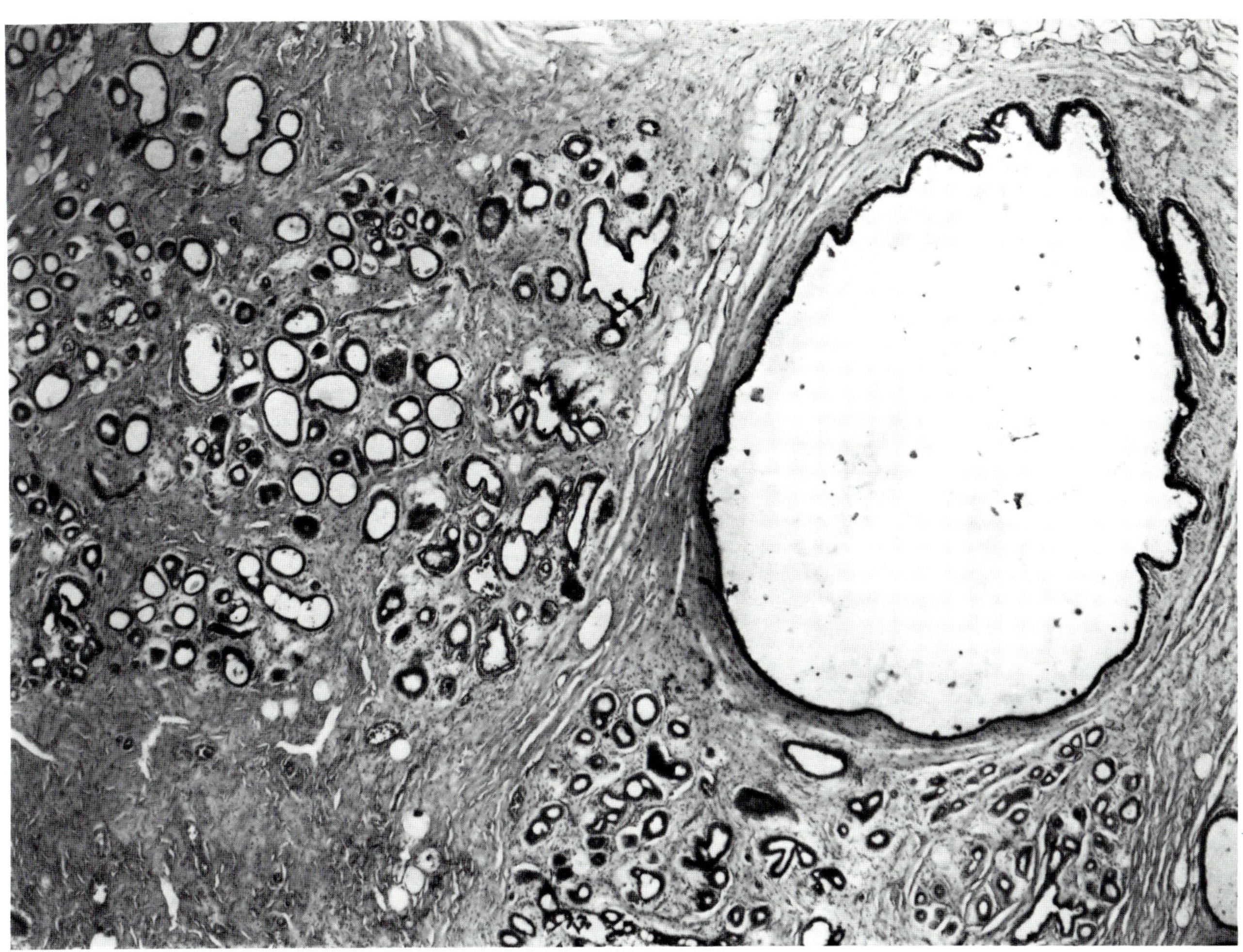

22 *Histology.* Dilated lactiferous duct (right side) with periductal fibrosis. Microcystic changes of acini. Enlargement and fibrosis of intralobular connective tissue with fragmentation of acini.

Congenital Anomalies

Accessory breast

Accessory breast parenchyma is common. It is found along the milk line but may also appear in the neck, chin, ear, trunk and upper arm. The most common location is the axilla, where it is almost always bilateral. Nipple and areola are absent most of the time. A lactiferous duct going directly to the skin may be present.

A 28-year-old patient had ectopic breast tissue in the left axilla with a lactiferous duct ending in this area. There was swelling of the parenchyma in the axilla during pregnancy. There was extensive secretion of milk during lactation from this accessory breast. Following the end of lactation, the secretion of milk and swelling of the accessory breast in the left axilla disappeared. Occasionally a minimal amount of secretion from the ectopic lactiferous duct was noted.

The accessory breast tissue is seen radiographically in the axillary extension (Fig **23**). Diseases appear in the accessory breast tissue in the same manner as in the normally placed breast. The accessory tissue reacts like the ordinary breast to hormonal changes (changes during menstrual cycle or during pregnancy).
It is believed that there is an increased tendency to tumor formation in the accessory breast. In two thirds of the cases, the tumor is a carcinoma; a fibroadenoma in the remaining third (Klose and Sebening, 1941). The therapeutic conclusion from these findings (Schwaiger and Herfarth, 1967) is that accessory breasts should be surgically removed in all cases.

Anomalies of the nipple and lactiferous ducts

Flat and inverted nipples are common and must be differentiated from the usually unilateral nipple retraction of carcinoma. The inverted nipple should have been present since early childhood to justify such a diagnosis. *Inward rotation of both nipples* is rare. It was seen only once in 13,000 examinations. This patient also had a pterygium colli (Fig **30**).

Hypertrophy

Hypertrophy of one or both breasts is found at an early age as an individual or familial maldevelopment, but also may occur with corpus luteum cysts of the ovary. Hormonal influence in idiopathic uni- or bilateral hypertrophy of the female breast has not been proven. In the mammogram, the glandular parenchyma is distributed as spotty opacities within the extensive fat tissue in the breast. Partial removal of the breast may be indicated as patients suffer psychologically from the hypertrophy and also complain about back pain and drawing pain in the axillae because of the increased weight of the breasts (Figs **29** a, b).

Hypoplasia

Reduction in size of one or both breasts may be idiopathic. It also can result from operative intervention between ages four and eight because of unilateral juvenile hypertrophy, from fibroadenomas between ages 12 and 16 (Figs **25**, **26**) and from juvenile cysts.

Ectopic lactiferous ducts

Normally 12 to 15 lactiferous ducts end at the nipple. If the retroareolar lactiferous sinuses join, there may be a smaller number. Occasionally there is only a single lactiferous duct present. But lactiferous ducts may end at the nipple as well as the areola.

In a 15-year-old patient, there was in the lateral region of the right areola an ectopic lactiferous duct with intermittent secretion. The secretion ceased for a few weeks. Subsequently a painless retroareolar nodule appeared, which consisted of a multichambered cyst corresponding to a rudimentary lobule. A lentil-size, blue-tinged hemangioma of the skin of the areola was incidentally noted next to the ectopic lactiferous duct (Figs **44**, **46**).

39-year-old female, left breast. Swelling of the left axilla (Figs 23–24).

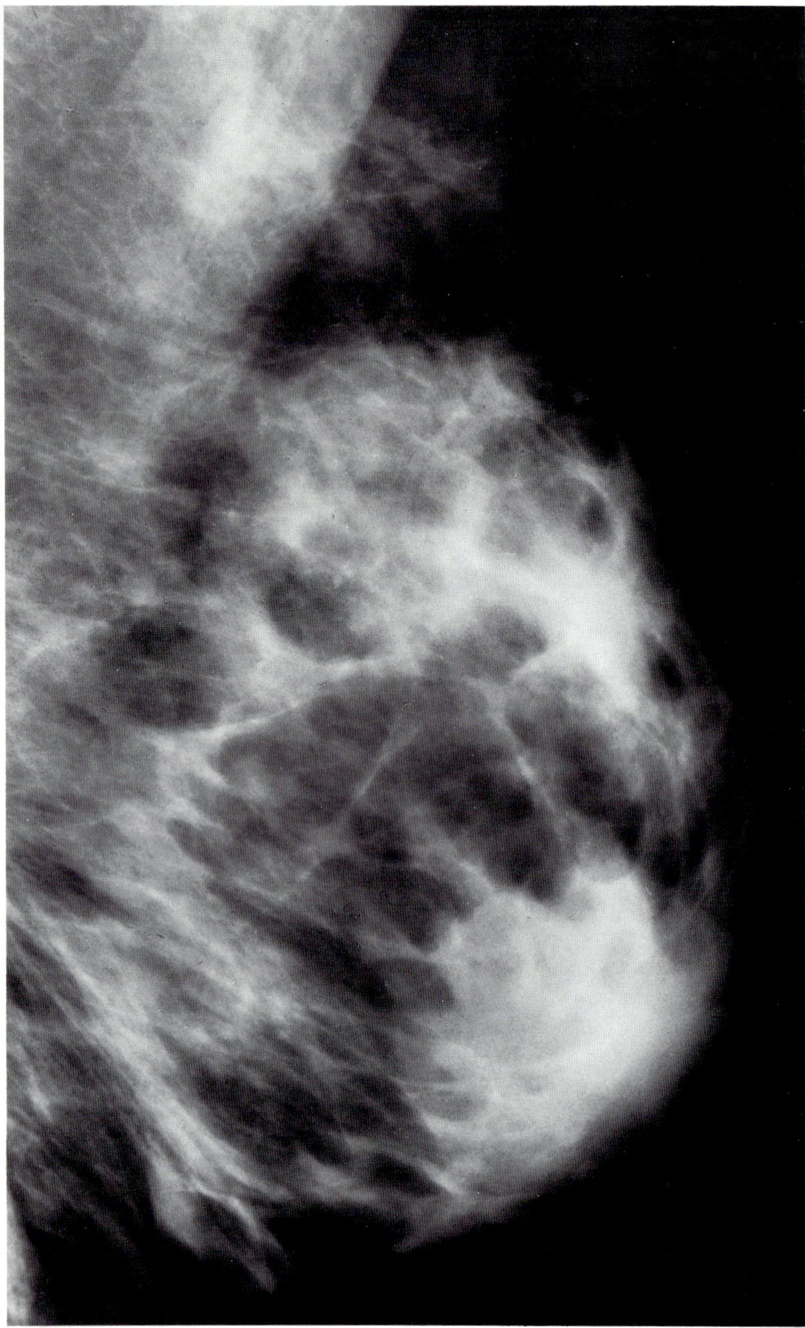

23

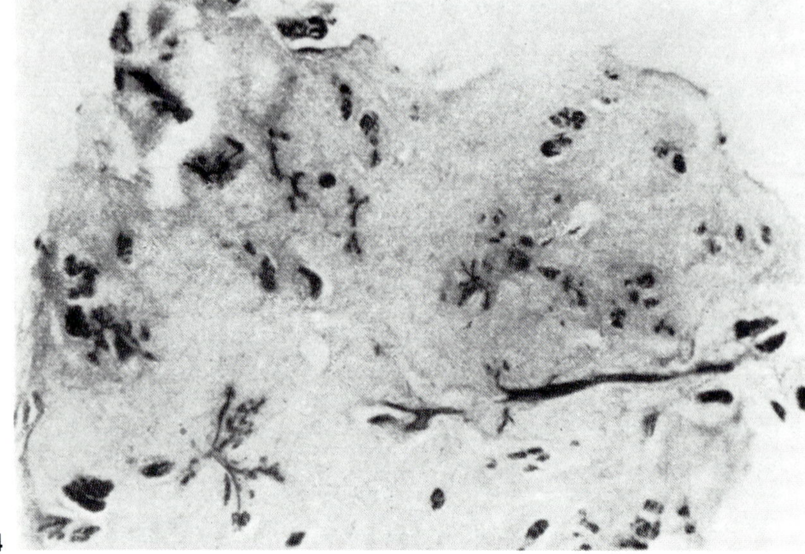

24

23 *Mammogram* (medio-lateral). Normal breast. Continuing into the axilla there are nonhomogeneous focal opacities indicating ectopic breast tissue. No evidence of malignancy.

24 *Histologic macrosection.* Poorly developed, small lobules of varying sizes. Longitudinal section of lactiferous duct. Interlobular fibrosis. (From Ingleby and Gershon-Cohen: Comparative Anatomy, Pathology and Roentgenology of the Breast. Univ. Pennsylvania Press, Philadelphia, 1960).

22-year-old female. Nodular masses in the breast were removed surgically at age 6 (apparently juvenile hypertrophy) (Figs 25, 26).

25 Left breast hypoplastic, about ⅓ the size of the right breast.

26 a, b. Bilateral *mammogram* (medio-lateral).
a) Right breast, normal. Lobules near thoracic wall are identifiable as very fine nodular opacities.
b) Left breast. Retroareolar, non-homogeneous, large opacity. No identifiable lobules.

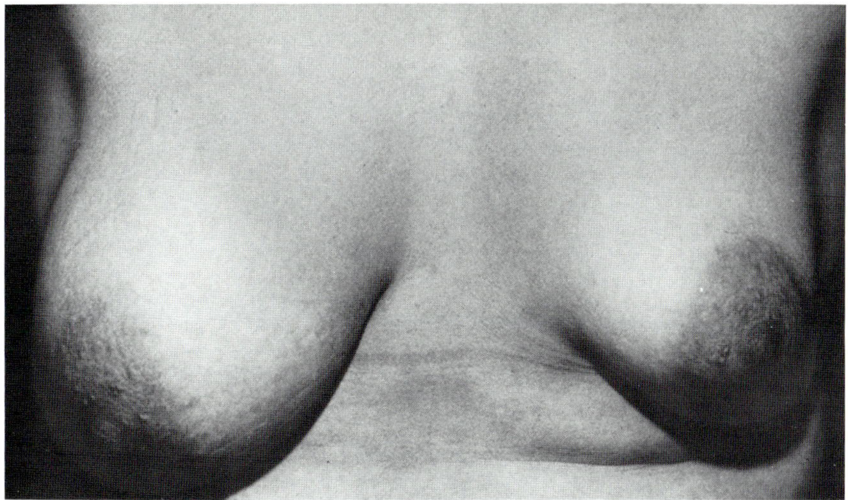

25

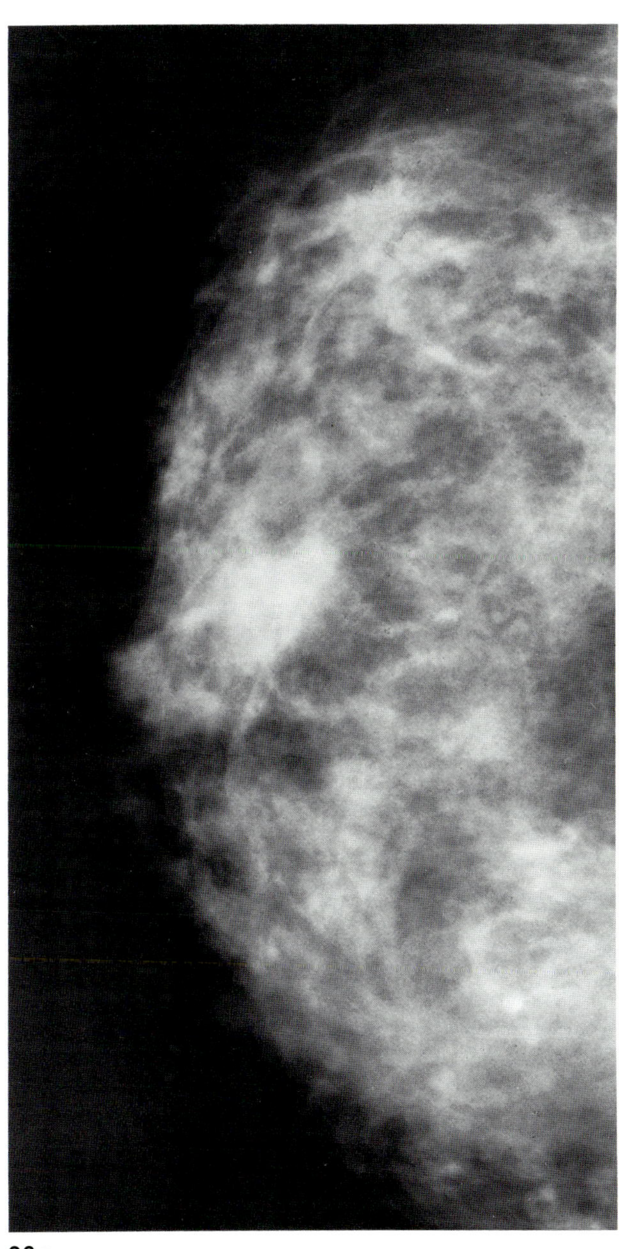

26a

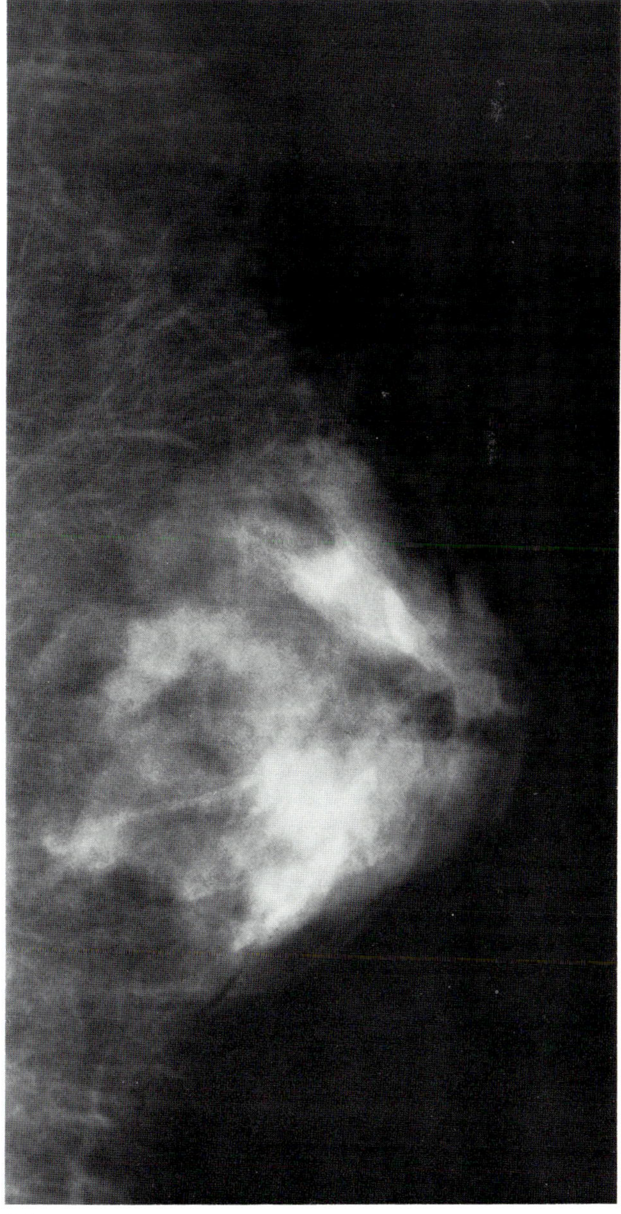

26b

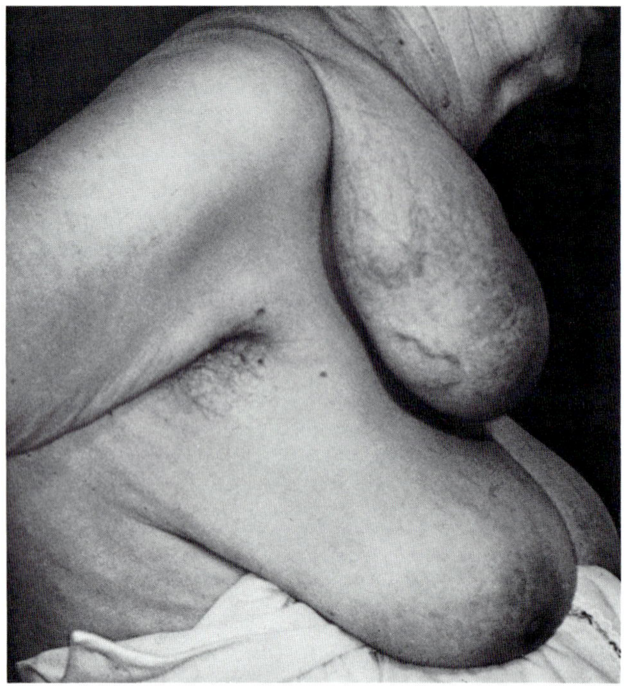

27

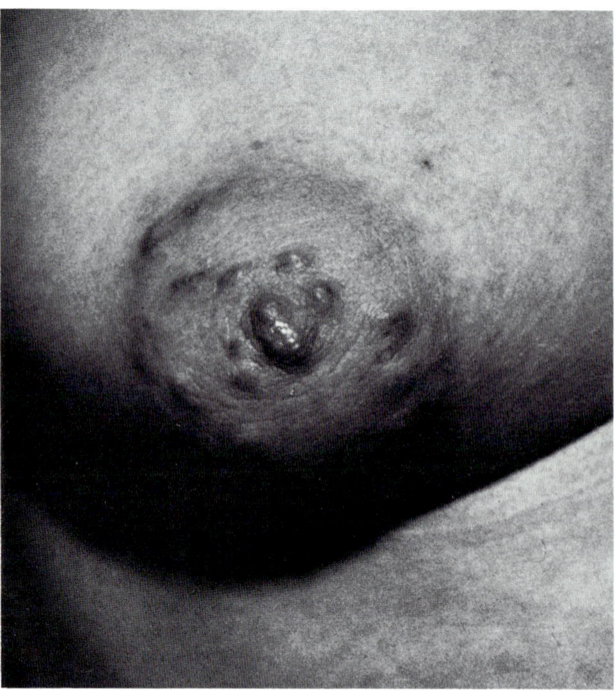

28

27 68-year-old female, lateral view. Pendulous tumor of right thoracic wall, the size of two fists, originating from the supraclavicular fossa. Slow growth over a period of 40 years. Histologically fibrolipoma.

28 Enlarged and coalescing sebaceous glands in the right areola of a 38-year-old female.

29 a, b. 27-year-old female. Continuous enlargement of breasts, marked hypertrophy bilaterally since age 18.
a) Before and
b) after plastic surgery to reduce size.

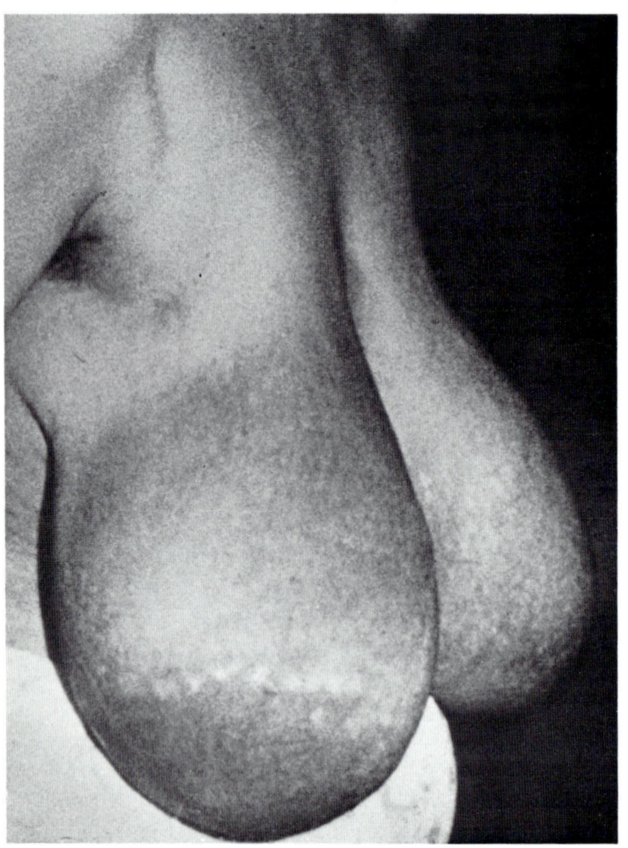

29a

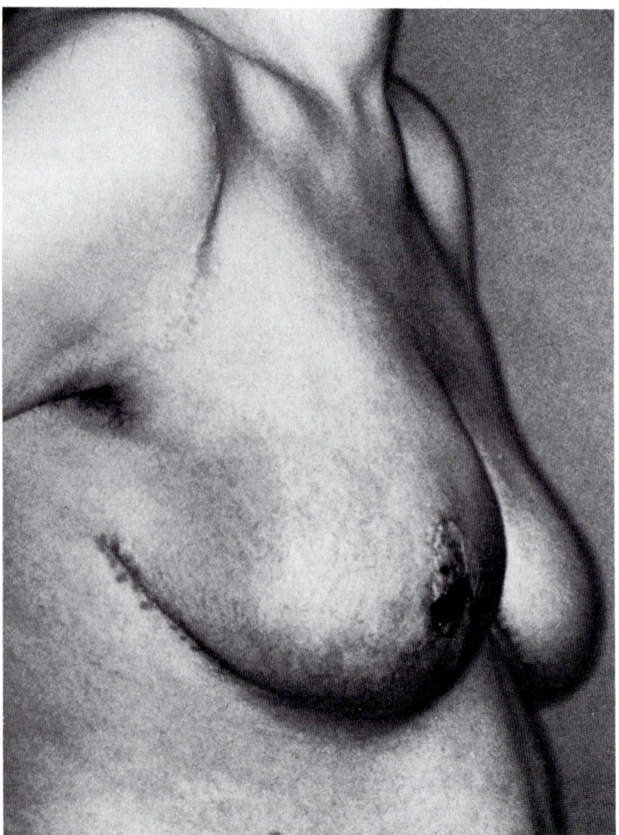

29b

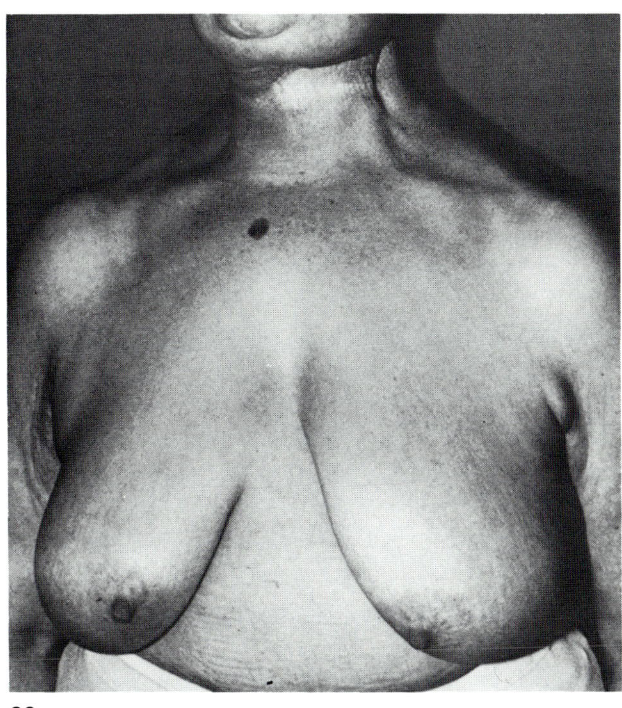

30

30 Inwardly rotated nipples of 57-year-old female. Normal mammogram. Pterygium colli.

31 a, b. 39-year-old female. Keratoma of right areola under nipple since childhood,

a) *Lateral view* of breast.

b) *Mammogram,* cranio-caudal. The keratoma simulates radiographically a benign retroareolar tumor.

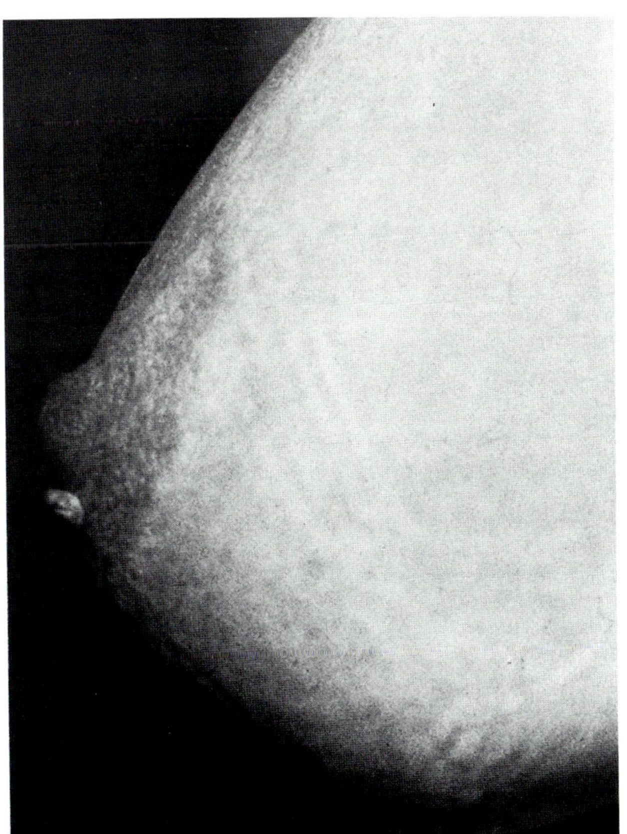

31a

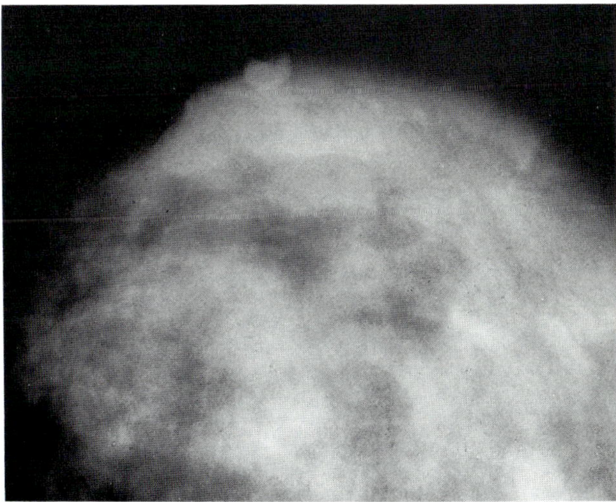

31b

Simple Benign Diseases of the Breast (Dysplasias)

Definition: The expression *dysplasia* is of Anglo-American origin and indicates simple benign changes of the breast.
Mastopathy, however, signifies complicated but also benign changes of the breast with numerous concomitant dysplastic changes.
The benign simple changes of the breast:
a) juvenile hypertrophy,
b) gynecomastia,
c) cysts,
d) fibroadenomas,
e) lipomas and fibrolipomas,
f) diseases of the lactiferous ducts (secretory disease) and chronic mastitis (plasma cell mastitis).

Juvenile hypertrophy

Juvenile hypertrophy rarely occurs before age 7 in girls. It is idiopathic. In boys hypertrophy rarely occurs prior to puberty.
Pathological hypertrophy may occur with tumors of the ovaries, the adrenal cortex, or the pineal gland (GERSHON-COHEN, 1970). Clinically there is a nodular bean- to cherry-sized uni- or bilateral enlargement. The nodule is retroareolar and easily moveable.
Juvenile hypertrophy appears radiographically as a round, nonhomogeneous, partially sharply defined (and partially unsharply), retroareolar opacity. Surgical removal of the hypertrophied rudimentary breast will result in a deformed breast following puberty (Fig **25**). Thin-needle biopsy should be done to exclude any chance of malignancy.

Gynecomastia

Gynecomastia is the minimal to marked enlargement of the male breast which may become as large as the female breast. Both breasts are usually involved but unilateral gynecomastia may occur. Incidence of gynecomastia in adult males is quoted to be less than 0.01% (WEBSTER, 1944).
HALL (1959) differentiates three grades:
Grade 1 is a palpable hyperplasia which is difficult to recognize mammographically. Directed towards the nipple are band-like retroareolar opacities separated by fat (Figs **32** b, **33** d).
Grade 2 is easily recognizable mammographically, usually shows a somewhat ill-defined, nonhomogeneous opacity behind the nipple (Figs **32** a, **33** b and c, **34**, **35**).
Grade 3 shows clinical and mammographic enlargement. The radiographic appearance is that of the juvenile female breast. This type of enlargement was seen in a 17-year-old with hormonally active testicular carcinoma (Fig **33** a).
Histological findings in all three stages are relatively uniform. There is increased periductal and interlobular connective tissue (Fig **36** a) with proliferations of the epithelium of the tubules. Lobules are not formed. The histological appearance of the gynecomastia is identical to the female breast during puberty (INGLEBY and GERSHON-COHEN, 1960; KLEY and KRÜSKEMPER, 1975).
The *aspirate* demonstrates multiple, solid, relatively large, epithelial colonies with uniformly small nuclei. Epithelium from the lactiferous ducts is occasionally aspirated (Figs **36** a, b). Cytology will differentiate it from a carcinoma of the breast (Fig **270** b).
Thermographically one or both breasts are hyperthermic. Warm nipples are common, so thermography is unreliable for excluding a carcinoma of the male breast.

Gynecomastia is related to:
local factors,
pituitary and other hormonal effects (steroids).

Increased sensitivity of the parenchyma of the male breast to normal hormonal blood levels is considered a *local* factor in gynecomastia.
Pituitary influence is exercised through somatotropic hormone (STH), gonadotropin, insulin and prolactin. The occurrence of gynecomastia in association with tumors of the hypothalamus and pituitary are additional confirmatory evidence in this respect. There is an increased incidence of gynecomastia with tuberculosis and sarcoidosis (TURKINGTON, 1972; FRIESEN and HWANG, 1973).
Gynecomastia may be medically induced by tranquilizers and antihypertensive drugs (phenothiazine, meprobamate, butyrophenone, α-methyldopa and rauwolfia alkaloids).
Absolute or relative increase of plasma estrogen is a hormonal factor. This is found with tumors of the adrenal cortex and of the gonads (Leydig cell tumor, seminoma, chorioepithelioma, teratoma).
An increase of estrogen relative to androgens is found with primary hypogonadism.
According to KLEY and KRÜSKEMPER (1975) the following diseases are prone to cause gynecomastia:

leprous orchitis,
mumps orchitis,
pseudohermaphrodism,
masculinization,
after-effects of irradiation of malignant tumors,
neurologic diseases (like FRIEDREICH's ataxia, muscular dystrophy, traumatic paraplegia and syringomyelia).

In conjunction with cirrhosis of the liver after digitalis and spironolactone administration, gynecomastia is also believed to be secondary to the estrogen effect.
KLEY and KRÜSKEMPER wrote an extensive review about the pathogenesis of gynecomastia in 1975.

Cysts

Cysts (Figs **37–40**) are the most common benign breast changes. They may be solitary or multiple in association with cystic fibrosis of the breast or mastopathy (see page 53).
Small cysts occur in almost all women above age 30. They may be associated with dilatation of the lactiferous ducts and with periductal fibrosis during involution of the parenchyma. This involution is a normal aging process since multiple cysts are found in the breast in senescence. KRAMER and RUSH (1973) found 89% solitary or multiple cysts in autopsies of 70 women over age 70 (whose cause of death was unrelated to breast carcinoma).
Solitary cysts are usually unilateral. Inflammation of the surrounding parenchyma may also be present, causing hyperthermia in the thermogram simulating a malignant tumor.
The pathogenesis of the solitary cyst is unclear. According to our own experience cysts almost always occur in lobuli following blockage of secretions and marked dilatation of terminal lactiferous ducts and acini. The formation of ridges and septa in the walls of cysts is also thus explained (Figs **40**, **45**).
The increased pressure in the cyst causes atrophy of the secreting epithelium of the cyst wall, found to be absent on histologic examination. Adenosis is commonly found next to the cyst (Fig **38** b). The cyst appears as a round or oval, sharply defined, homogeneous opacity in the *mammogram*. A radiolucent halo may separate cyst wall from surrounding fat. The sharp configuration of the cyst edge is commonly absent due to superimposition of fibrous breast tissue. The breast, however, is larger on this side as compared to the opposite breast and more radiopaque.
Solitary cysts may grow rapidly. It is commonly stated by the patient that the nodule occurred "over night." This is important in differential diagnosis, as the slowly growing *solid tumors* (fibroadenoma, cellular malignancy), have a similar mammographic appearance.
Incompletely filled cysts may not be palpable.
The *therapy* of the solitary cyst is *complete* aspiration. Aspiration may be unsuccessful if the cyst wall consists of dense fibrous tissue. If the cyst is incompletely filled, the dense wall may move with the needle tip, and perforation of the cyst wall can then only be accomplished with a brisk forward thrust of the needle.
The *pneumocystogram* permits evaluation of the cyst's inner wall and excludes intracystic epithelial proliferations. Stellate carcinomas or microcalcifications are easily identifiable in the cyst wall after the filling of the cyst cavity with air.
The *cyst aspirate* is either serous, milky or gray-green. Inflamed cysts have a cloudy aspirate or contain pus. Cytological examination should always follow.
On the smear there are protein sediments and degenerated epithelium (commonly foam cells). With associated inflammation there are leukocytes, lymphocytes and histiocytes. Intracystic papillomas appear as small solid epithelial conglomerates (Fig **161** b). Atypical cells point to malignant transformation.
Papillomas in a cyst have to be removed surgically in any case in order to be examined histologically as potential malignant infiltration of surrounding tissue cannot be excluded by pneumocystogram or cytological examination.
Of aspirated cysts 80% regress within 8 weeks of aspiration. Palpation usually reveals slight induration at the site of the regressed cyst; thin-needle biopsy will then demonstrate histiocytes, foam cells and proliferating ductal epithelium. The cell structure is irregular, so in at least 10 cases after cyst regression, we have recommended that tissue biopsy of the cyst remnant be performed. A carcinoma, however, could not be found on the histological examination done subsequently. In case the cyst is incompletely aspirated, it will regress to the size of the residual liquid content. Although significantly smaller, the cyst is still palpable. Subsequent aspiration to remove residual content is necessary to achieve complete regression of the cyst.
Surgical removal of the cyst is indicated

a) for intracystic epithelial proliferations diagnosed by the pneumocystogram and/or cytological smear,
b) for bloody fluid in the cyst (excluding iatrogenic bleeding secondary to injury of a vessel),
c) for stellate opacities or localized microcalcifications in the wall or next to the cyst,
d) for failure of cyst to regress despite multiple aspirations.

After pneumocystogram incompletely aspirated cysts may simulate a pulmonary cavity with an air-fluid level in a roentgenogram of the chest (Fig **41**).

Fibroadenoma

Proliferation of intralobular connective tissue and lactiferous ducts may cause formation of fibroadenomas (Figs **53** a, **54**). They commonly occur as solitary tumors in girls and young women during increased hormonal activity (GERSHON-COHEN, 1970). They are most common between ages 25 and 30.

The tumor is anatomically very firm with a smooth surface. Usually it can be relatively easily dissected (Figs **52**, **56**), although there is vascular bridging to the surrounding breast. Common in larger fibroadenomas is necrosis which may calcify (Fig **76**) or liquefy, resulting in large defects in the tumor's center (Fig **52**).

Histologically there is proliferation of lactiferous ducts and of intralobular tissue; connective tissue elements (fibroadenoma) or epithelium (adenofibroma) may predominate. An intracanalicular type is differentiated from a pericanalicular type.

Radiographically there is a homogeneous, smoothly defined opacity. Vascular and tissue bridging to surrounding parenchyma will cause unsharpness at the fibroadenoma's edge. Necrotic liquefaction cannot be seen radiographically. Extensive irregular calcifications may be present in older women (Figs **53** b, **109**). Microcalcifications may occur and may simulate comedocarcinoma in breasts rich in stroma (Fig **82**).

Most commonly fibroadenomas are poorly vascularized and appear in the *thermogram* usually as a "cold spot" (Fig **47** b). Very cellular adenofibromas, however, can also have hypervascularization and may then exhibit hyperthermia. The difference in temperature between adenofibroma and normal breast parenchyma is 0.5 to 1 °C which is considerably less than the temperature difference between the normal breast and nodular cellular carcinomas (Fig **185**).

Cytologically in fibroadenomas are found distinctly multiple cords of epithelium with small round and oval nuclei and a thin rim of cytoplasm. Cell structure is uniform. Many small cells with naked nuclei are identifiable between the epithelial layers; because of their peculiar oval shape, these have been named "bipolar naked nucleated cells" by ZAJICEK (1974). These epithelial cells occur with fibroadenoma and adenofibroma. Apparently this is a myoepithelium (Fig **49**, **55** b).

In addition to epithelial layers and naked nucleated bipolar cells, there may be small particles of connective tissue in the smear. The number and overall appearance of cells may vary with the fibroadenoma. Commonly there are many epithelial layers. The nuclei are larger and more polymorphous producing an irregular cytological picture. Duct epithelium, foam cells and mucus indicate the regressive changes of a fibroadenoma.

Differential diagnosis from solid and medullary cellular carcinomas growing in nodular form is relatively easy with thin-needle biopsy (Fig **181** b). Differentiation from mucinous carcinoma, however, may be difficult (Fig **182** b).

Lipoma and fibrolipoma

According to HAMPERL (1968) lipomas are encapsulated fatty tumors which appear radiographically as sharply-defined round- or oval-shaped radiolucencies.

Palpation of lipomas reveals soft, easily movable nodules; they are most common in middle-aged patients after the menopause. Patients state that the nodule has remained unchanged for a long period of time. This differentiates the lipoma from a solid tumor or a cyst. Thin-needle biopsy will differentiate the lipoma from another solid tumor in dense breasts. There is abundant fatty tissue in the cell-free smear.

It should, however, be mentioned that fatty changes commonly surround scirrhous carcinomas. The clinical-cytological diagnosis of a lipoma without mammography may therefore be in error. Connective tissue also may grow within the lipoma. It is then morphologically called a fibrolipoma.

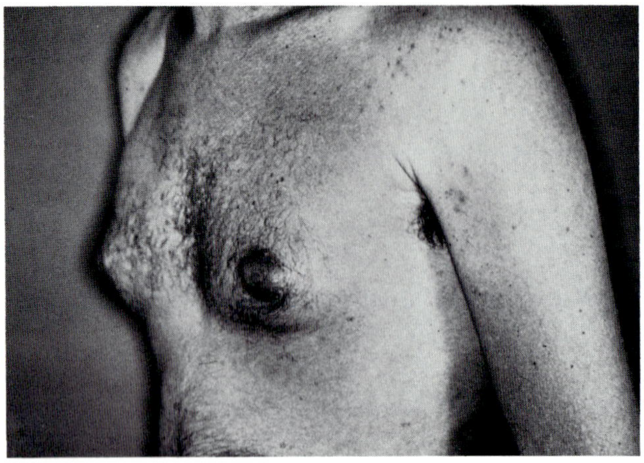

32 a

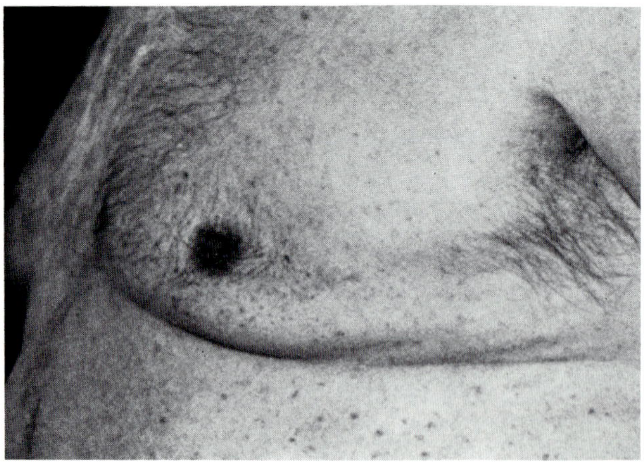

32 b

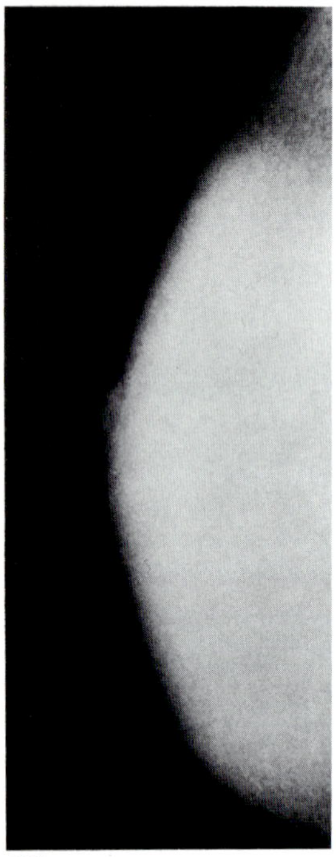

33 a

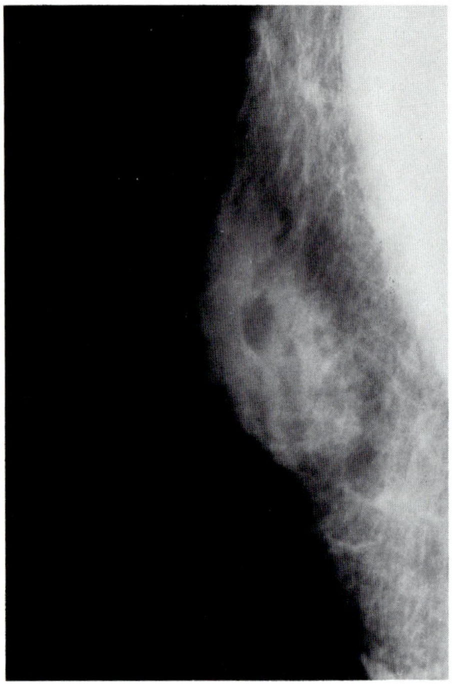

33 b

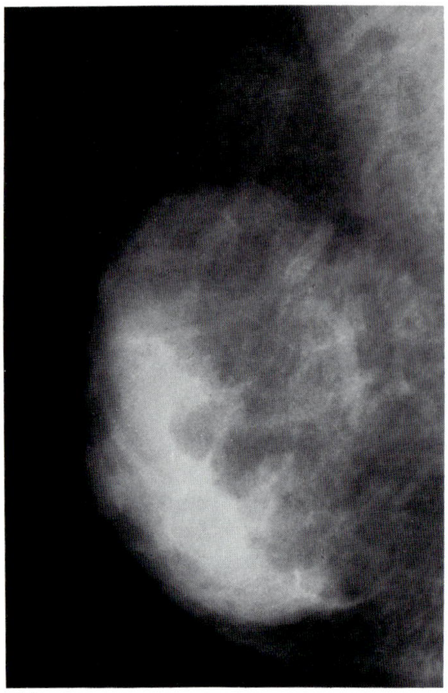

33 c

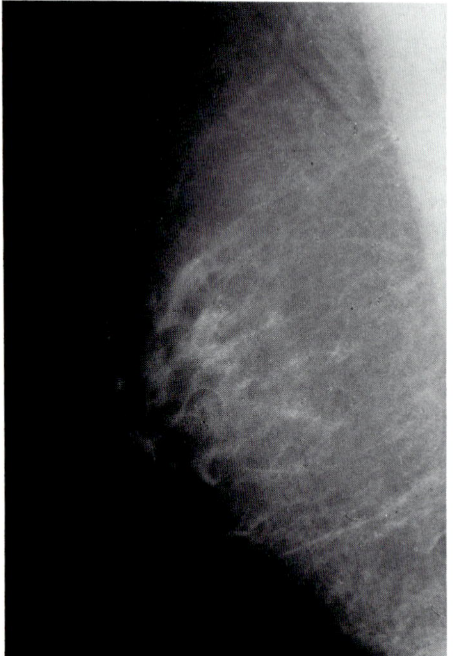

33 d

32 a, b. *Clinical history and appearance.*

a) 28-year-old male. Chorionepithelioma of the left testis. Regression of gynecomastia following removal of the testicular tumor.

b) 73-year-old male, on digitalis for 6 years.

33 a–d. *Mammogram* (medio-lateral).

a) Homogeneous increased density of the breast, 25-year-old male with testicular tumor.

b) Retroareolar, nonhomogeneous, ill-defined opacity. Mammogram of same patient as in Fig 32a.

c) Tangerine-sized retroareolar radiopaque breast. More radiolucent near chest wall. Increased vascularity. 35-year-old male with cirrhosis of the liver treated with spironolactone.

d) Delicate band-like retroareolar opacities. Mammogram of same patient as in Fig 32b.

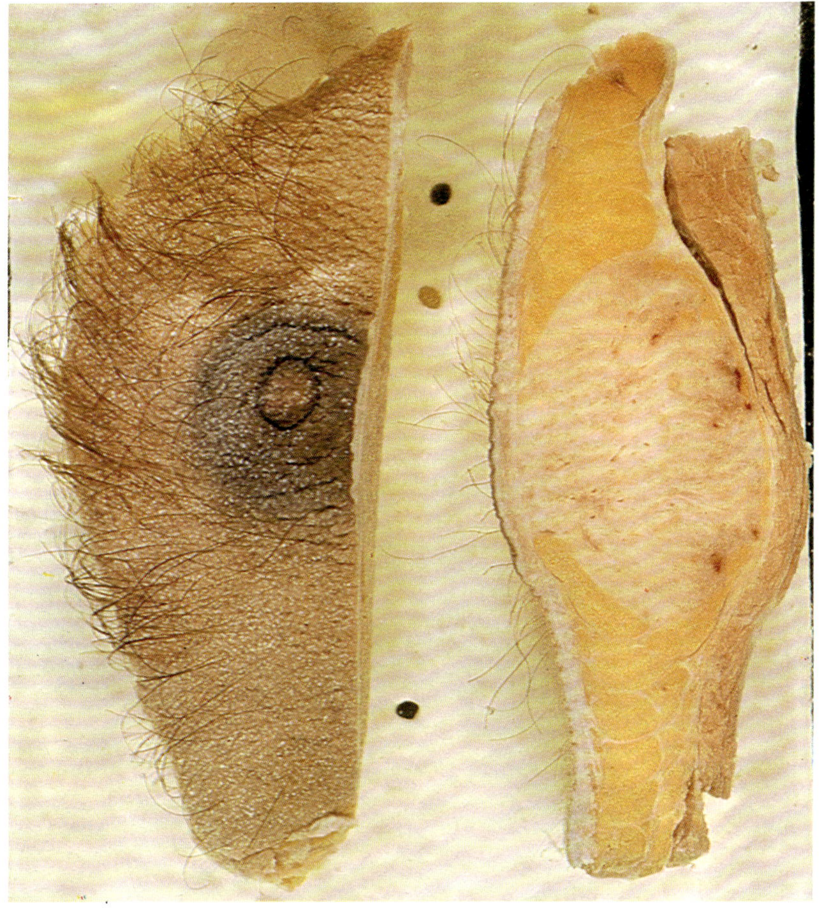

34

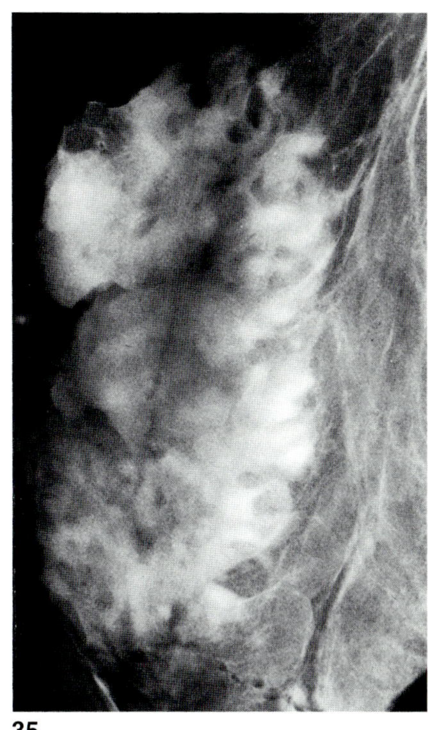

35

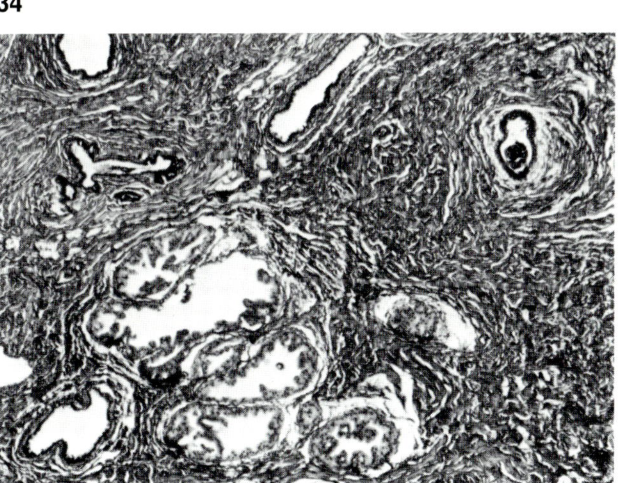

36a

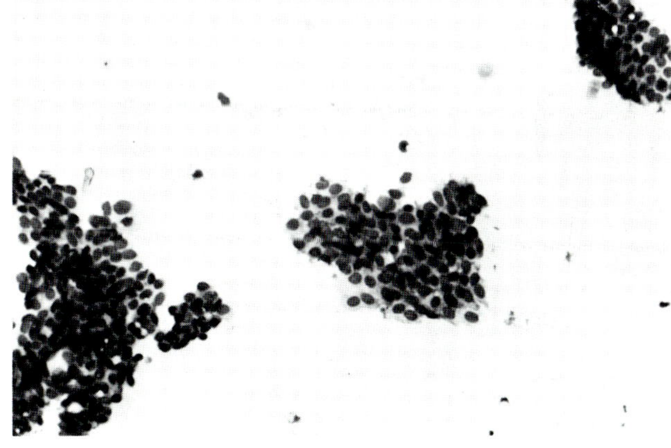

36b

34 *Anatomical specimen* of gynecomastia. Nodular retroareolar tumor. Irregular border toward the pectoralis muscle; sharp, smoothly-defined border toward fatty tissue cranially and caudally.

35 *Specimen radiograph.* Nonhomogeneous multilobular radio-opacities surrounded by delicate stromal septa extending into surrounding fatty tissue.

36 a, b. *Histology and cytology.*
a) Histology, magnif 80×. Dilated lactiferous ducts with extensive periductal fibrosis. Several dilated ducts with benign papillary epithelial proliferations.
b) Cytology, magnif 80×. Several solid epithelial layers with uniform epithelium and multiple bipolar cells with naked nuclei (myoepithelium). The latter also occur separated from the epithelial layers.

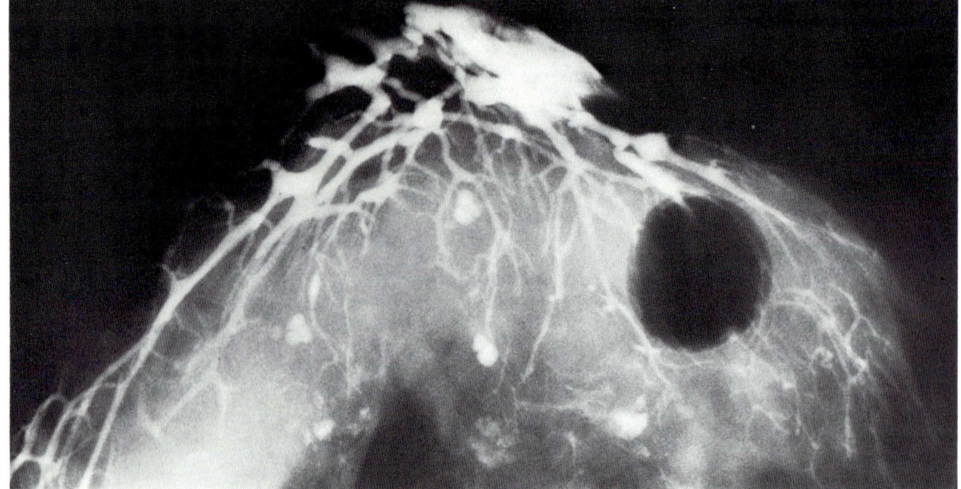
37

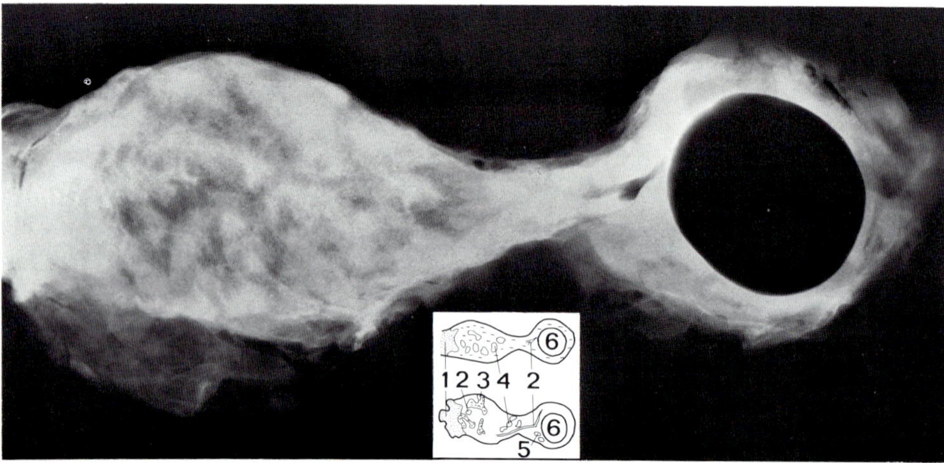

38a

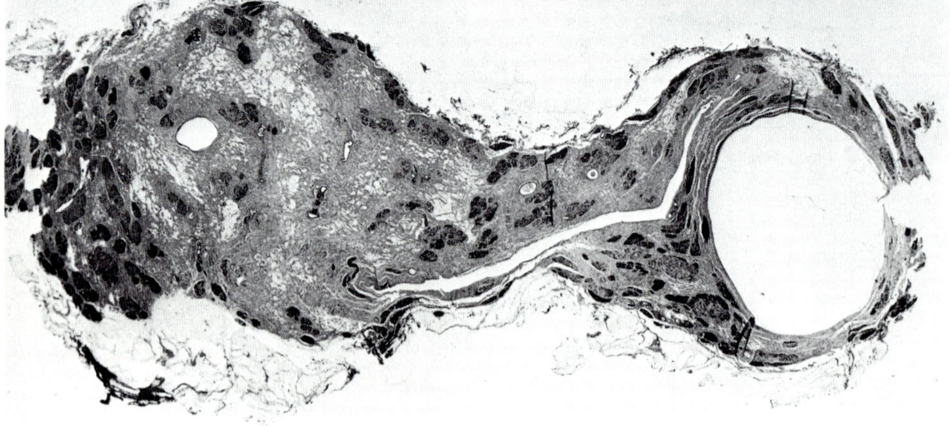
38b

37 37-year-old female, left breast. After aspiration of a cyst of the inner quadrant. Secreting breast. Galactography and pneumocystogram: retroareolar ectatic lactiferous ducts filled with contrast medium. Multiple peripherally located cysts filled with contrast medium. Large palpable cyst caused by obstruction of secretions. Smooth walls.

38 a, b. *Radiological-histological comparison.*
a) Specimen radiograph. Smoothly defined cyst (6). Dilated lactiferous duct (2) at left edge of cyst, disruption of contiguity to the cyst. Multiple small nodular opacities in remaining parenchyma indicating mastions (4,1) (lobule and perilobular [interlobular] connective tissue = mastion).
b) Histological macrosection. Smooth-walled cyst. Next to cyst and in remaining parenchyma of the gland are proliferating and enlarged lobules (adenosis) with surrounding perilobular connective tissue. Ectatic and fibrotic lactiferous ducts.

39 a, b. 42-year-old female. Cyst of the outer upper quadrant.
a) *Mammogram.* Homogeneous, smoothly defined opacity. Otherwise normal breast.
b) Pneumocystography. Smoothly defined cyst cavity.

40 Anatomic cross section of a cyst. Smooth shiny inner wall. Sharply defined septum. Remaining cyst fluid at bottom of cavity.

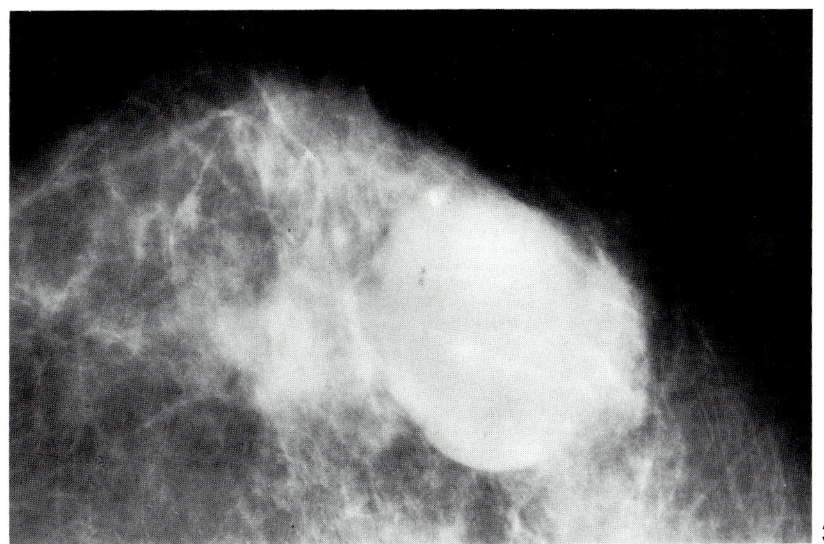

39a

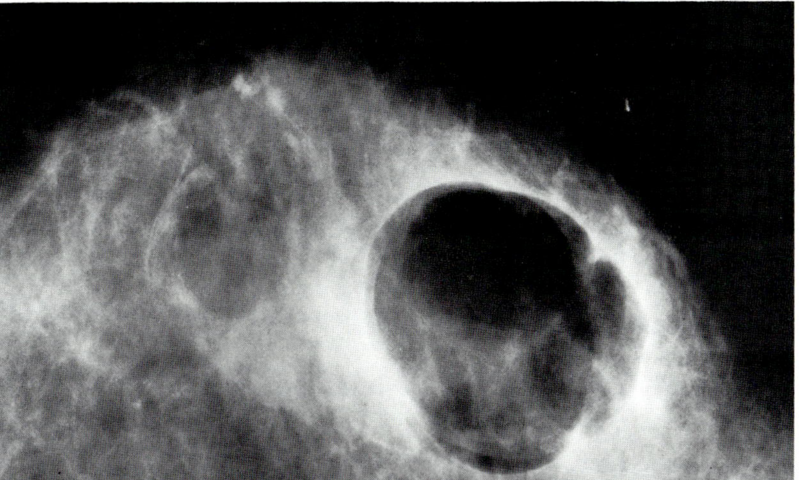

39b

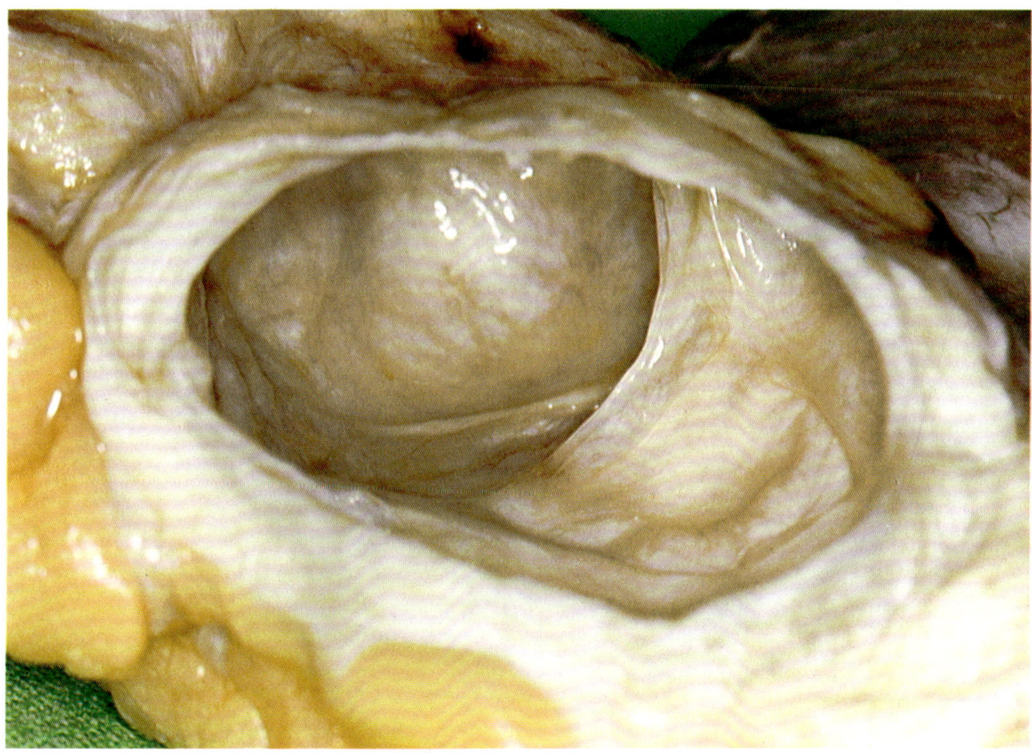

40

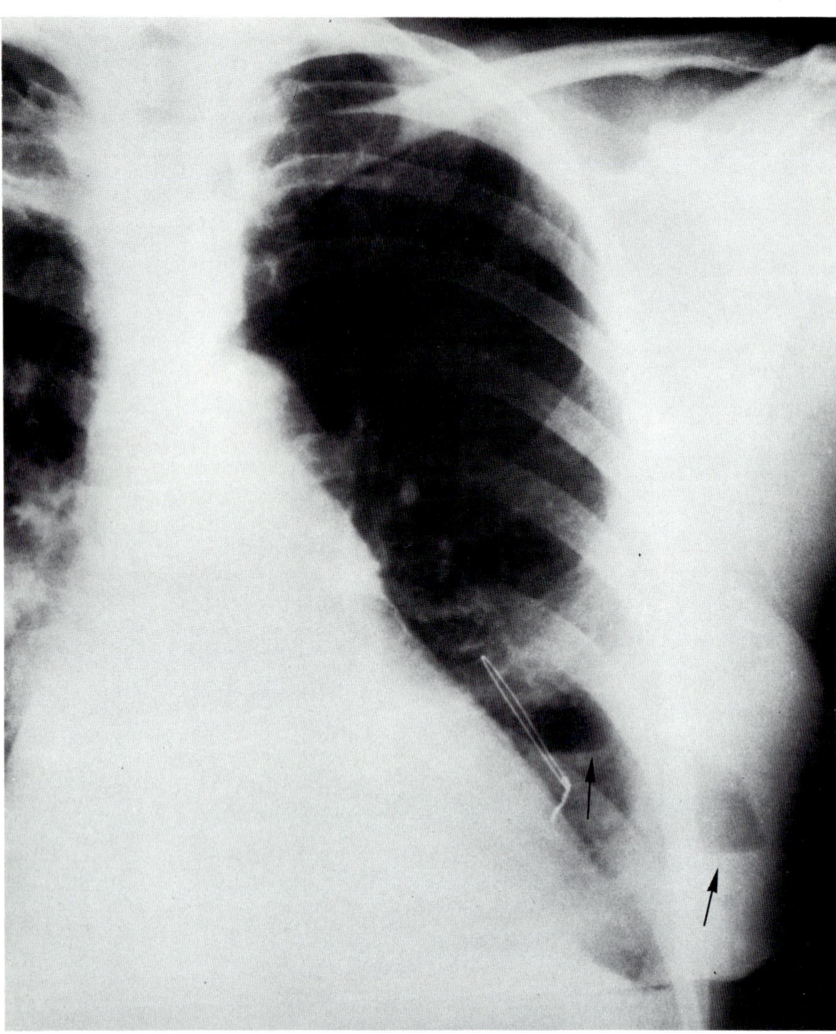

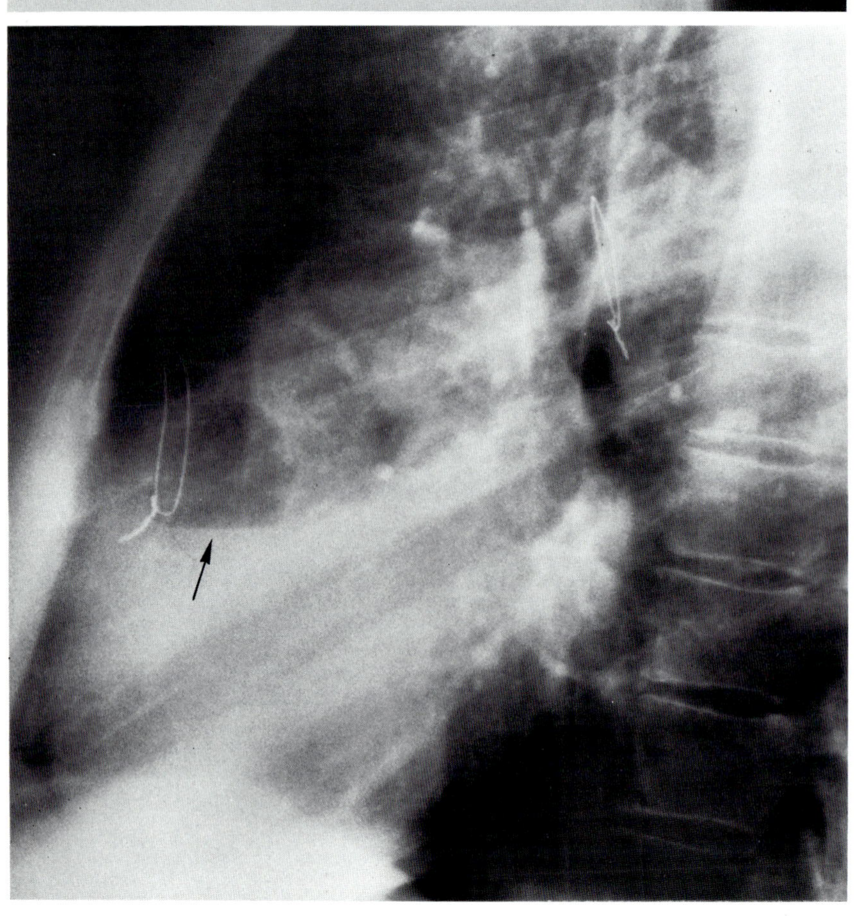

41 a, b. 52-year-old female. After surgery for mitral stenosis, wire sutures in anterior thoracic wall. After incomplete aspiration of two cysts of left breast. Lateral view of pneumocystogram demonstrates air-fluid levels in the cyst from the remaining fluid. The air-fluid level projected over the lung parenchyma simulates a pulmonary cavity (arrow).

a) Chest posterior-anterior. Round "lucency" in left lower lung field with an air-fluid level; similar changes in left breast outside lung fields (arrow).

b) Chest, lateral. Simulation of a pulmonary cavity with an air-fluid level (arrow).

A 48-year-old patient had an approximately fist-sized tumor in the left breast. This tumor had existed for 30 years but remained unchanged for the last 15. The left breast was twice as large as the right. Radiographically there was a large radiolucent tumor surrounded by a delicate fibrous capsule with multiple dense foci in the center (Fig **57** a).
A patient with paraffin implanted in her breast for cosmetic reasons had a similar mammogram (Fig **58**).

A large area of fibrosis in a fibrolipoma may appear in the mammogram as an ill-defined opacity so similar to a stellate growing carcinoma as to make differential diagnosis difficult. Thin-needle biopsy will be necessary to differentiate a fibrolipoma from a carcinoma.
Lipomas are *thermographically* similar to surrounding tissue; there is no typical vascular picture or hyperthermia.
Lipomas and fibrolipomas also occur on the trunk and extremities.

An extremely large fibrolipoma was found in a 62-year-old woman in the right infraclavicular fossa. The tumor size was over two fists and hung along the anterior chest wall appearing as a "third breast" (Fig **27**).

Secretory disease and chronic mastitis

Acute mastitis must be differentiated clinically from chronic mastitis. Acute infectious mastitis during lactation will not be discussed here; its development and course are so typical, there are no differential diagnostic problems.
Outside of lactation acute mastitis may be secondary to exacerbation of a chronic mastitis.
Chronic mastitis is also called *plasma cell mastitis* because of the large number of plasma cells and lymphocytes in the inflammatory cell infiltrate. Plasma cell mastitis occurs in older women. The lactiferous ducts are dilated and filled with debris and secretions (Figs **59**, **60** b). Lymphoplasma cellular infiltrates are present in the wall of the lactiferous ducts and periductally (Fig **61** b). It is assumed that the chronic mastitis is a so-called "chemical mastitis" secondary to secretions entering the periductal connective tissue (Hoeffken and Lanyi, 1977).
Microabscesses surrounding lactiferous ducts are common and may lead to fistulas between the lactiferous system and the skin (Fig **61** a). Passage of secretions into periductal tissue leads to round cell infiltration followed by periductal fibrosis (Baessler, 1970).

Fibrosed lactiferous ducts appear *mammographically* as retroareolar, band-like opacities (Fig **60** a). Periductal fibrosis may cause *retraction of the nipple*. Forty percent of patients with chronic mastitis have secretions (Ingleby and Gershon-Cohen, 1960; Barth et al, 1975).
The affinity of intraductal debris for calcium salts causes deposition of typical needle-like calcifications in lactiferous ducts. They may be localized or distributed diffusely over the entire breast and can be recognized radiographically (Fig **98**). Formation of macroabscesses in a 36-year-old patient with plasma cell mastitis was noted.

The history was typical. There was bilateral spontaneous recurrent secretion from both breasts over a period of three years. The secretions were watery-serous. The patient complained of localized recurrent pain in different areas of both breasts, independent of menstrual cycles.
One day, the secretion from the right breast stopped. Four days later, a tumor developed in this breast which, after eight days, was hard and very tender to palpation. The skin was reddened, the nipple retracted. Clinically and cytologically, there was an acute abscess. Lancing revealed 50 cc of cream-like, foul-smelling, yellow-green pus (Figs **63**, **64**).
What is typical about this observation is the fact that the abscess developed after obstruction (of lactiferous ducts by debris or inflammatory wall infiltrates) had caused cessation of secretion. This led to accumulation of secretions in lactiferous ducts and hence acute exacerbation of the chronic mastitis with subsequent formation of an abscess. With accumulation of secretions (without inflammation in the parenchyma) only a simple cyst would have resulted.

The *subchronic* stage of a case of mastitis was followed clinically and mammographically in a 62-year-old patient.

A slowly (over a period of four months) growing, retroareolar tumor was found in the right breast. This tumor had become harder and had finally reached the size of a tangerine. The tumor was only relatively tender. Nipple *secretion* was serous with lymphocytes and a few leukocytes.
The breast showed an increased homogeneous density radiographically The discrepancy between palpation and veil-like opacity in the mammogram was striking. The cytological smear following *thin-needle biopsy* revealed multiple granulocytes, lymphocytes and multinucleated histiocytes. It was interpreted as subchronic mastitis. After anti-inflammatory treatment with oxyphenbutazone and antibacterial therapy with tetracycline, there was complete regression of the palpable tumor and veil-like opacities in the mammogram (Figs **65**, **67**).

Increased radio-opacity of inflammatory fatty tissue over normal fat can also be demonstrated microradiographically (Fig **66** a).

49-year-old female, left breast. Palpable retroareolar small nodule (Figs 42, 43).

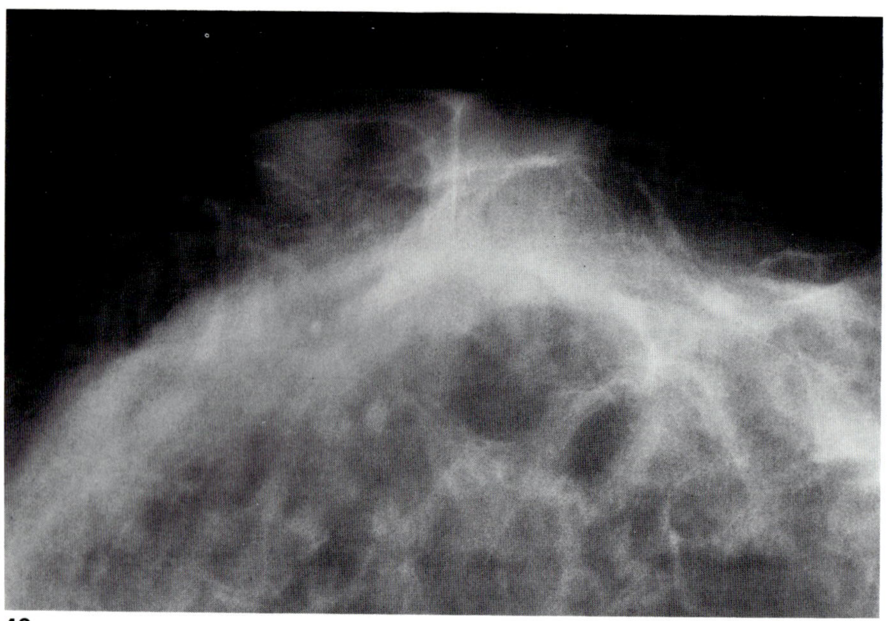

42 a

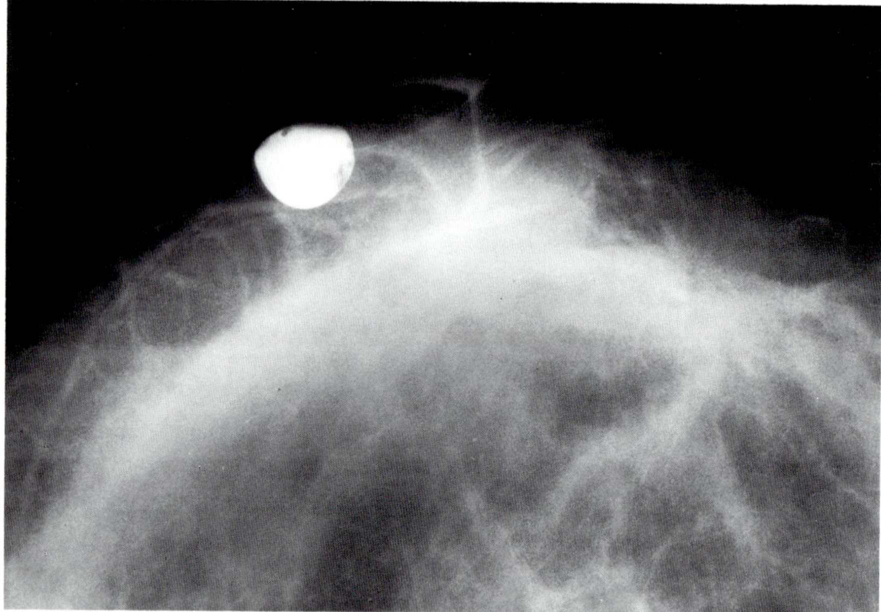

42 b

42

a) *Mammogram.* Round, partially smooth, partially ill-defined homogeneous opacity behind lateral portion of areola.

b) After aspiration of the cyst and injection of contrast medium into the cavity. Irregular filling defects along cyst wall.

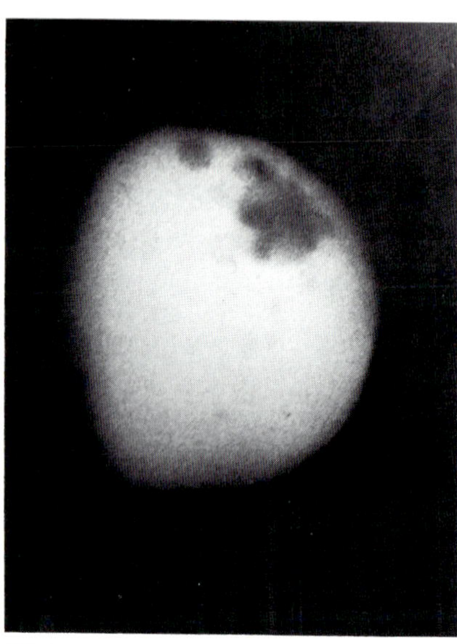

43 a

43 b

43

a) Contrast filled cyst, magnif 5×. Lobulated-nodular filling defects.

b) The anatomic specimen exhibiting polypoid, papillary, benign tumor at bottom of opened cyst.

16-year-old female, right breast. Since childhood bluish discoloration of areola laterally with ectopic, intermittently secreting, lactiferous duct. No secretion for three weeks. Palpable retroareolar nodule for eight days. No tenderness to palpation. Aspiration of 5 ml serous fluid from the nodule (Figs 44–46).

44 Right breast. Hemangioma of the areola. The ectopic lactiferous duct is not identifiable.

45 *Pneumocystogram.* Multiple communicating cysts. Cyst pattern suggests cystically dilated terminal ducts of a dysplastic lobule.

46 *Cytology* of aspirate. Clusters of so-called "foam cells."

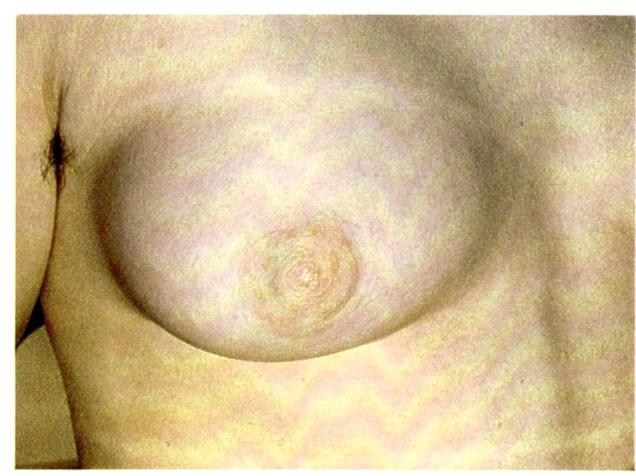

44

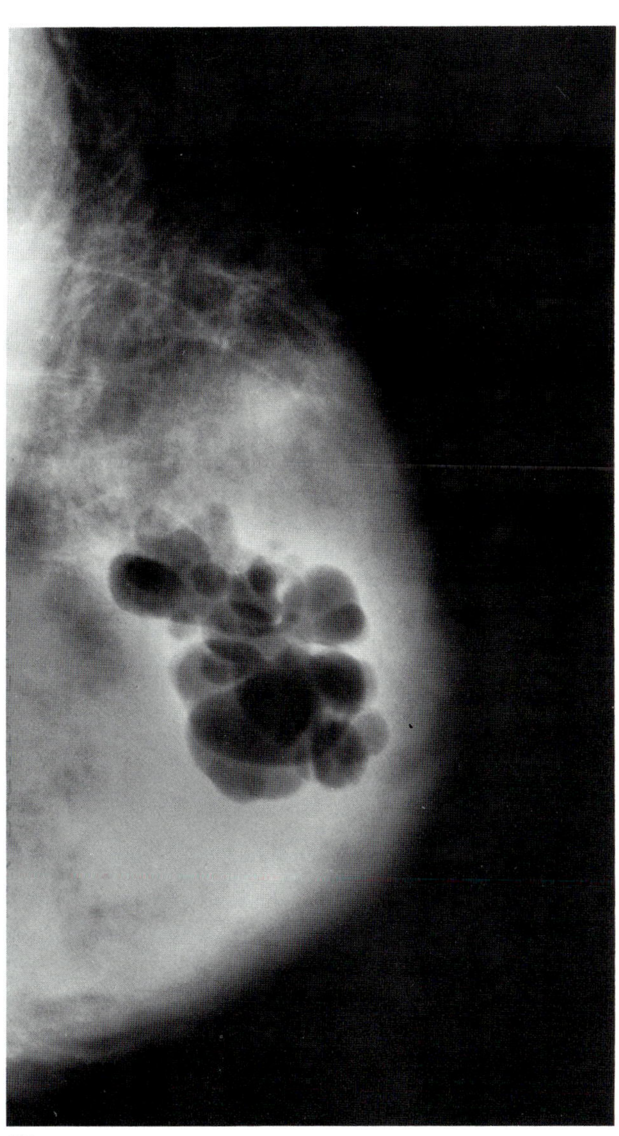

45

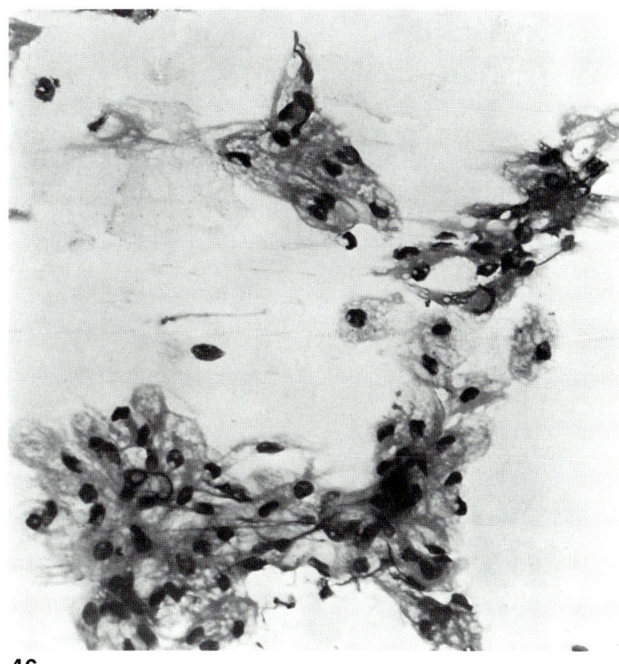

46

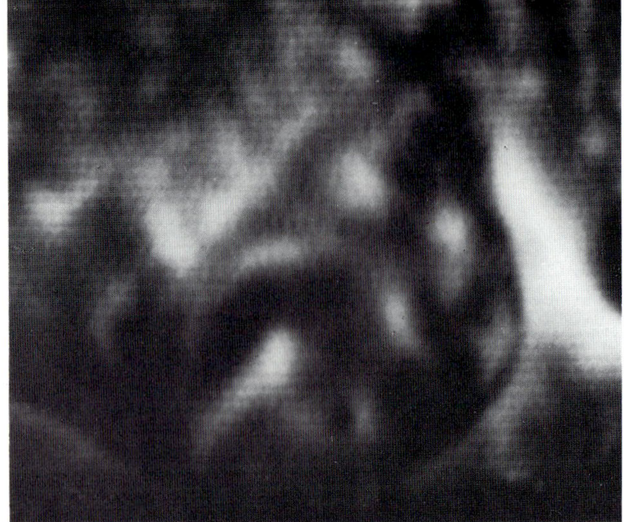
47 a

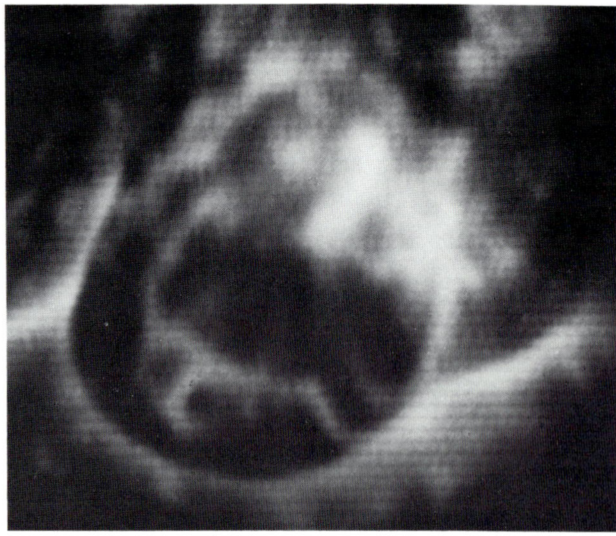
47 b

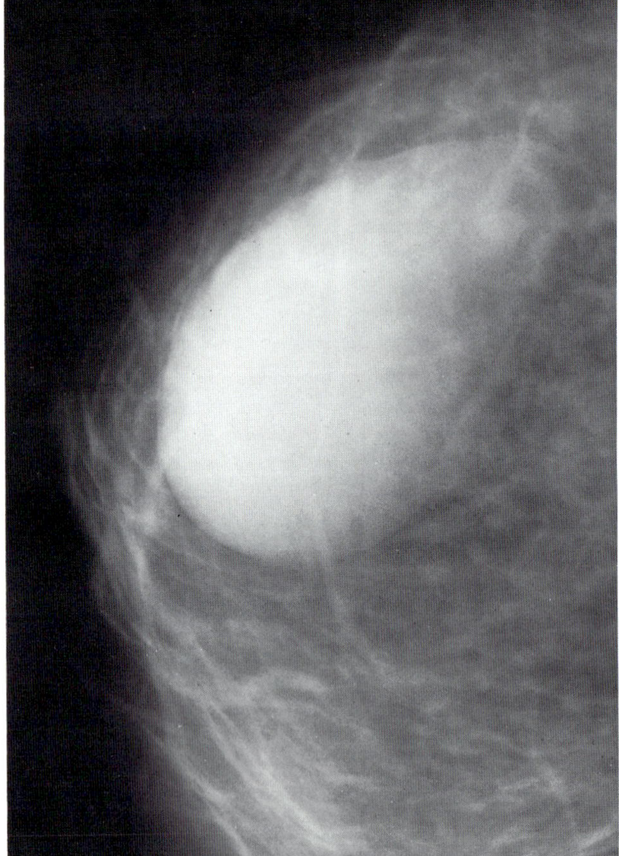
48

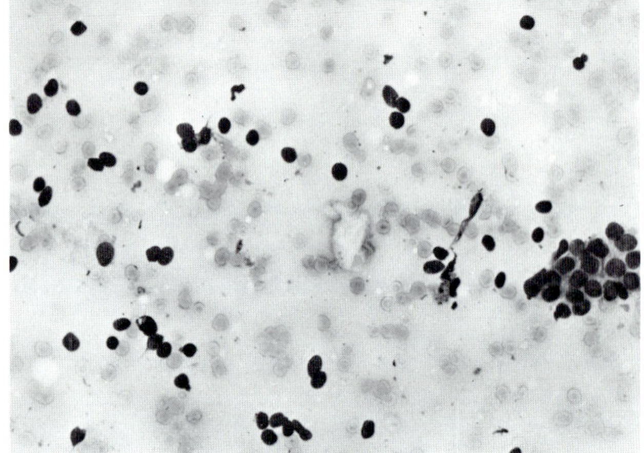
49

29-year-old female, left breast. Nodule enlarging for one year in upper-outer quadrant. Markedly accelerated growth the last four weeks (Figs 47–52).

47 a, b. *Bilateral electronic thermovision.*
a) Right breast. Normal vascularity. Cold nipple.
b) Left breast. Decreased vascularity (so-called "cold spot") with displacement of vessels in region of palpable nodule in upper-outer quadrant. Cold nipple.

48 Large, oval, mostly smoothly defined opacity becoming ill-defined near chest wall.

49 *Thin-needle biopsy.* Small, apparently normal epithelial layers. Multiple so-called "bipolar cells" with naked nuclei (myoepithelium or basket cells). Magnif 160×.

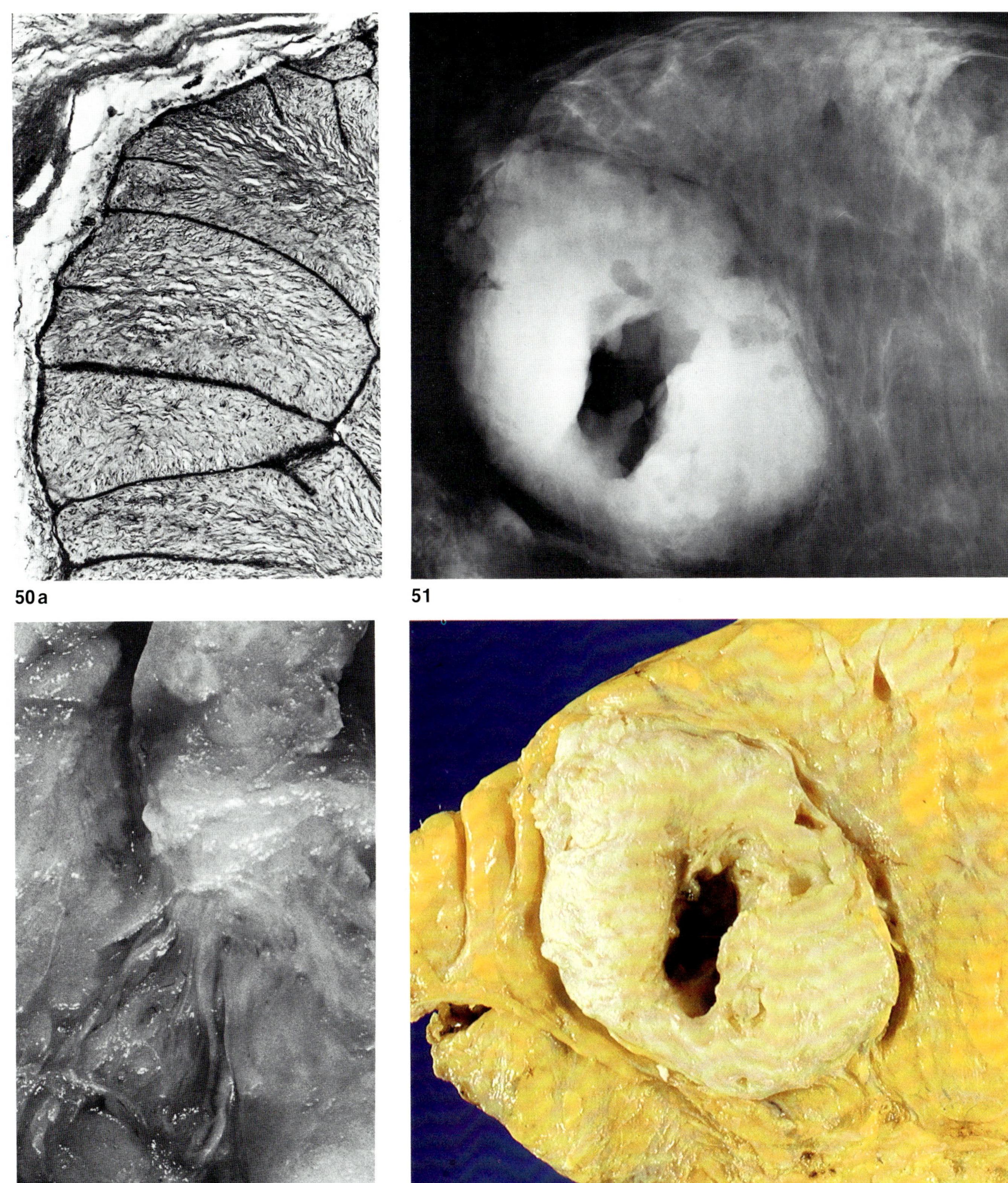

50
a) *Histology.* Intracanalicular fibroadenoma. Plump branching papillae from abundant fibromyxoid connective tissue. Papillae are covered by normal epithelium and fill the lumen of a markedly dilated lactiferous duct. Multiple basket cells between epithelium and stroma. Above-left: compressed breast stroma. Magnif 80×.
b) A vascular stem supplies nodule and connects it intimately with breast. This portion of tumor is ill-defined in mammogram. Magnif 3× over Figs 51, 52.

51 *Specimen radiograph* of fibroadenoma with central necrosis and liquefaction.

52 *Cross section of specimen* from same case. Smoothly defined tumor nodule with vascular basilar stem. Central necrotic cavity.

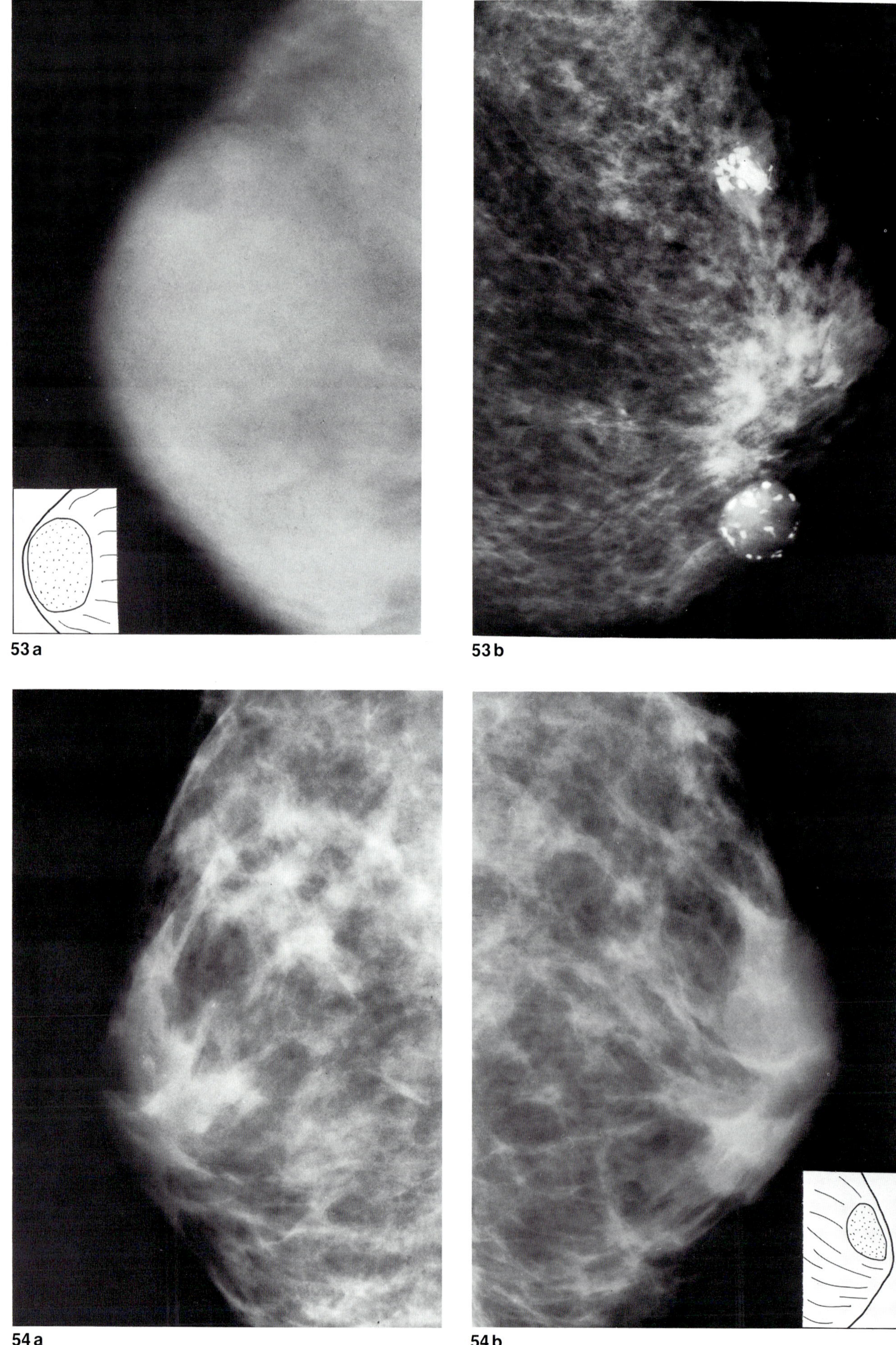

53a

53b

54a

54b

55
a) *Histology* of case shown in Fig 54b. Pericanalicular fibroadenoma. Multiple branched lactiferous ducts covered with normally arranged epithelium. Loose connective tissue. Increase in number of subepithelial basket cells. Smooth border of surrounding breast parenchyma (right). Magnif 80×.
b) *Cytology*. Multiple small epithelial layers. Numerous dissociated bipolar naked nucleated cells in between. Some mucus in center of field. Magnif 180×.

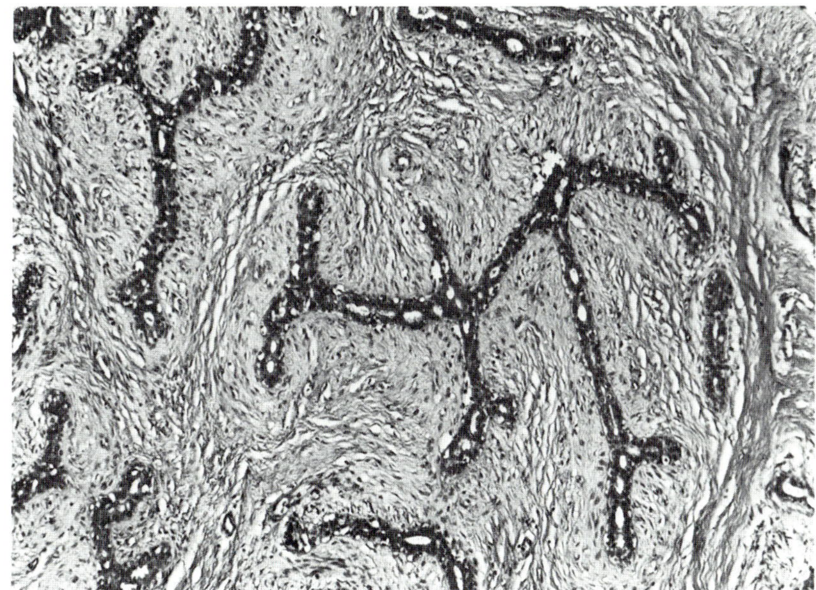

55a

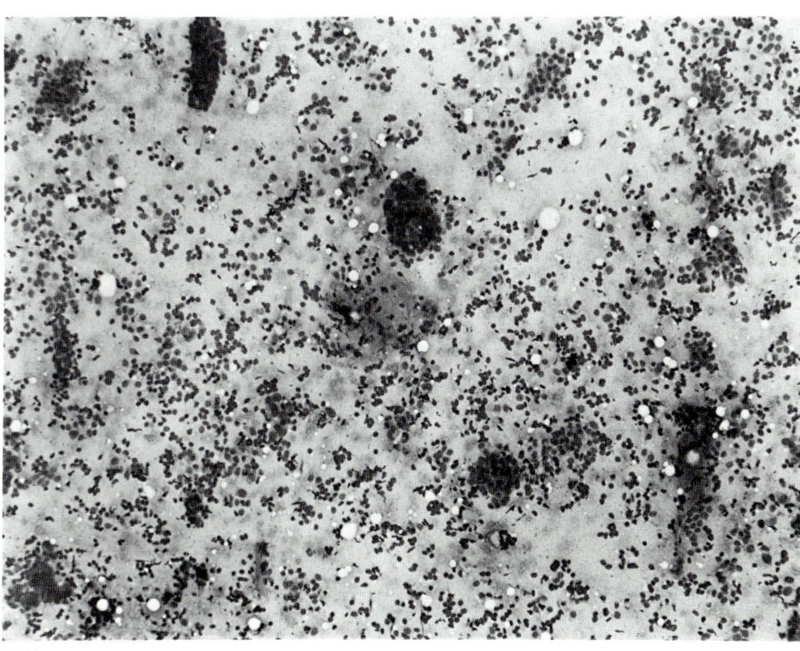

55b

◁ **53**
a) 18-year-old female with tangerine-sized nodule in left breast. No radiographic difference between fibroadenoma and dense breast.
b) 79-year-old female. Cherry-sized nodule below nipple for 30 years. In the mammogram there is periductal fibrosis with two smoothly-defined fibroadenomas. Extensive coarse calcifications.

◁ **54** a, b. 20-year-old female with cherry-sized nodule above the nipple of the right breast.
Mammogram.
a) Left breast. Normal. Lobules identifiable near the thoracic wall.
b) Right breast. Same appearance. Irregular, retroareolar, nonhomogeneous opacity.

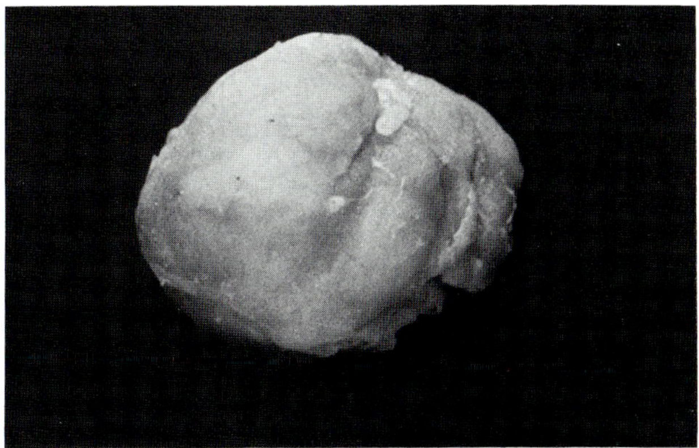

△
56 Nodule excised from breast of Fig 54b. Smooth, lobulated surface.

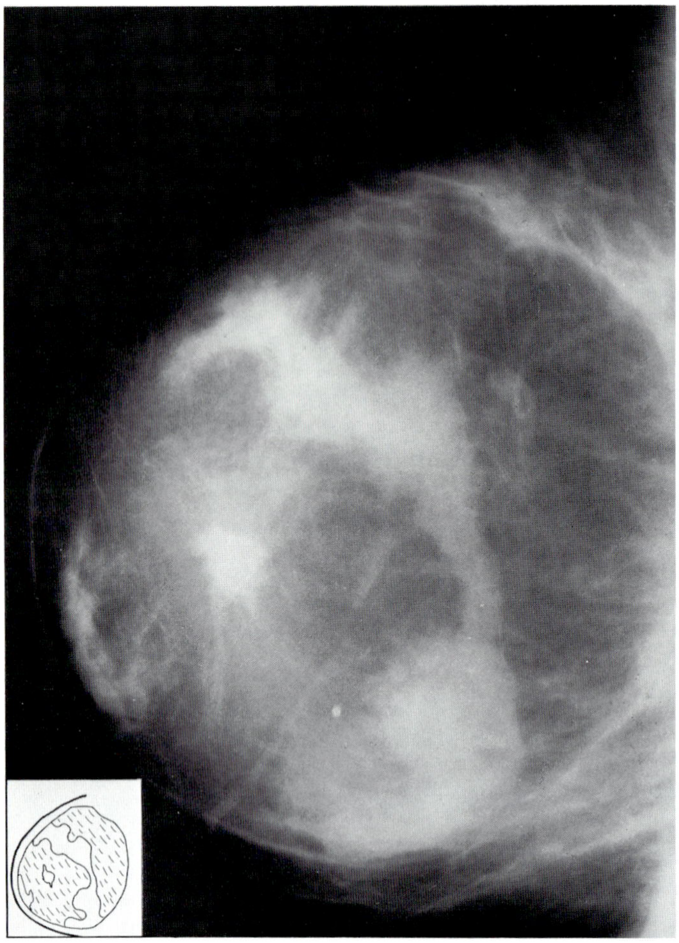

57 a

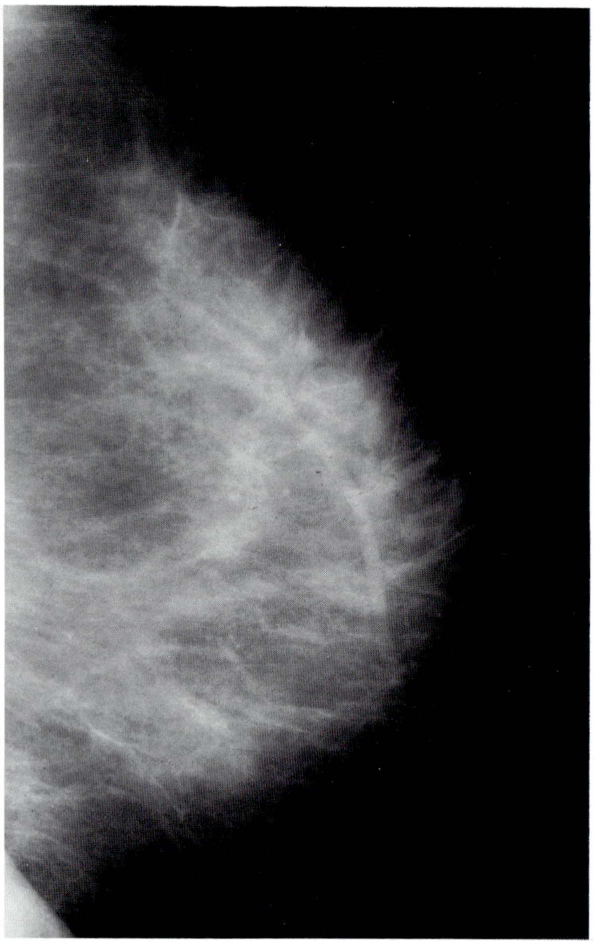

57 b

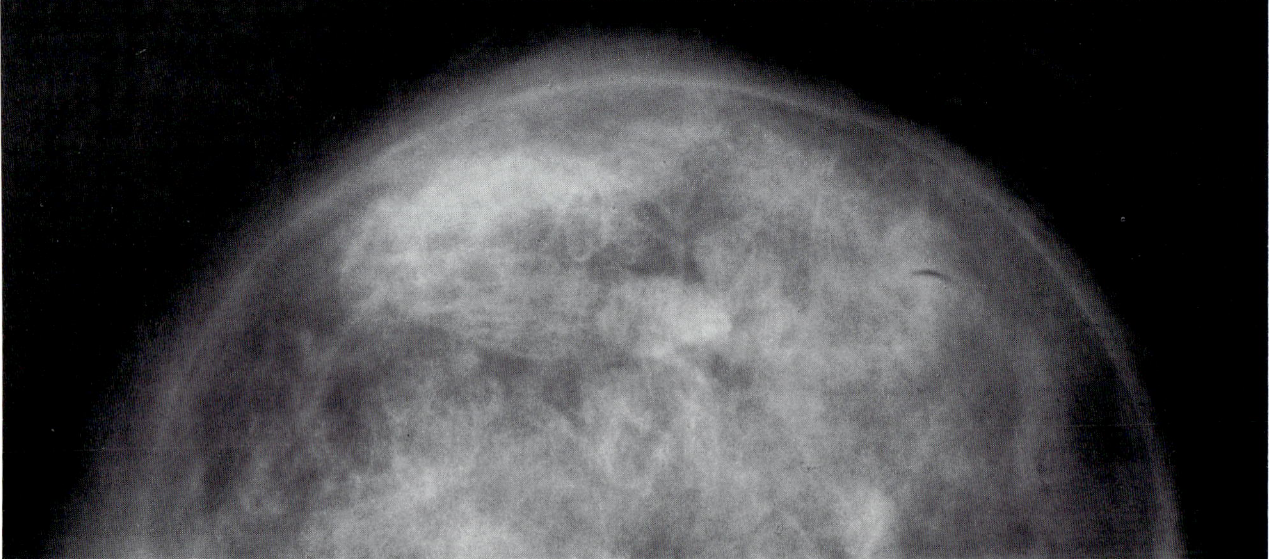

58

54-year-old female. Fist-sized soft tumor of left breast for 30 years (Fig 57).

57
a) *Mammogram left* (medio-lateral). Large, sharply defined tumor. Increased radiolucency. Broad, poorly defined opacities within tumor.
Histology: fibrolipoma.
b) *Mammogram right.* Normal breast.

58 32-year-old female. After cosmetic surgery with paraffin implant.
Mammography (cranio-caudal): Density of nonhomogeneous paraffin is sharply defined against compressed, condensed breast parenchyma. Radiographic findings similar to fibrolipoma, but edge of paraffin prosthesis is sharper.

61-year-old female. Recurrent, bilateral, serous secretions present for many years (Figs 59–62).

59 *Cut section of anatomical specimen.* Retracted nipple. Retroareolar, markedly dilated, lactiferous ducts and sinuses filled with debris. Stromal septa with dilated ducts in upper portion. Large amount of fat.

60 a, b. *Radiological-histological comparison.*
a) Specimen radiograph. Retracted nipple. Band-like, retroareolar opacities continuing cephalad into breast. Markedly dilated, retroareolar, lactiferous ducts and sinuses filled with debris exhibiting double contour (increased radiolucency of debris).
b) Histological macrosection. Markedly ectatic lactiferous ducts (1) and sinuses. Periductal fibrosis. Retraction of nipple. Circumscribed inflammatory periductal infiltrate (3). Sebaceous glands in areola (2).

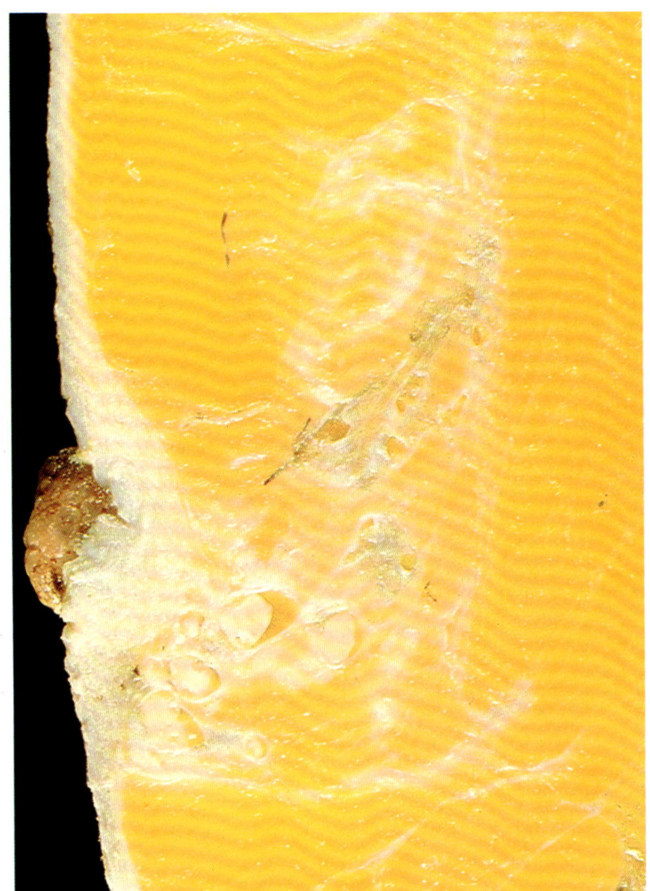

59

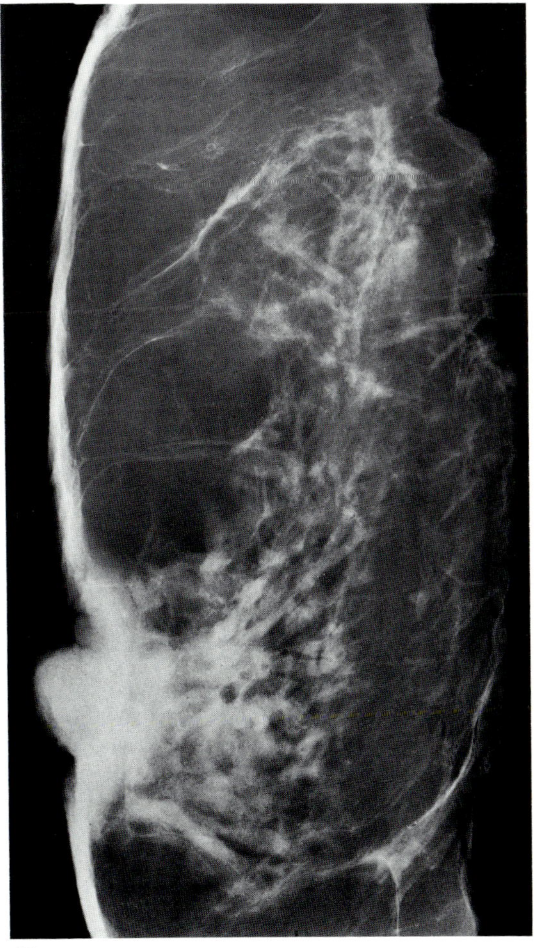

60a

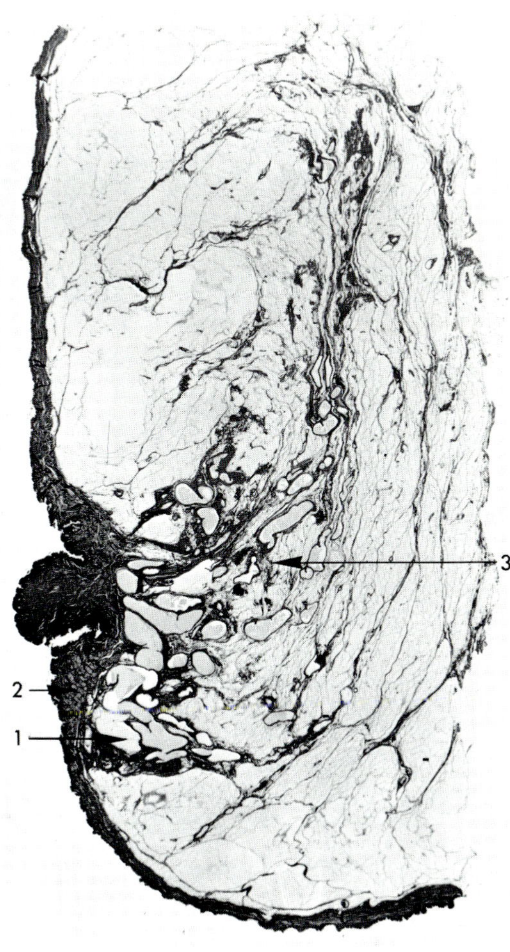

60b

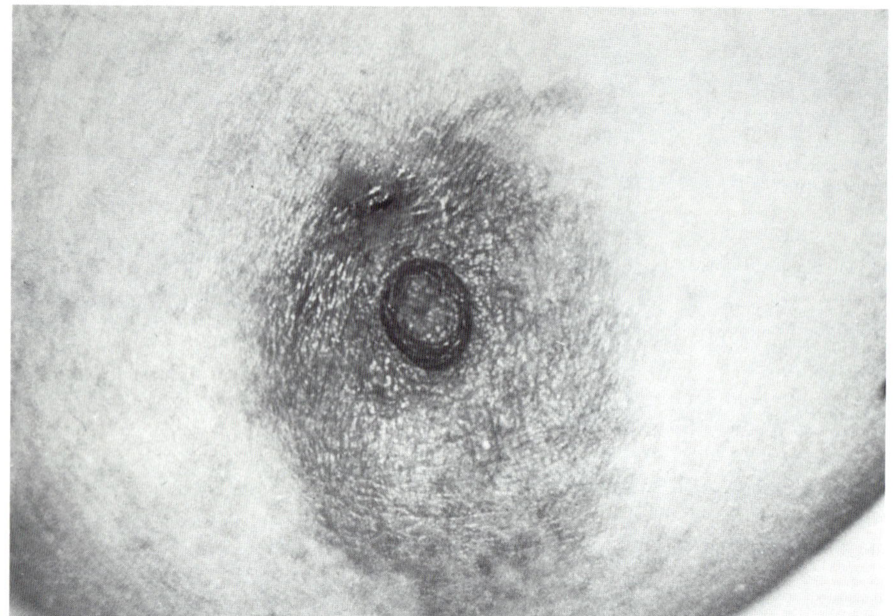

61a

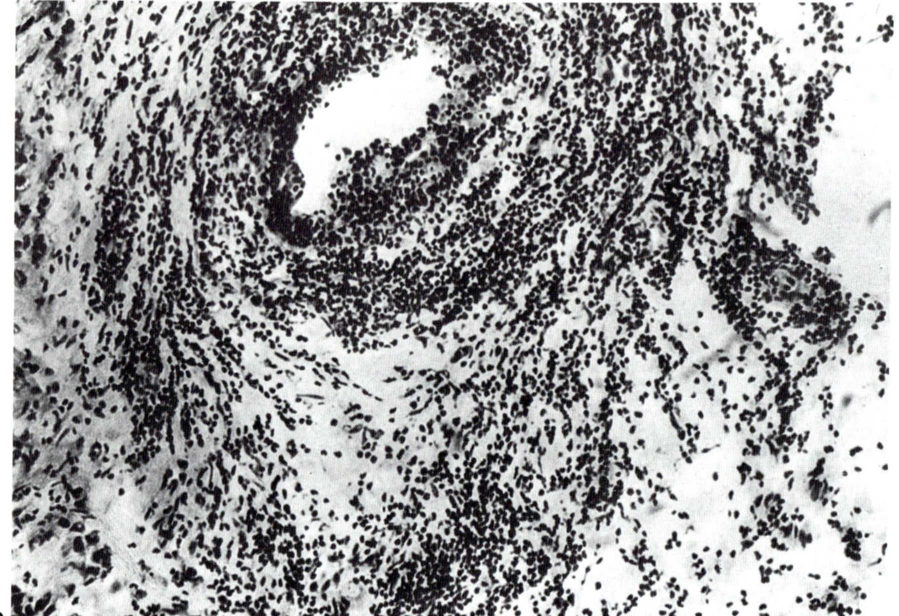

61b

61 a, b. Chronic mastitis with microabscesses and spontaneous perforation toward skin. Chronic fistula formation.

a) Nipple with fistula opening (delicate normal lactiferous ducts in the galactogram).

b) *Histology* of a lactiferous duct. Dense round cell infiltrate (lymphocytes and plasma cells) in duct wall and periductal stroma. Inflammation destroys lactiferous epithelium. Inflammatory cells in lumen of duct.

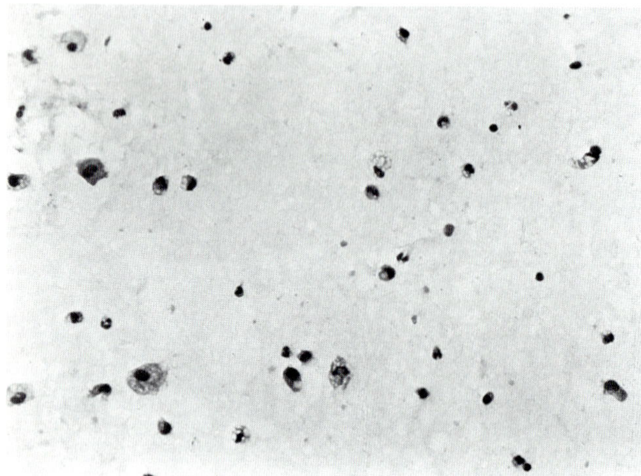

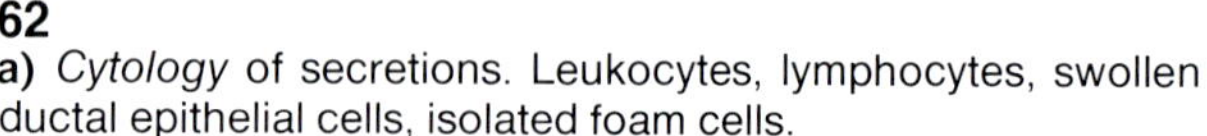

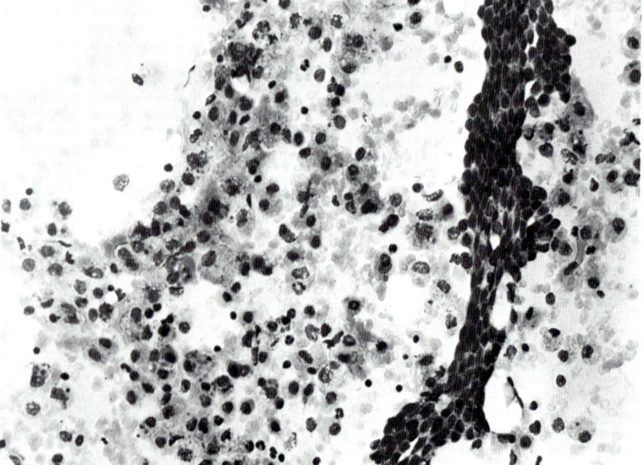

62

a) *Cytology* of secretions. Leukocytes, lymphocytes, swollen ductal epithelial cells, isolated foam cells.

b) Retroareolar *thin-needle biopsy*. The cytological smear shows multiple lymphocytes, leukocytes, duct epithelium and foam cells in addition to normal cell layers (right). Chronic mastitis.

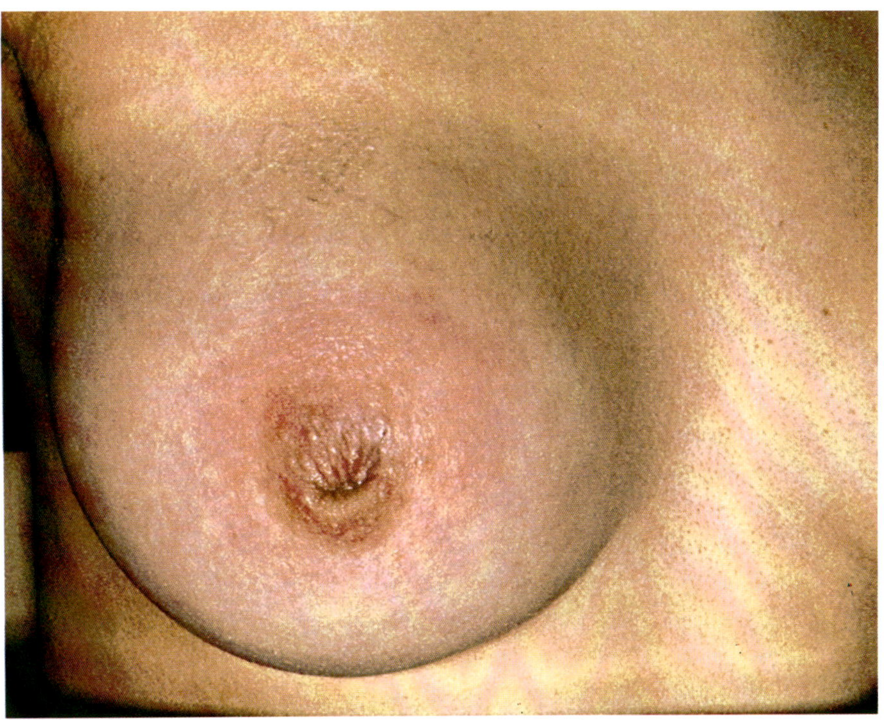

63

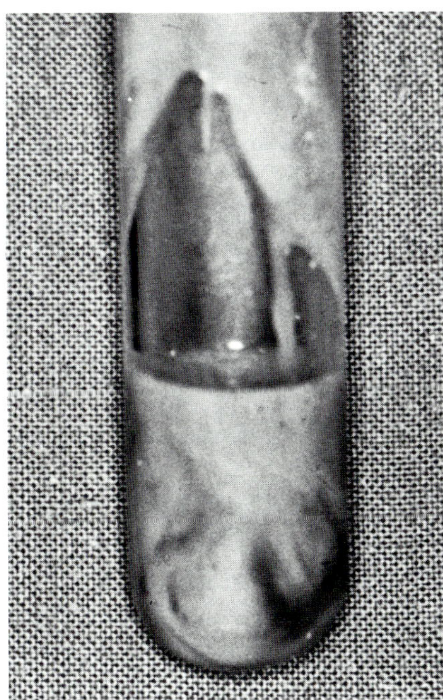

64 a

64 b

36-year-old female, right breast. Bilateral secretion for years. No secretion from right for 14 days. For 8 days increasing swelling of right breast. Marked pain. Mammographically there is a homogeneous, nonseparable opacity. Palpation reveals a dense, nodular, poorly movable tumor (Figs 63–64).

63 Right breast. Nipple retraction. Marked periareolar erythema of skin of breast.

64
a) *Thin-needle biopsy.* Aspiration of 20 ml cream-like, foul-smelling, gray-green pus.
b) Numerous granulocytes and cell debris (abscess) in *cytological smear.*

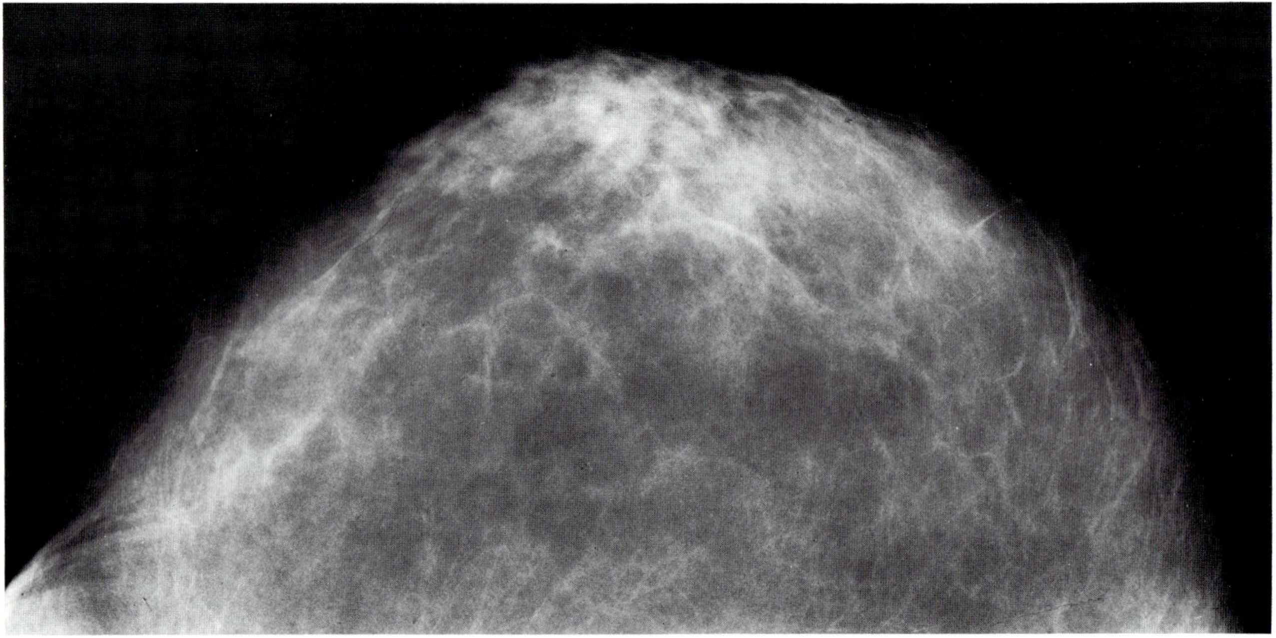

65

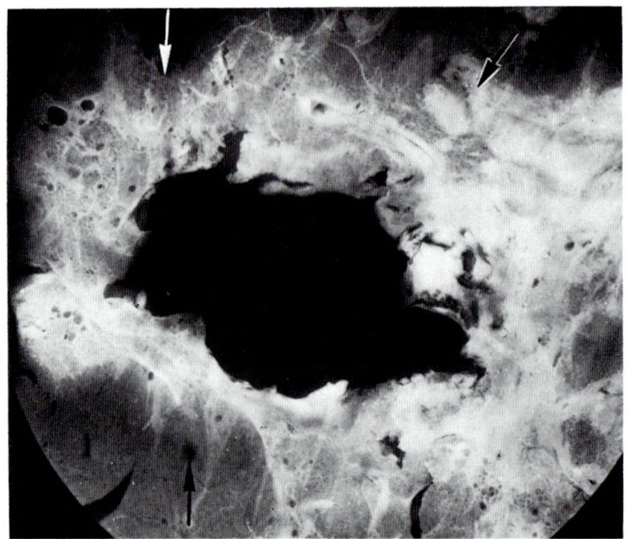

66a

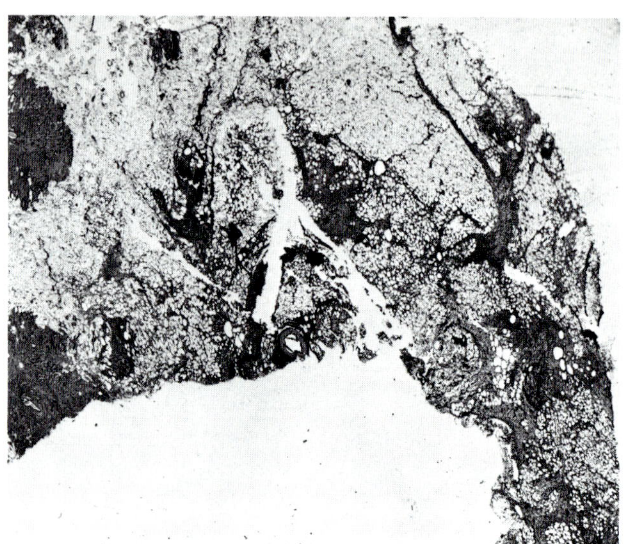

66b

62-year-old female, right breast. Slight secretion from both breasts for many years. For 3 months tangerine-sized, poorly movable, firm, retroareolar tumor of right breast. Slightly tender to palpation. No nipple or skin changes. Thermographically slight, diffuse temperature difference: right breast 0.5 °C warmer than left. (Figs 65–67).

65 *Mammogram,* left. Increased density of retroareolar lactiferous ducts; otherwise normal.

66 a, b. *Microradiographic-histological comparison.*
a) Microradiograph. Central abscess cavity. Perifocally decreased radiolucency of inflamed fatty tissue (arrows).
b) Abscess cavity surrounded by fat and islands of parenchyma. Inflammatory infiltration of fat. Magnif 5×.

67
a) *Mammogram,* right. Retroareolar, markedly thickened, lactiferous ducts with marked increase in density of breast and surrounding fat. No calcifications.
b) *Mammogram.* Follow-up examination 3 months after anti-inflammatory treatment. Practically complete regression of ground-glass-like opacification of breast tissue and fat. Regression of increased duct pattern. Mammogram as in Fig 65a after additional 6 months. No further secretions.
c) *Cytology.* Smear of secreting breast. Protein-rich secretions with several epithelial layers. Nuclei are hyperchromatic with granulocytes between them. Magnif 240×.
d) *Thin-needle biopsy* of nodule of right breast. Numerous granulocytes, a few degenerated epithelial cells, a large number of lymphocytes, many histiocytes and macrophages with large cytoplasm. Next to them (right) a large number of multinucleated giant cells (subacute to subchronic mastitis). Magnif 180×.

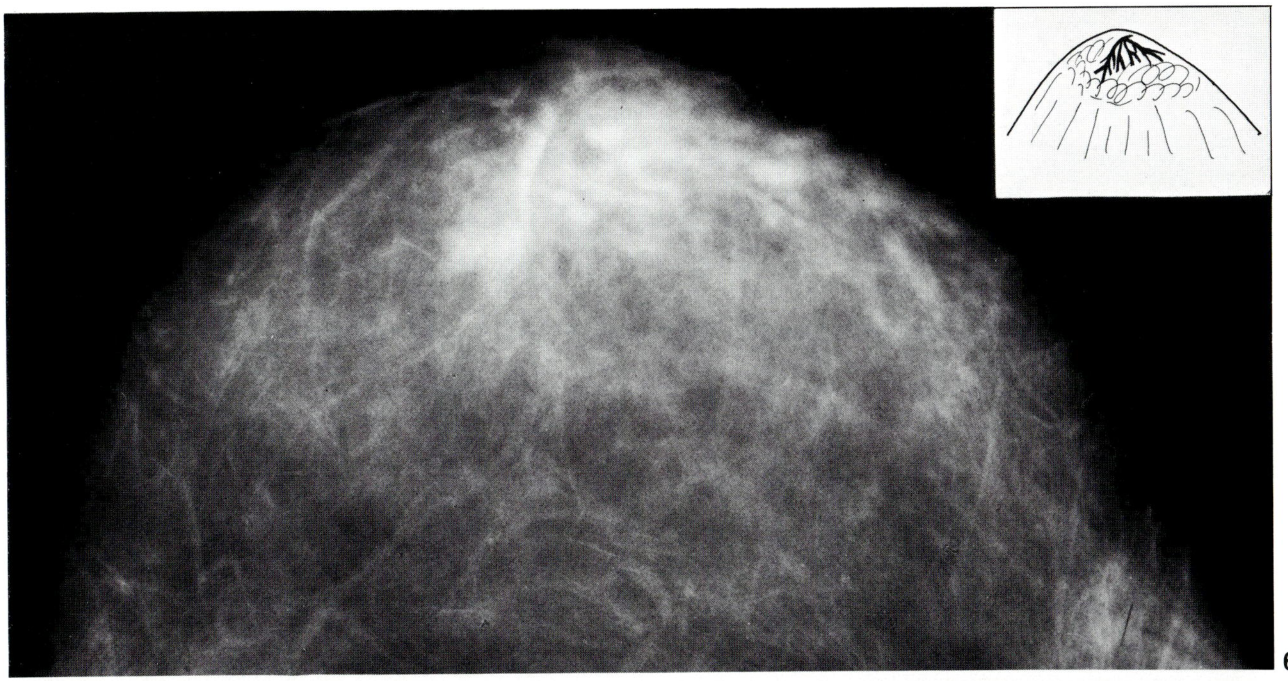
67 a

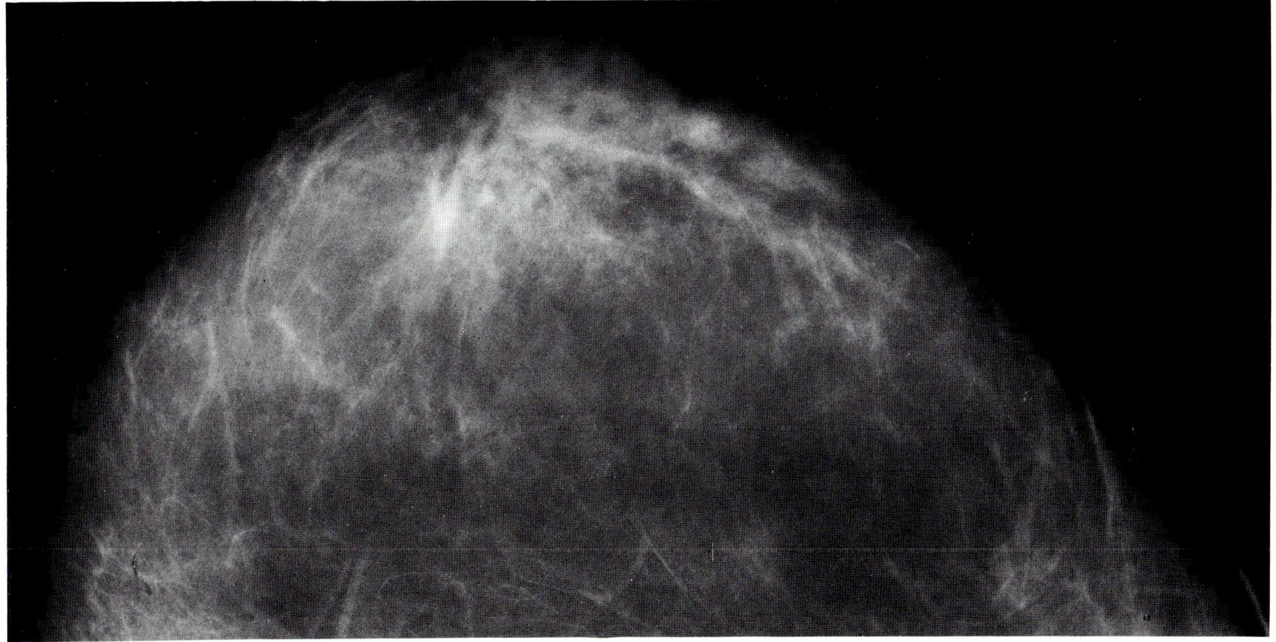
67 b

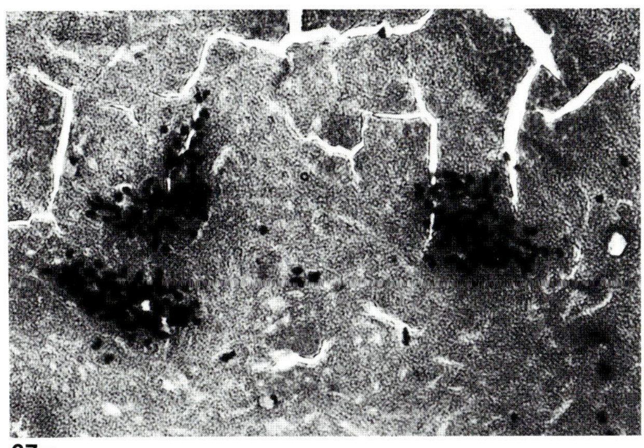
67 c

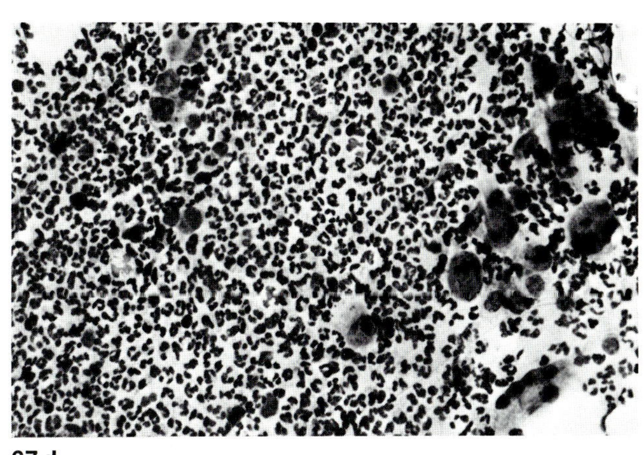
67 d

Mastopathies

Mastopathy is a *general term* for a heterogeneous group of proliferating and fibrosing lesions of the breast.

Fibrotic mastopathy is a premature change with atrophy of the lobules, disappearance of the intralobular connective tissue and hyalinization of the perilobular connective tissue. After disappearance of the intralobular tissue, the atrophic lobules lie within the sclerotic perilobular tissue (RAHN, 1972).

Cystic mastopathy indicates dilated lactiferous ducts and/or cystic lobule changes.

Both forms of mastopathy may occur concomitantly. The changes from fibrous to cystic mastopathy are gradual, so it is unimportant radiographically which predominates. It is only important to recognize the typical radiographic changes of mastopathy and thence to make the diagnosis. According to DOERR and ULE (1970), progression, regression and proliferation of the epithelium (layering of epithelium and formation of papillae) dominate the histology of mastopathy. These changes are demonstrated in Fig **68**.

Regressive changes

There is regression of lobules with fibrosis and hyalinization of intralobular tissues. By occlusion of lactiferous ducts with secretion and proliferation of the wall of the lactiferous duct, there is *dilatation of the duct system* and *formation of cysts* in the lobules (mastopathia fibrosa cystica). The basal membrane of acini and ductules becomes thicker.

Secretions and debris lie in the cysts and dilated lactiferous ducts. Debris consists of desquamated and necrotic epithelium and may be rich in lipoids (Fig **98** c). There is a marked affinity of degenerated epithelium for calcium salts; hence comes deposition of calcium. According to KOEHL et al (1970), 23% of all benign proliferations of epithelium tend to become calcified. Cell debris and calcium particles may be rubbed off or squeezed out from a fresh cut section of a specimen of fibrocystic mastopathy (so-called comedomastitis).

Formation of cysts is the most important change of fibrocystic mastopathy (BÖHMIG 1964, HAMPERL 1968 and 1975, BAESSLER et al 1971, HAAGENSEN 1971, PRECHTEL 1971 and 1974). There are apocrine, secretory

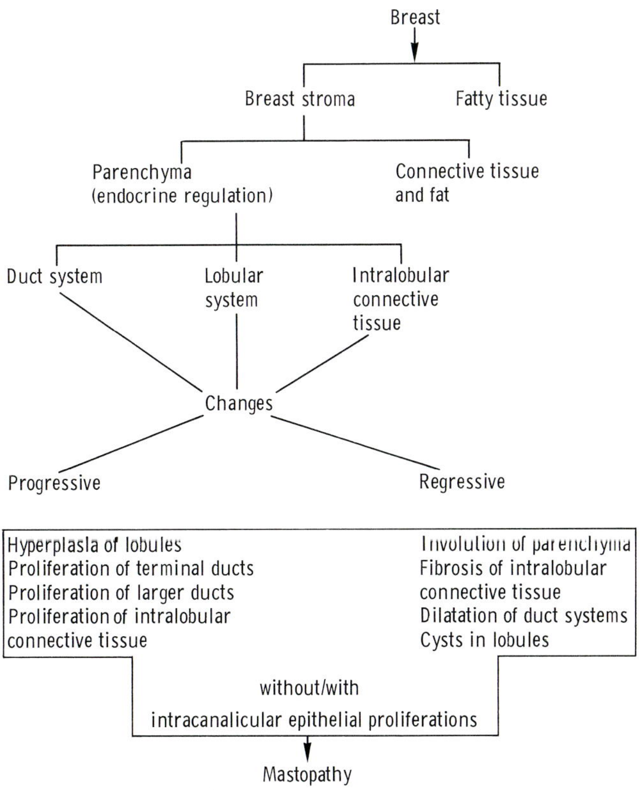

68 Regressive and progressive changes in breasts with mastopathy. (From Prechtel, K.: Fortschr. Med. 92:374, 1974)

and papillary cysts (INGLEBY and GERSHON-COHEN, 1960). The papilloma of the papillary cyst seems to originate from a lactiferous duct which has become cystically dilated by the growing secreting tumor (Figs **159**, **202** b).

Localized, tender induration of the breast may suddenly occur in many females with fibrocystic mastopathy. The underlying cause is a conglomerate of smaller cysts which swell acutely and thereby become painful. Individual cysts within the conglomerate are a few millimeters in diameter. If the cyst conglomerate is surrounded by fat, mammography may demonstrate a polycyclic opacity (Fig **70** a, b). Individual cysts may become very large in a short period of time, but 80% regress spontaneously after aspiration. Increased intracystic pressure apparently destroys secreting epithelium, stopping secretion and after-secretion in an aspirated cyst.

Cystic changes occur mostly during the fourth and fifth decades. Absolutely or relatively increased serum estrogen levels seem to be the underlying cause. Large doses of estrogen stimulate cyst formation. It has been said that ovulation-depressing drugs with high estrogen content may cause the formation of cysts and proliferation of epithelium (LANG and co-workers, 1972).

Changed progesterone metabolism is observed to result from stress, ovarectomy, hysterectomy and disease of the thyroid gland (COWIE and FOLLEY, 1961). The menstrual cycle may be regular. There is excessive and very painful swelling of the breasts premenstrually.

Many women with cystic changes also have diseases of the pelvic organs. There is a 7% incidence of uterine fibroids; in 3% there is a concomitantly enlarged thyroid gland (INGLEBY and GERSHON-COHEN, 1960; BREZINA and HERNUSS, 1975).

If painless, the multiple large and small cysts in cases of mastopathy are of no significance but must be differentiated radiographically from other pathologic entities (fibroadenoma, medullary carcinoma). More important is adenosis of the lobules which (according to INGLEBY and GERSHON-COHEN, 1960) always occurs in the area of cysts (Fig **38** b). There is no tendency to malignant transformation of adenosis and fibrocystic mastopathy. SILVERBERG et al (1972) found an incidence of fibrocystic mastopathy of 39.4% in 398 breast cancers. This rate is identical to that of the normal population free of cancer (the author also noted that carcinomas in fibrocystic mastopathy are smaller and axillary lymph node metastases are less common than with breast cancer unassociated with cystic changes).

Progressive changes

Hyperplasia of lobules

Hyperplasia of lobules with preservation of their basic structure is a common finding with mastopathy (Figs **72**, **84** b, **88**). Proliferation of acini with associated reaction of intralobular connective tissue outside the duct system is called *adenosis*. It occurs commonly in a cystic area.

Adenosis is a very common change in the female breast. It occurs bilaterally but may involve one breast more than the other. Adenomatous foci may be circumscribed or diffuse. The enlarged lobules are identifiable in the mammogram and microradiograph, if there is only a small amount of interlobular connective tissue in the mastion and breast. Markedly reactive enlarged lobules consistent with adenosis were found surrounding a multilocular polymorphous cellular carcinoma in a 32-year-old woman (Figs **193** a, **197**).

In the *mammogram* the foci of adenosis appear as irregular, ill-defined, homogeneous opacities. The opacities may become confluent to form extensive densities. Conglomerate adenomatous foci may be palpated as coarse, easily movable nodules in the breast.

Abundant cellular material may be obtained from the nodule with *thin-needle biopsy*. This consists of proliferating epithelial layers and multiple bipolar cells with naked nuclei. The cell pattern cannot be differentiated from a fibroadenoma.

Proliferation of the epithelium

Intraductal epithelial proliferations are of great importance as they may precede a carcinoma. In 30% of all mastopathies there are, according to PRECHTEL (1974), epithelial proliferations of varying sizes in large and small lactiferous ducts.

Two thirds show normal cells; one third shows atypical changes in structure of cell layers, in cells and in nuclei. *According to* BÄSSLER *(1975), however, to call the fibrocystic mastopathy precancerous is not justified.* A significant risk for malignant transformation exists only with proliferating atypical epithelium. Retrospective studies by BLACK et al (1972) on biopsy specimens of 332 patients showed that the chance of malignant transformation is five times higher with atypical proliferation of epithelium in lactiferous ducts than with ordinary epithelial proliferations.

Mastopathia cystica fibrosa shows the greatest spectrum of epithelial hyperplasia of varying degree. The intraductal proliferation consists commonly of a large cluster of epithelial cells, commonly without stroma, leaving small openings by obliterating the duct lumen (Fig **89** d). Other cell proliferations are traversed by stromal papillae containing blood vessels which finally form villous-like epithelial and stromal papillae also called ductus papillomas (Fig **73** a, c, d). Solid, glandular and papillary intracanalicular growths may be distributed over the entire breast in cases of mastopathy. They may also occur as isolated lesions such as the *solitary papilloma of the lactiferous duct* with the bleeding breast (HAMPERL, 1968) (Figs **91**, **92** a). This occurs particularly after the 40th year.

Transformation of a papilloma to a carcinoma is rare. Because of the large number of papillomas and papillary proliferations with mastopathy and the rarity of papillary carcinomas with mastopathy, it is not justifiable to consider all papillary tumors precancerous (BÄSSLER, 1975). Especially in the elderly female, proliferating

lactiferous epithelium is commonly seen. KRAMER and RUSH (1973) did autopsies on 70 females over 70 years of age and examined their breasts which had been considered normal clinically. Their findings were as follows: 62 cystic dysplasias, 56 apocrine metaplasias, 40 adenoses, 15 small papillomas and 48 intraductal hyperplasias of the epithelium in which atypical epithelium occurred 7 times and malignant transformation 4 times.
Extensive epithelial proliferation in a lactiferous duct may cause marked duct dilatation. As tumor cells are less dense than the fibrotic wall of the lactiferous duct, double contours may be noted in the mammogram. The double contour is *not* conclusive evidence of extensive cell proliferation. *Debris* in the dilated lactiferous ducts may also cause a double contour as the debris often has a high (30%) content of lipid and is therefore less dense than the fibrotic surrounding tissue (Fig **69**). Extensive filling of multiple lactiferous ducts with debris may produce a "negative galactogram."
Microcalcifications may occur with intraductal proliferation of epithelium. Some calcifications may have the size of psammoma bodies—too small to be identifiable mammographically. However, they may be seen in the enlarged radiograph and microradiograph (Figs **77–81**). Calcifications must have a diameter of 0.2 mm to be visible in the mammogram. It is not possible to determine radiographically the significance of microcalcifications in mastopathy. An intraductal carcinoma is more likely if calcium deposits are more localized, numerous and irregular (Figs **101**, **102**).

Increased branching of lactiferous duct systems

Large lactiferous ducts and small branches normally have a straight course and show little peripheral branching, but in mastopathy there is marked branching in the system.
Multiple anastomoses running across to surrounding ductules may be present and may be shown on a *galactogram* after filling with contrast material (Fig **71**c).
Branched lactiferous ducts filled with debris and proliferating epithelium are better shown in a microradiograph than in histological sections (Fig **71**a, b).

Proliferation of intralobular and periductal (interlobular) connective tissue

Proliferation of intralobular tissue and increase of periductal tissue appear mammographically as

a) solitary and multiple, round, homogeneous, well-defined opacities (with and without calcifications) of fibroadenomas (Fig **76**),
b) ill-defined, nonhomogeneous opacities between thickened and fibrotic lactiferous ducts caused by sclerosing adenosis (Fig **76**),
c) band-like, irregular, broad opacities along lactiferous ducts (increased periductular stroma) (Fig **75**).

Proliferation of intralobular and perilobular tissues as listed causes an irregular, radiating, nonhomogeneous pattern of mastopathy in the radiograph. In two-dimensional mammograms the projection of the extensively branched, dilated, lactiferous duct system and the surrounding connective tissue causes band-like and focal opacities (Figs **77–79**).

Regressive and progressive changes in the galactogram

Incidence of secretions excluding lactation is quoted differently (NYIRJESY, 1968, 0.76%; VETTER, 1974, 0.89%; FLEMING, 1974, 50%).
Five percent of our patients had spontaneous or stimulated increase in secretion from one or more lactiferous ducts.
A locally proliferating process in the parenchyma is the underlying cause of secretions in two thirds of all patients. In the rest the secretion is drug or hormonally induced (BARTH, 1975).
In those cells which are characteristic of apocrine metaplasia, dome-like or tongue-shaped projections of cytoplasm are commonly found in dilated ducts and cysts. The cytoplasm shows fatty degeneration. A peculiarity of this type of secretion is occasional inclusion of the nucleus in the production of secretions. In typical apocrine secretion, portions of the cytoplasm adjoining the lumen are desquamated and then appear in the secretion as spherules of varying size.
Foam cells found in the smear of the secreting breast are either desquamated, fatty, degenerated epithelial cells or histiocytes engulfing fat (Fig **89**b) (HAMPERL, 1975; PRECHTEL, personal communication). They correspond to degenerated epithelial cells which may cover the inside of cysts (Fig **89**a). The secretion may be watery, brownish-green or milky. Milky secretion is not identical with normal milk (VETTER et al, 1974).
The *galactogram* showed cysts in the region of the terminal lactiferous ducts and lobules in 31.6% of 558 patients with secreting breasts (Fig **37**). The cyst conglomerates are predominantly near the thoracic wall—the dominant location of the lobules.
Ectasia of a lactiferous duct with a diameter of over 3 mm could be demonstrated in 11.8% of 588 examinations. Ectasia occurs alone or in combination with cysts (BARTH et al, 1975).
Circumscribed filling defects of contrast-filled ducts in the galactogram may be caused by *papillomas* (Fig **90**). We found 74 such cases in our patients (13.4%).
Elongated filling defects in the contrast medium (Fig **154**b) or marked general dilatation of lactiferous ducts are suggestive of carcinoma (Fig **96**). This occurred in 1.2% of our patients.

Histologic examination of 81 galactrographic irregularities of the ductal system showed 37 atypical or papillary epithelial proliferations with cystic mastopathy, 20 benign papillomas of lactiferous ducts and 7 intraductal carcinomas. Four of the carcinomas were recognized on the mammogram by microcalcifications or circumscribed tumor shadow (Fig **154** a). Galactography therefore detected 3 occult carcinomas in 558 patients which were clinically, mammographically and thermographically occult except for secretion (BARTH et al, 1975). The number of carcinomas diagnosed *exclusively* by galactography is low when there is *little preselection* of patients. Our results and those of other examiners are compared in Table 4.

Table 4. Number of satisfactory galactograms compared with biopsies and carcinomas found *exclusively* by galactography. Comparison of results of several examiners.

Author	Galactography	Biopsy	Carcinoma
Nunnerly and Field (1972)	21	8	0 (0%)
Threatt and Appelman (1973)	54	20	4 (7.4%)
Rummel and co-workers (1969)	75	45	5 (6.6%)
Quimet-Oliva and Hebert (1974)	265	127	7 (2.7%)
Grünberg et al. (1974)	59	10	1 (1.7%)
Menges and co-workers (1974)	80	14	4* (5.0%)
Barth et al. (1975)	558	81	3 (0.5%)
Tabar et al. (1973)	53	20 (?)	3 (5.6%)

* Inclu. two in situ carcinomas.

Drugs and hormones also may produce breast secretions. This explains the normal galactogram in 35.4% of 588 patients with secreting breasts (BARTH et al, 1975). The causes of galactorrhea are:

a) *accompanying symptoms of endocrinological abnormalities* such as pituitary tumors, Cushing's syndrome, hyperthyroidism, myxedema, inflammatory or malignant tumors of the ovaries, menstrual abnormalities, premenopause and menopause, status post oophorectomy, diabetes mellitus,
b) *drugs* such as sedatives, antihypertensives, tranquilizers,
c) *mental illnesses* such as schizophrenia and other psychoses.

(SACHS, 1971; VETTER et al, 1974).

A pituitary tumor with unilateral enlargement of the sella turcica in a nulliparous patient caused marked galactorrhea from all lactiferous ducts of both breasts for three years. The galactorrhea stopped within three weeks following the administration of a prolactin-blocking drug (2-brom-alpha-ergocryptin). The galactorrhea recurred within one week after the drug was discontinued.
The galactogram was normal bilaterally (Figs **93–95**).
In addition to the galactorrhea the patient had hirsutism with a tendency to beard growth.

Diagnosis of mastopathy in the radiograph

"Mastopathy" can be diagnosed radiographically when typical changes of mastopathy are present in the mammogram and/or galactogram. This diagnosis will become difficult when these structures are embedded in a large amount of interlobular connective tissue and can no longer be differentiated with certainty radiographically.
There are no definite statements as to how much regressive and/or progressive change must be present to justify the term "mastopathy." Our own opinion based upon findings in 13,000 examinations is that at least one finding of each regression and progression in the mammogram should be present to make the diagnosis of mastopathy. The clinical examination supported by the cytological examination of aspirates and secretions may confirm the diagnosis.
It is incorrect to diagnose mastopathy exclusively by increased x-ray absorption. Density in the mammogram is predominantly caused by connective tissue which has no significance in the development of carcinoma (juvenile breasts consist of 90% connective tissue) (Figs **11–14**).

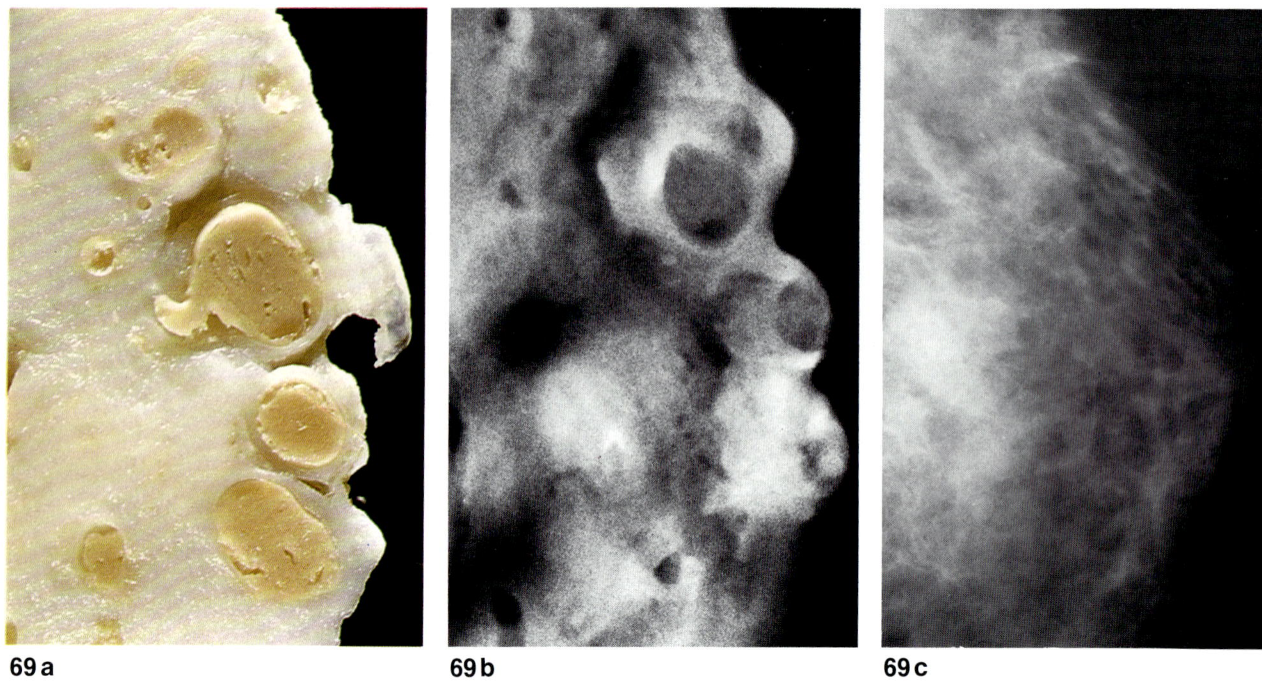

69 a 69 b 69 c

69 a–c. Dilatation of lactiferous ducts by debris.

a) *Cut section of anatomic specimen.* Multiple, markedly dilated ducts filled with yellow-brown plugs of debris. Fibrosis of surrounding gray-white breast parenchyma.

b) *Specimen radiograph.* Fibrosed duct wall is radiopaque. Debris is radiolucent.

c) *Mammogram.* Ectatic, debris-filled ducts are retroareolar and show double contour.

70 a–c. Cyst formation.

a) Cyst conglomerate. Surgical specimen of a painful nodule.

b) *Specimen radiograph.* Confluent, small, nodular, smoothly defined, nonhomogeneous opacity (cyst conglomerate). Surrounding fat radiolucent.

c) *Galactography.* Contrast-filled ducts and cysts of varying sizes.

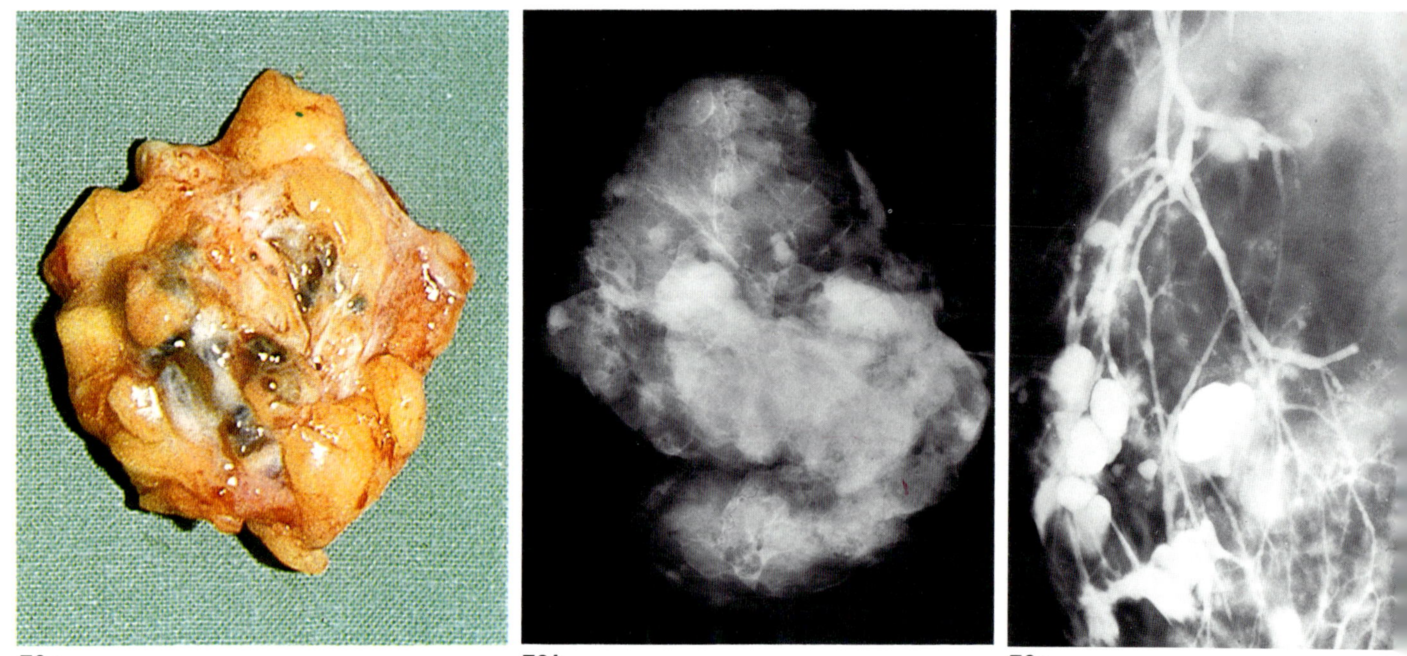

70 a 70 b 70 c

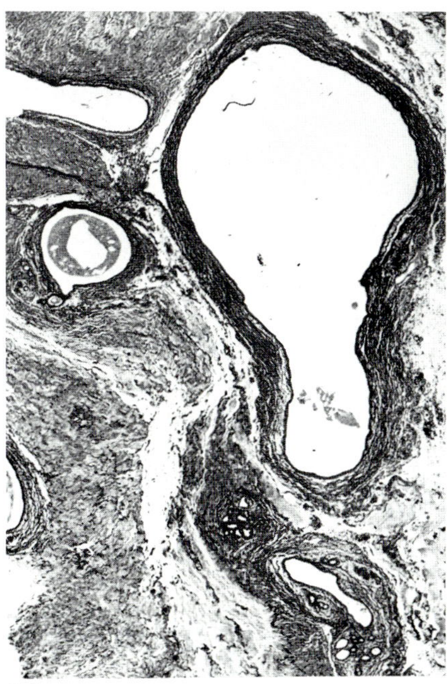
71 a

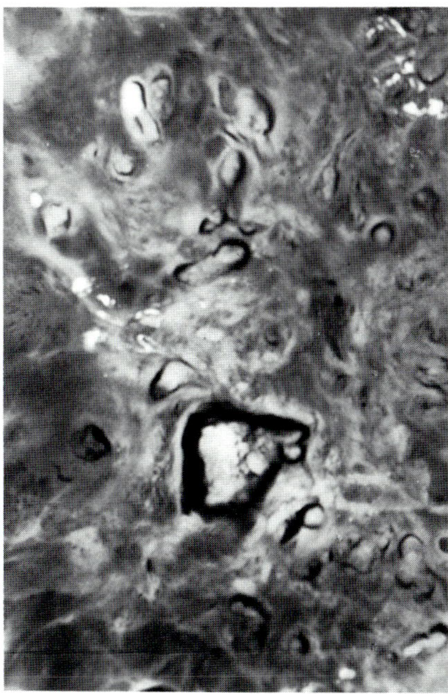
71 b

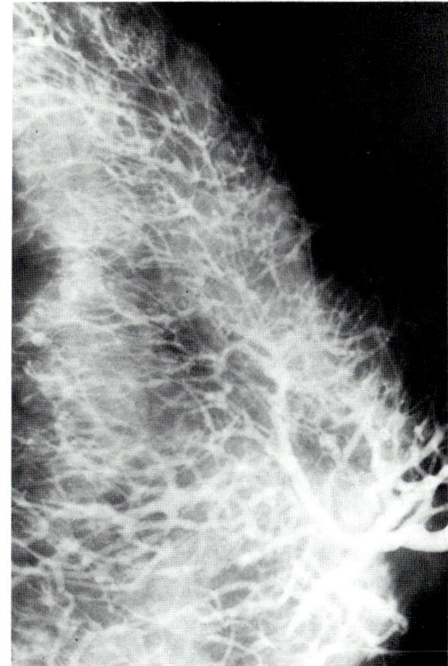
71 c

71 a–c. Branching of lactiferous ducts.
a) *Histology.* Multiple, sometimes markedly ectatic ducts with periductal fibrosis, of varying caliber. Magnif 120×.
b) *Microradiograph.* Multiple portions of lactiferous system next to a larger duct (below center of picture). All lactiferous ducts are blocked with debris. Microcalcifications above on right. Magnif 80×.
c) *Galactography.* Markedly branched lactiferous duct system with small cysts in terminal ducts.

72 a–c. Lobular hypertrophy.
a) *Histology.* Multiple lobules of varying sizes with proliferating acini (adenosis). Perilobular connective tissue absent. Magnif 80×.
b) *Microradiograph.* Oval opacities of varying sizes with delicate, mesh-like opacities produced by intralobular and perilobular connective tissue. Smaller lactiferous ducts are shown in the center in longitudinal and cross-section. Magnif 80×.
c) *Mammogram.* Multiple tiny opacities from hypertrophied lobules.

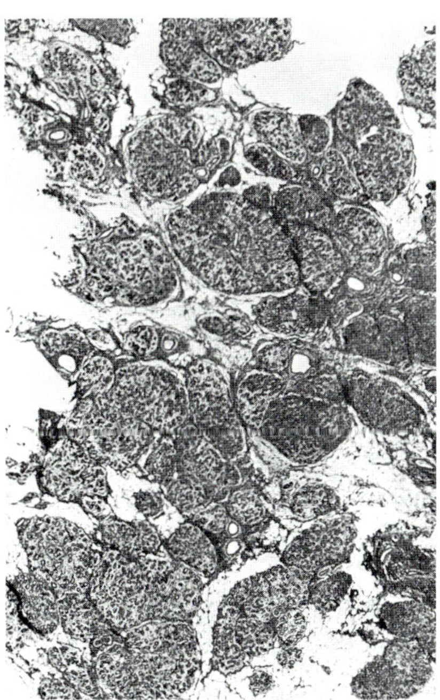
72 a

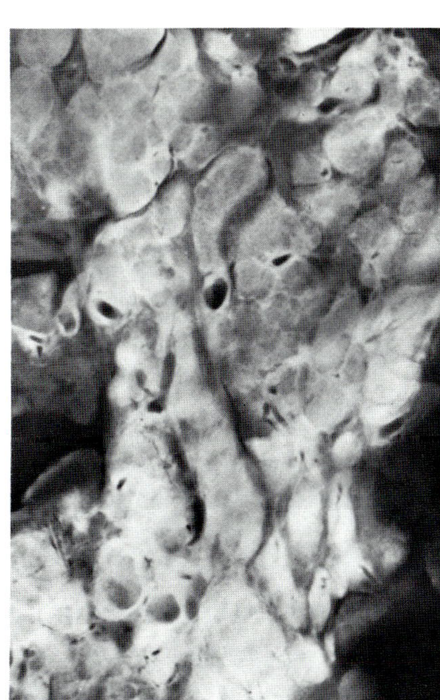
72 b

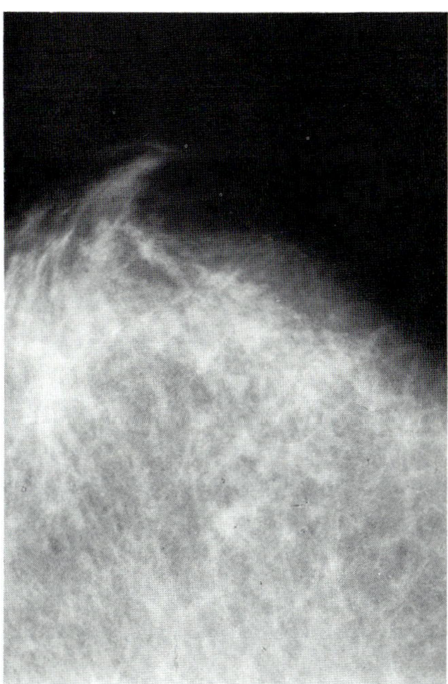
72 c

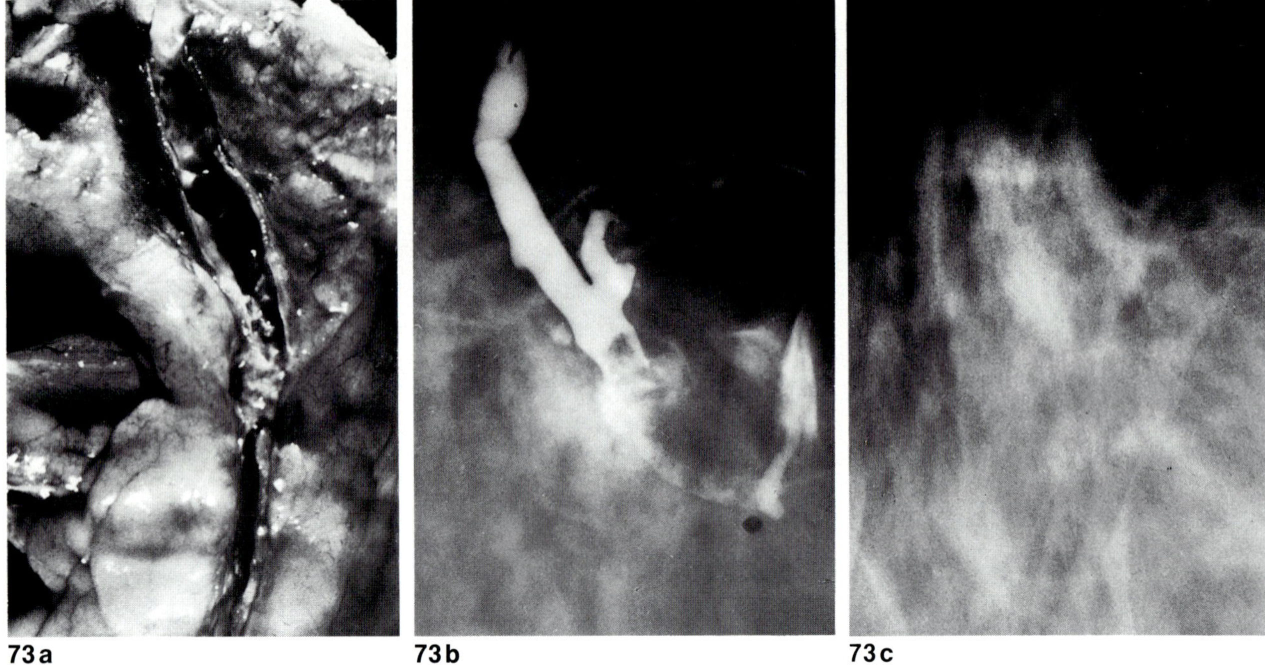

73 a 73 b 73 c

73 a–c. Proliferation of epithelium of lactiferous ducts.
a) *Anatomic representation.* Lactiferous duct open. Partial occlusion of duct lumen by papillary lesions. Histologically: papillomatosis. Magnif 5×.
b) *Galactography.* Dilated duct filled with contrast medium. Interruption of contrast column by papilloma of duct. Magnif 5×.
c) *Mammogram.* Section of retroareolar area with thickened and dense lactiferous ducts.

74 a–c. Epithelial proliferations with calcifications.
a) *Histology.* Dilated acini and terminal lactiferous ducts with single layer of epithelium. Circumscribed proliferations of epithelium. Calcium deposits of varying sizes in lumen, between epithelial layer and basal membrane and in the interstitium. Magnif 80×.
b) *Microradiograph.* Partially interstitial, partially intraductal microcalcifications. Calcium particle in lactiferous duct along the wall (above) (in the epithelium or between epithelium and basal membrane). Magnif 80×.
c) *Specimen radiograph.* Dust-like calcium deposits in breast parenchyma. Magnif 5×.

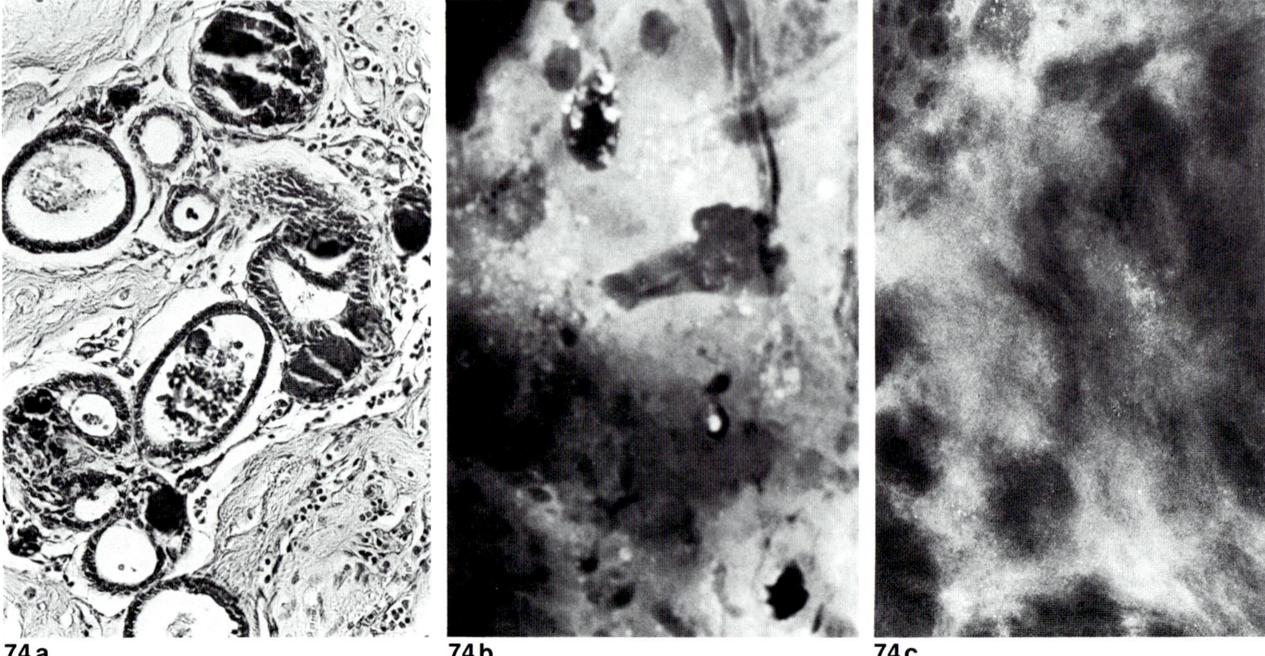

74 a 74 b 74 c

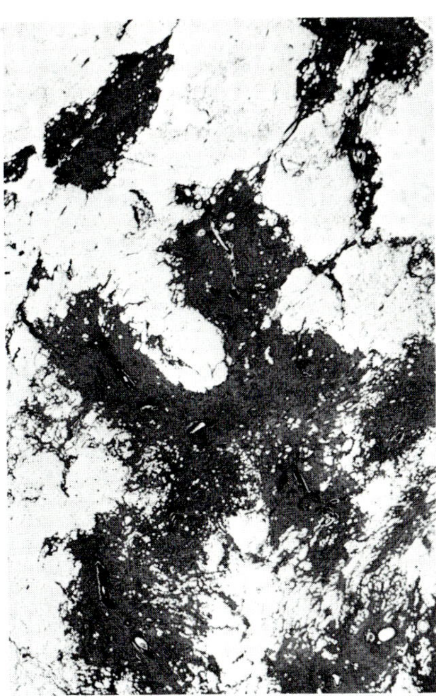

75 a

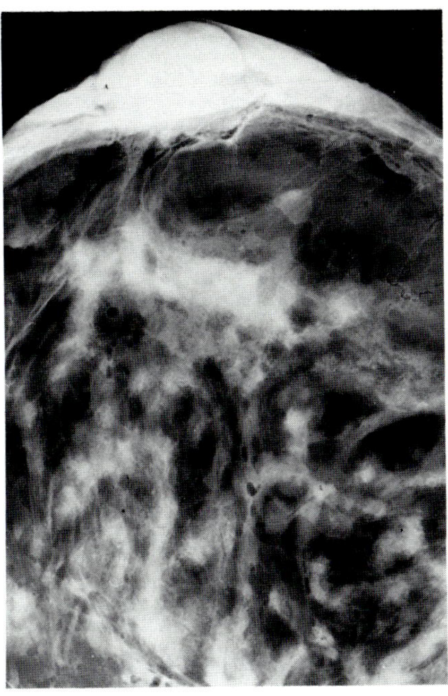

75 b

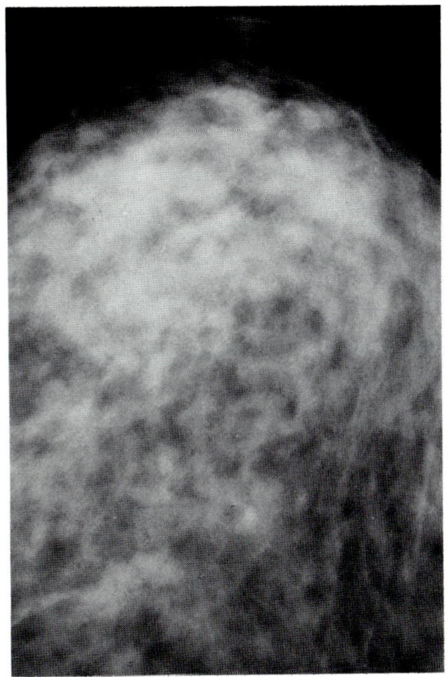

75 c

75 a–c. Proliferation of periductal intralobular connective tissue.
a) *Histology.* Lactiferous ducts cut obliquely with surrounding broad rim of connective tissue. Border with fatty tissue is not sharp. Magnif 90×.
b) *Specimen radiograph.* Periductal nonhomogeneous opacities with unsharp borders.
c) *Mammogram.* The ductal opacities shown in Fig 71b add up to partially band-like and partially small spot-like opacities (two-dimensional picture of branched duct system).

76 a–c. Proliferation of intralobular connective tissue.
a) *Histology.* Fibroadenoma with hyalinized and partially calcified stroma (lower portion of nodule). Coarse calcium in remaining nodule. Magnif 90×. Focal fibrosis with dilated lactiferous ducts and atrophic lobules. Proliferating acini with growth of intralobular connective tissue (sclerosing adenosis).
b) *Cut section of anatomic specimen.* Smoothly defined fibroadenoma above. Lighter oval area in lower portion of nodule (necrosis with calcification). Below nodule are small parenchymal foci within fatty tissue (fibrosis and sclerosing adenosis).
c) *Specimen radiograph.* Above, fibroadenoma with coarse bizarre calcifications. Below, unsharp nonhomogeneous fibrosis and sclerosing adenosis (cannot be differentiated radiographically).

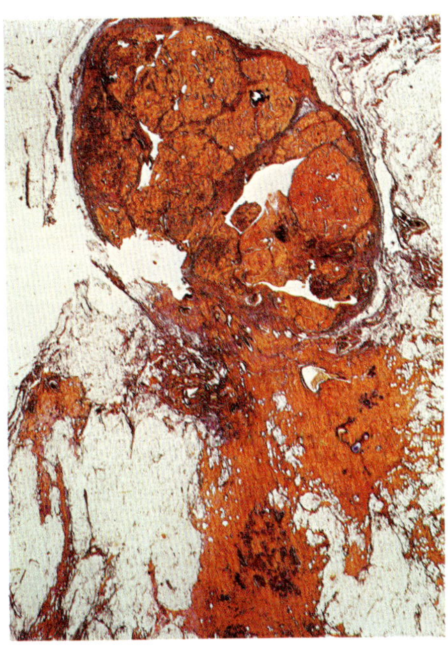

76 a

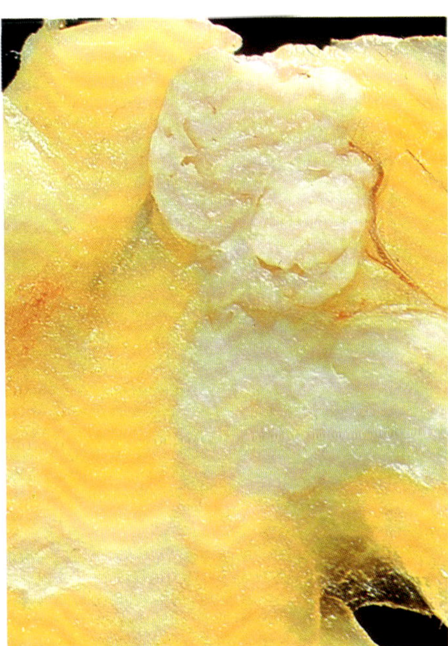

76 b

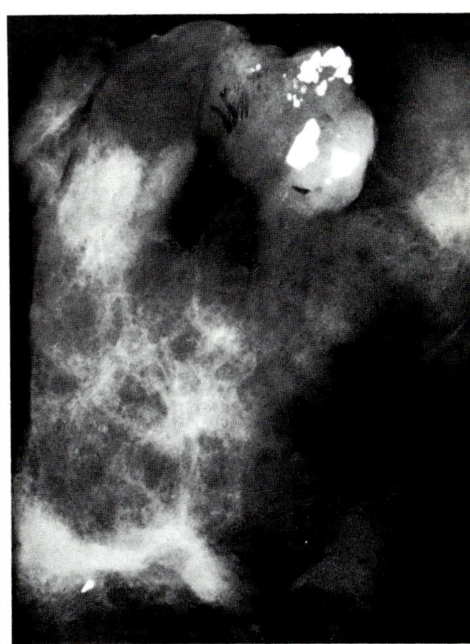

76 c

61-year-old female, left breast. Repeated radiographic examinations in past six months. No abnormal findings. The patient worries about her left breast (Figs 77–81).

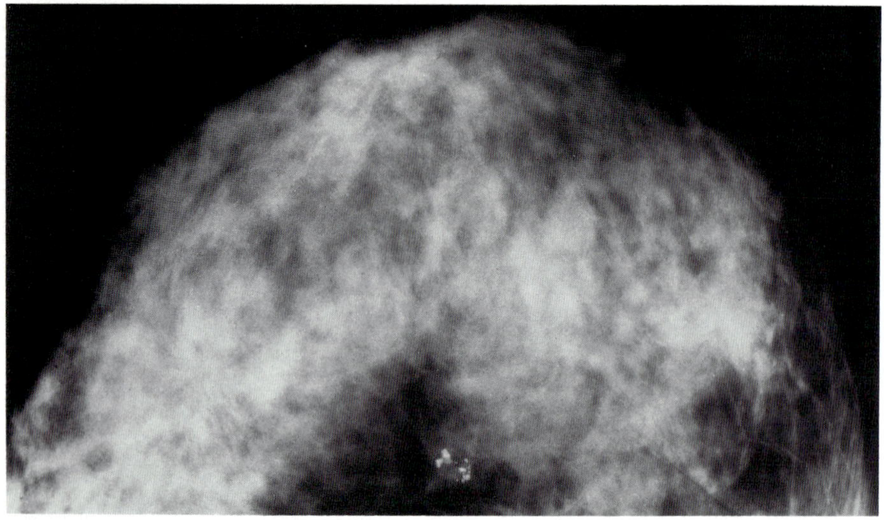

77

77 *Mammogram* (craniocaudal). Fibrous mastopathy with band-like and small spot-like opacities along lactiferous ducts. Stellate carcinoma of lateral quadrant (Figs 123, 124). Next to thoracic wall, between both upper quadrants, fibroadenoma with coarse calcifications (Fig 76).

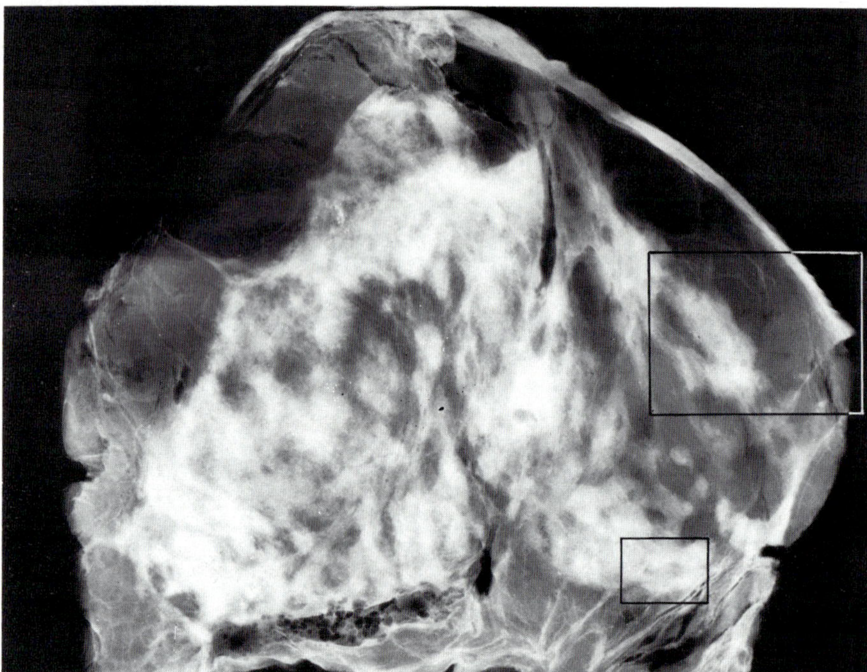

78

78 *Specimen radiograph.* Band-like and small spot-like opacities partially confluent. Retroareolar on left, some microcalcifications.

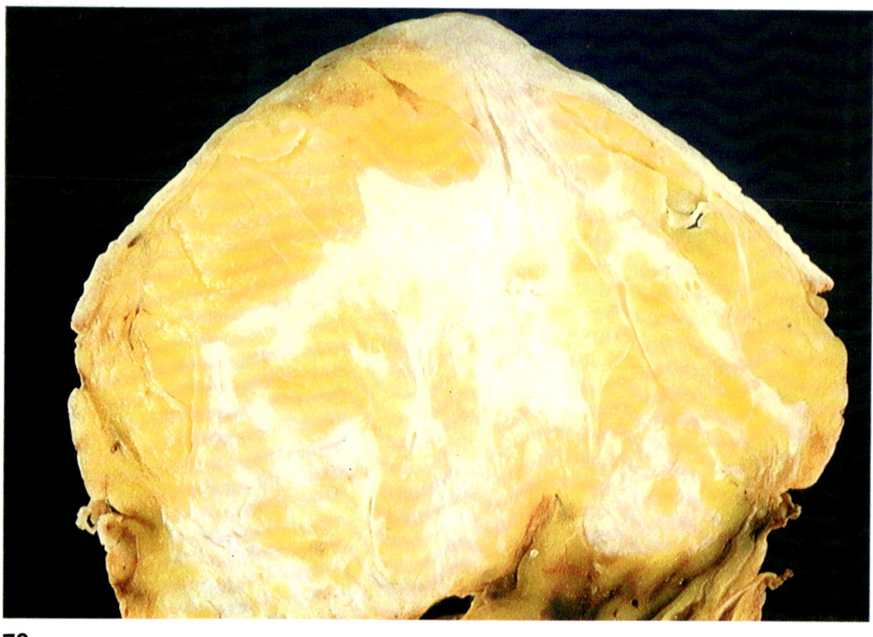

79

79 *Cut section of anatomic specimen.* Coarse and spotty nodules, partially band-like, surrounded by fatty tissue. Histology: see Fig 75.

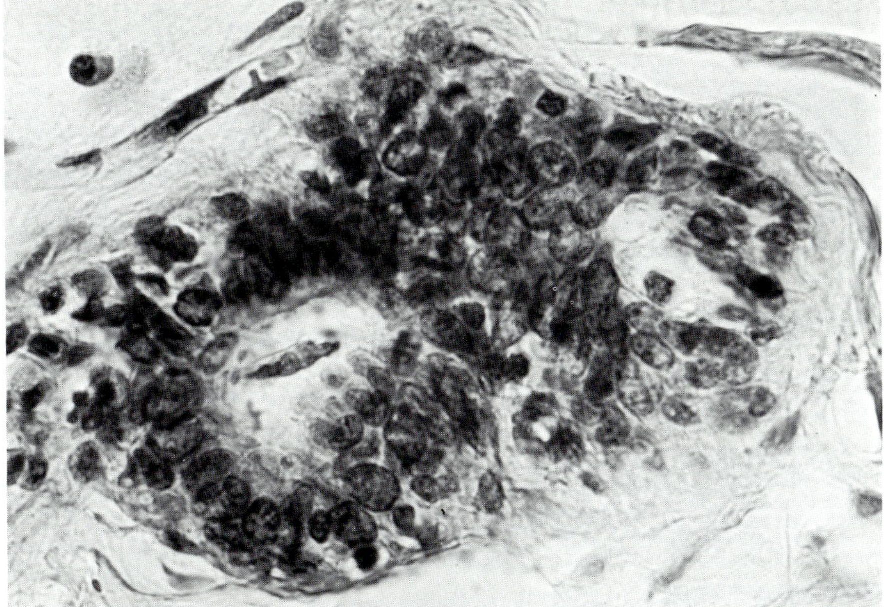

80 Epithelial proliferations. Proliferating ductal epithelium, several layers with atypical nuclei of varying size. Intact basal membrane. Magnif 160×. (See also Fig 74a.)

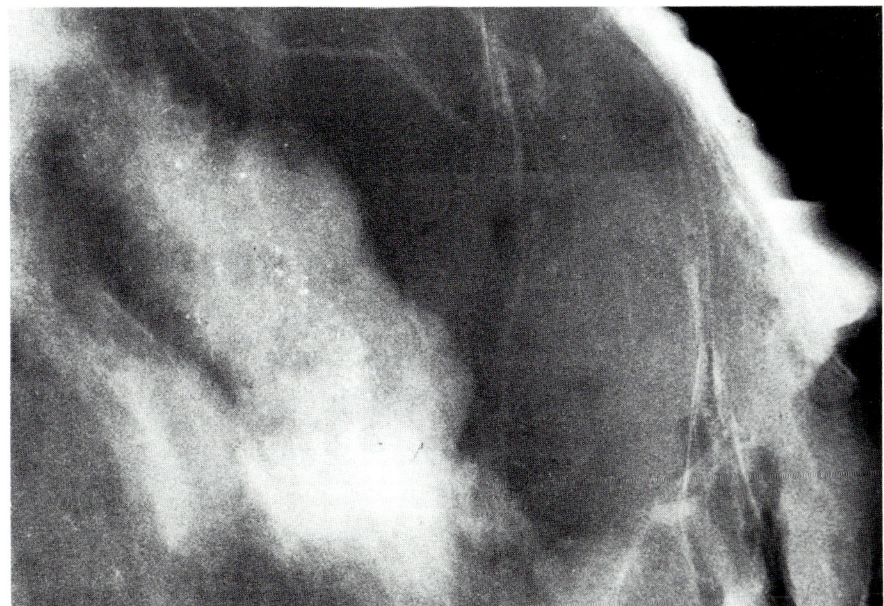

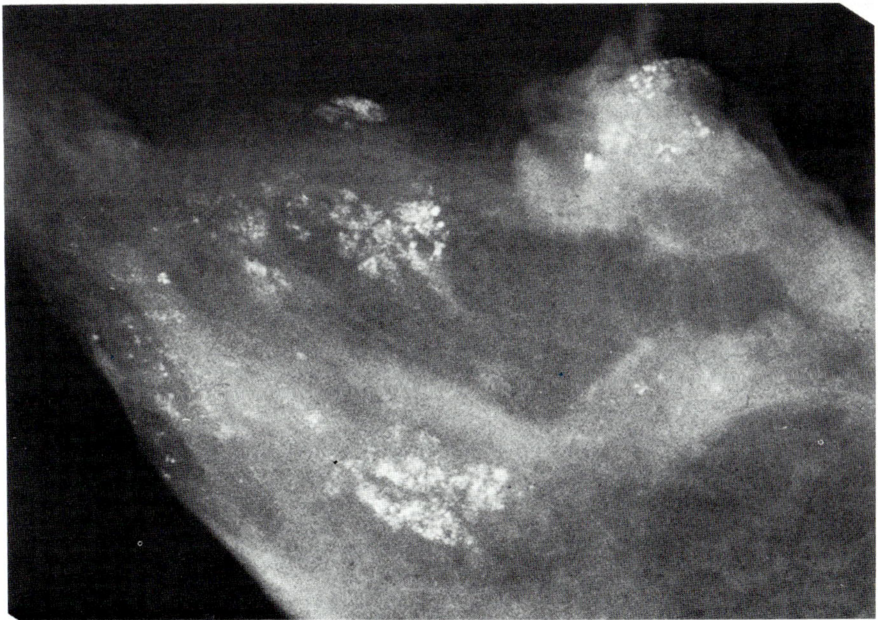

81 a, b. Magnification 5× of portions of Fig 78.
a) In a nonhomogeneous area of multiple groups of microcalcifications, coalescing.
b) Coarse microcalcifications in an additional portion. This type of calcification is found in the entire breast with magnification. The calcium particles cannot be seen in the mammogram (Fig 77) because of their small size.

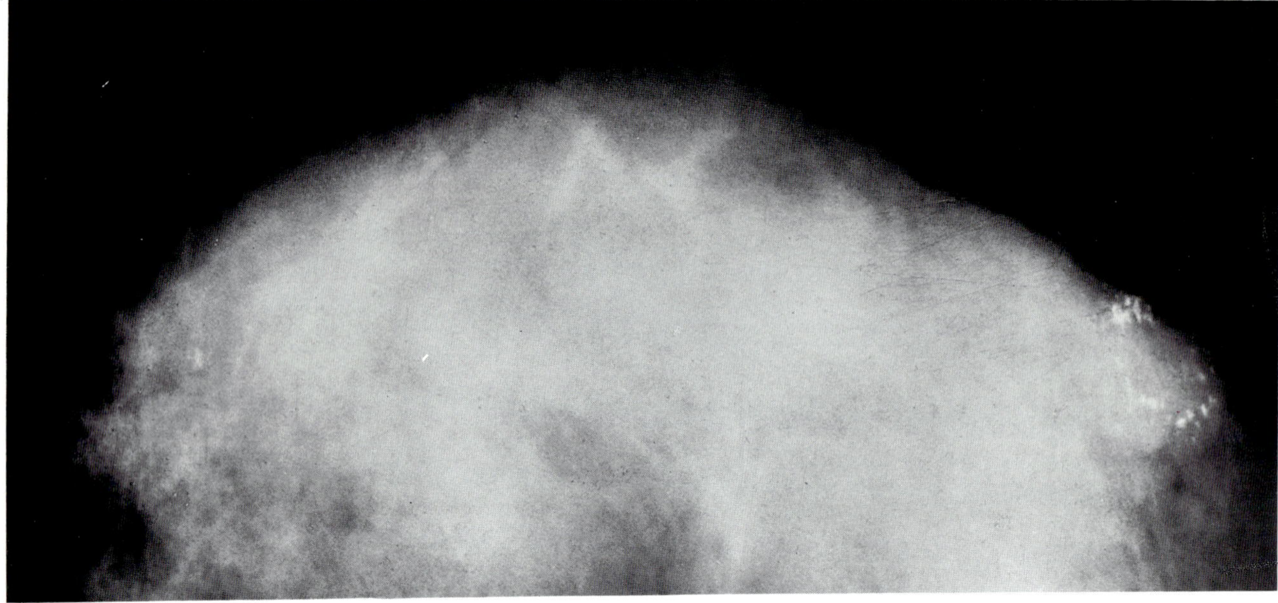

82

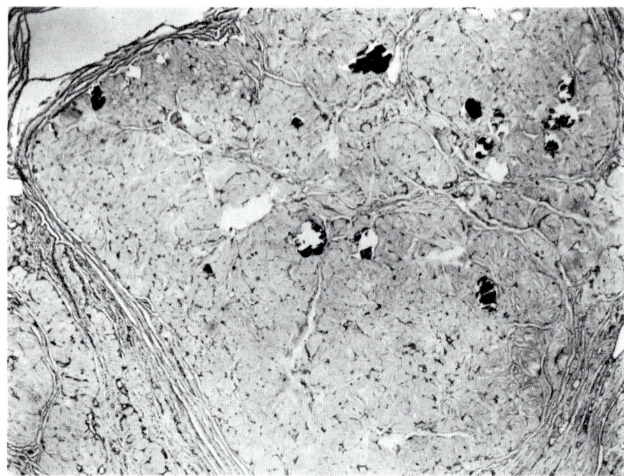

83a

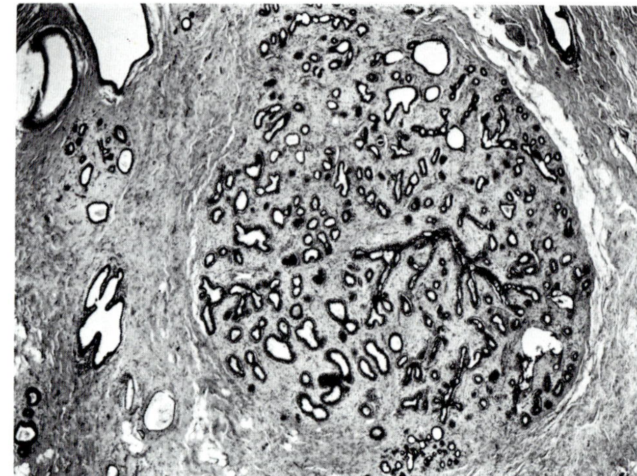

83b

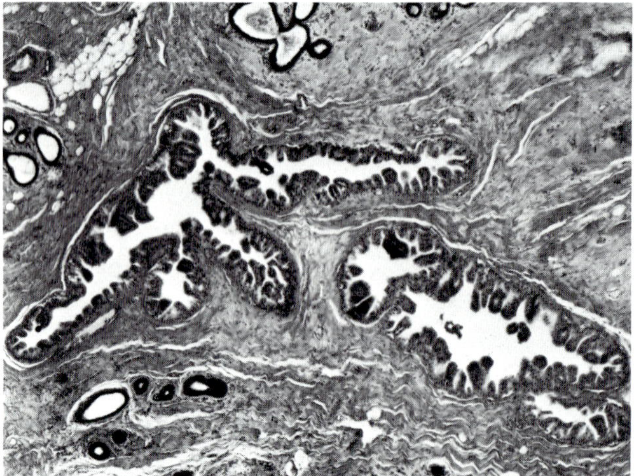

83c

34-year-old female, left breast. Previous right mastectomy. Left mastectomy also performed because of difficulty in early detection of possible carcinoma (Figs 82–85).

82 *Mammogram* (cranio-caudal). Dense, nonhomogeneous, minimally radiolucent breast with a nodular area left and lateral showing microcalcifications and macrocalcifications (fibroadenoma? comedocarcinoma?).

83 a–c. *Histological structures* of this breast.
a) Fibroadenoma with extensive degeneration of epithelium and multiple calcium particles of varying sizes in dilated lactiferous ducts of varying sizes. Magnif 80×.
b) Proliferation of intralobular connective tissue and acini (fibroadenomatosis, beginning fibroadenoma). To the left are seen ectatic ducts and a cystically degenerated, atrophic lobule. Magnif 80×.
c) Dilated ducts with cupola-like, epithelial proliferations. No atypical cells. Not indicative of carcinoma.

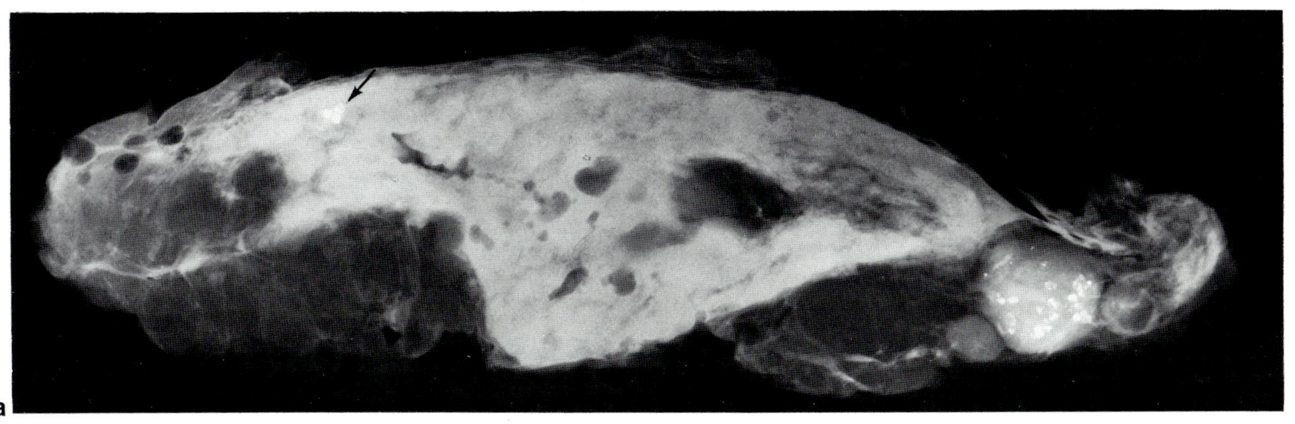
a

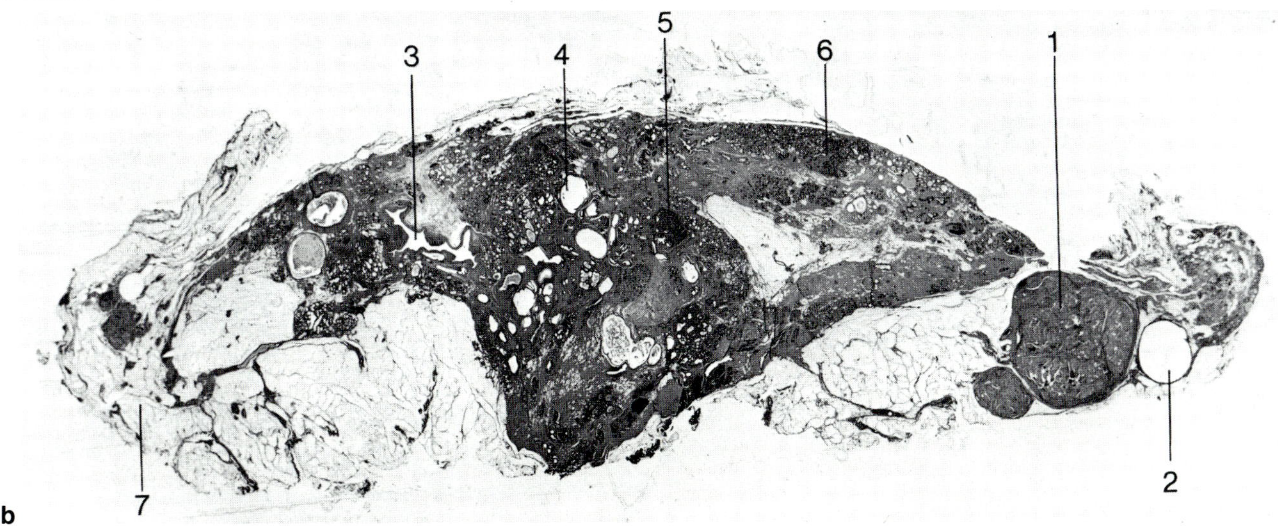

b

84

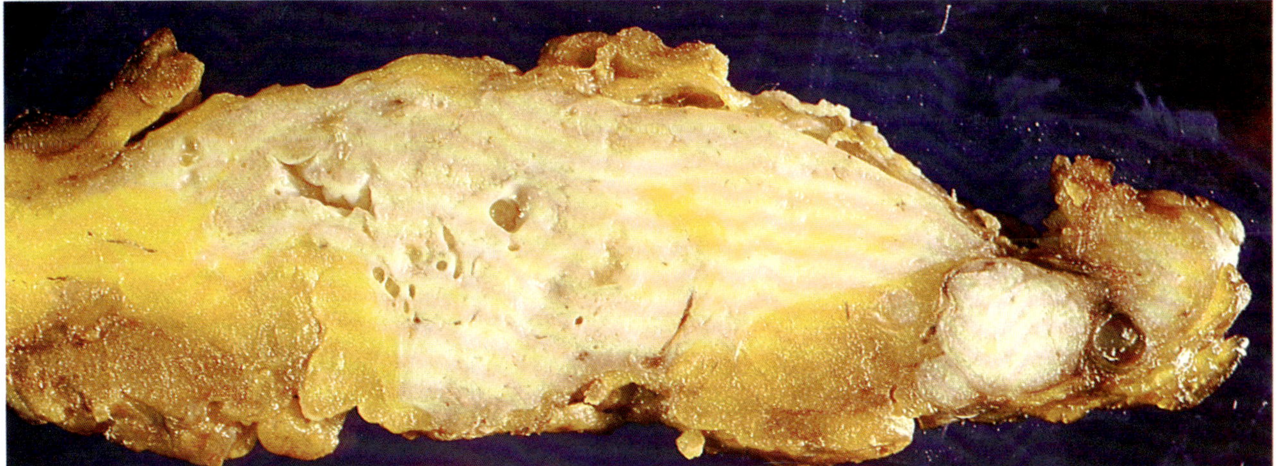

85

84 a, b. *Radiological-anatomic comparison.*
a) Specimen radiograph. Right fibroadenoma with multiple microcalcifications. Next to it an additional adenoma without calcification and a small cyst. Multiple small radio-opacities in remaining portion (foci of adenosis and fibrosis). In between, dilated ducts and cysts. Coarse calcifications are noted in a cyst in right outer portion (arrow).
b) Histological macrosection. Fibroadenoma with calcification (1). Next to it a smaller fibroadenoma with a cyst (2). In the remaining breast dilated lactiferous ducts (3), cysts (4), adenosis (5), and fibroadenomatosis (6). In surrounding fat (7) stromal septa with blood vessels.

85 *Cut section of anatomic specimen.* Fibroadenoma right. Additional fibroadenoma and smaller cysts nearby. Gray-brown breast with dilated lactiferous ducts and cysts. Surrounding yellow fat.

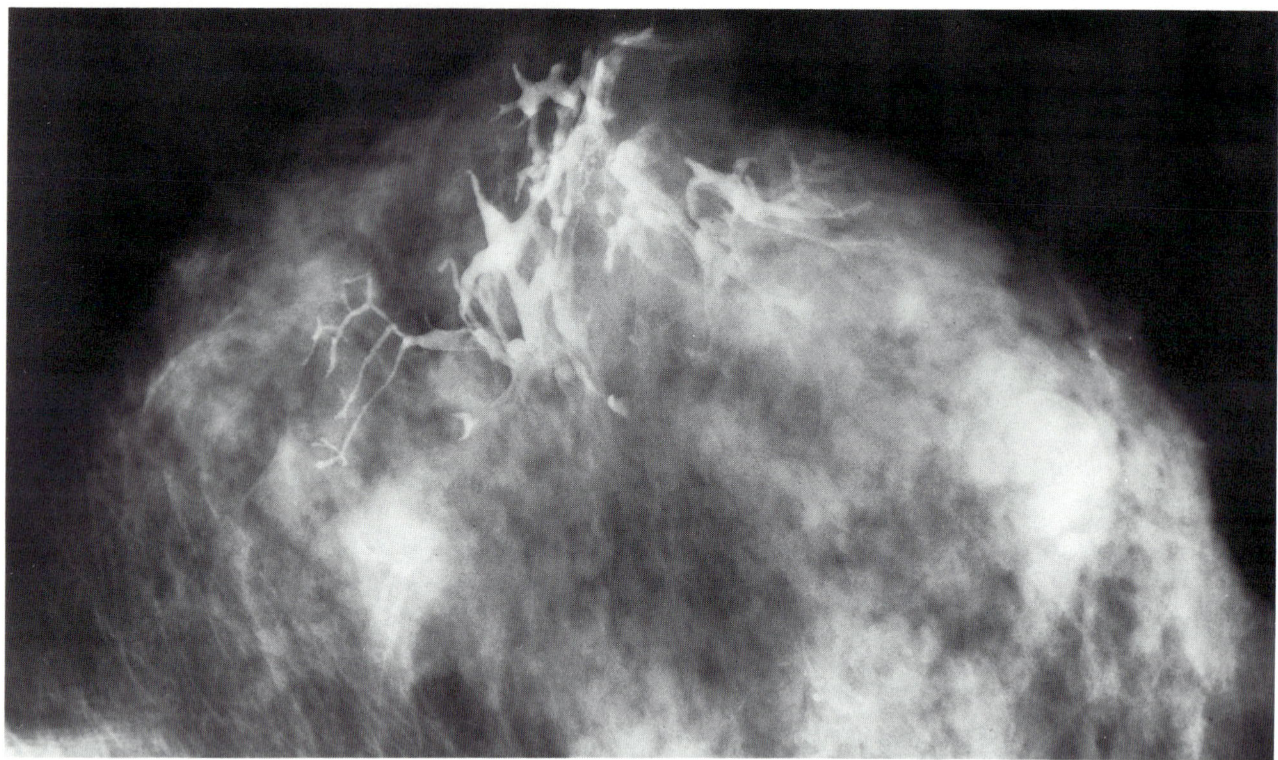

86

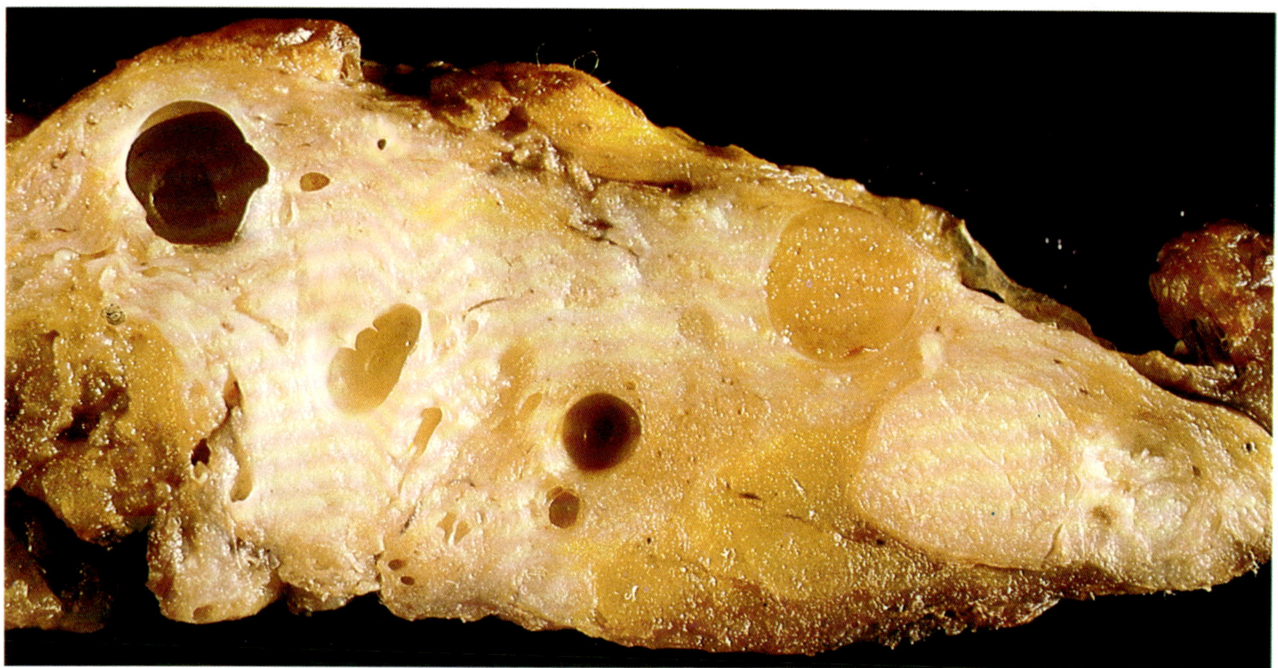

87

33-year-old female, right breast. For years marked, green-brown bilateral secretions. Multiple previous cyst punctures. Subcutaneous mastectomy with Silastic prosthesis.

86 *Galactography.* Partially contrast-filled, ectatic, lactiferous ducts. Small and large opacities. Coarse calcifications.

87 *Cut section of anatomical specimen.* Smooth fibroadenoma right. Above and left, cyst with thickened, gelatinous, yellow-brown content. Ectatic ducts and cysts of varying sizes in remaining breast.

88 *Histological macrosection* (from another portion of the breast). Multiple cysts of varying sizes (2). Cystically degenerated lobules (4). Multiple foci of adenosis with proliferation of the intralobular connective tissue (3). Fat (1).

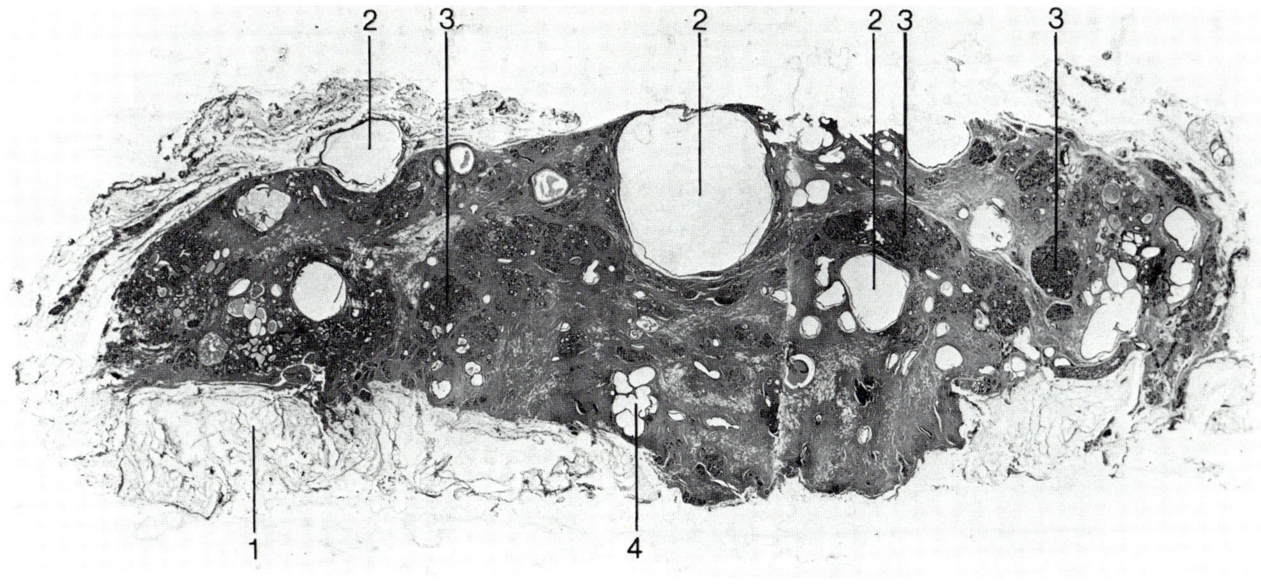

88

89 a–d. *Histological structures* in cystic mastopathy. Magnif 80×.

a) Cysts. Multiple layers of foam cells in the lumen. Cell debris in center of duct. Periductular fibrosis with infiltration of round cells (chronic mastitis).

b) So-called foam cells are found in breast secretion and in aspirate of cysts with degenerated epithelium and inflamed wall. Below and right, foreign-body giant cell.

c) Proliferation of intralobular connective tissue and dilatation of excretory ducts and acini. Left, cysts with proliferation of epithelium, partly multilayered (above), partly papillary (below), partly degenerated (center).

d) Dilated ducts with partly solid, partly cribriform epithelial proliferations. Intact basal membrane. Left above, an enlarged lobule with proliferating epithelium. The change from intraductal and intralobular eptheliosis into so-called carcinoma in situ is gradual.

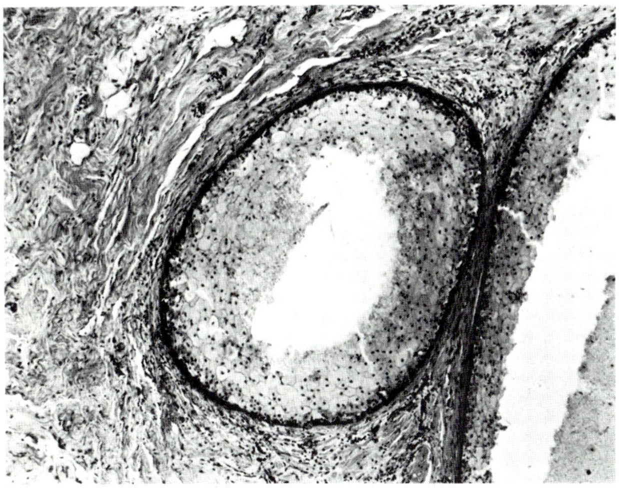

89 a

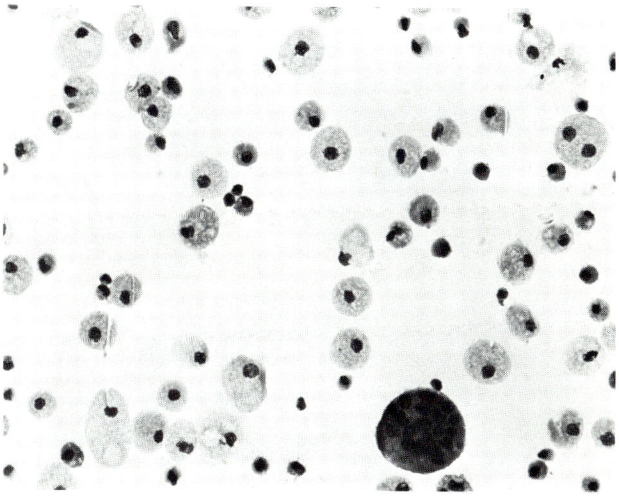

89 b

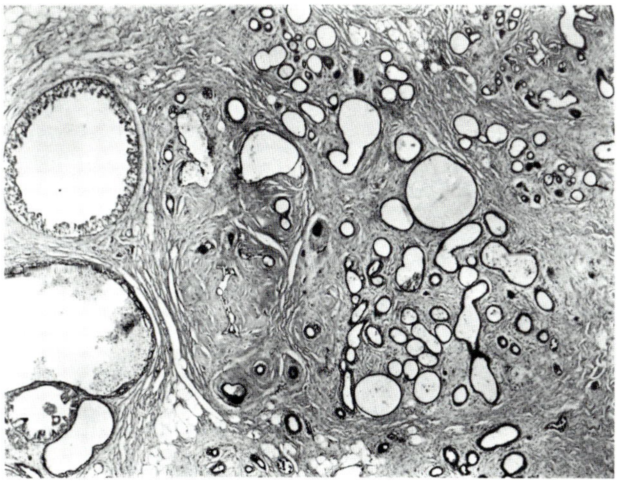

89 c

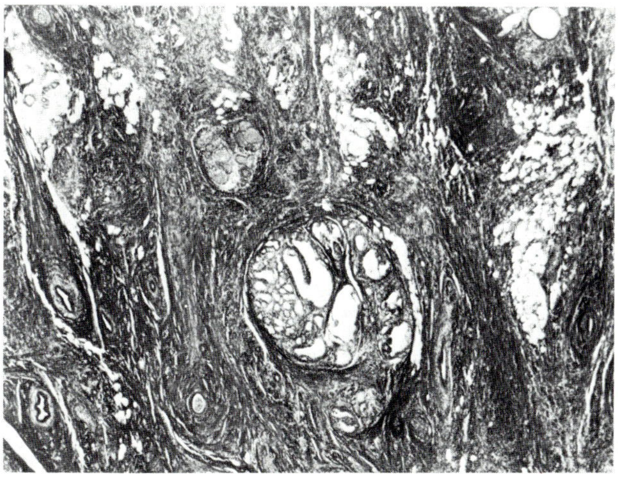

89 d

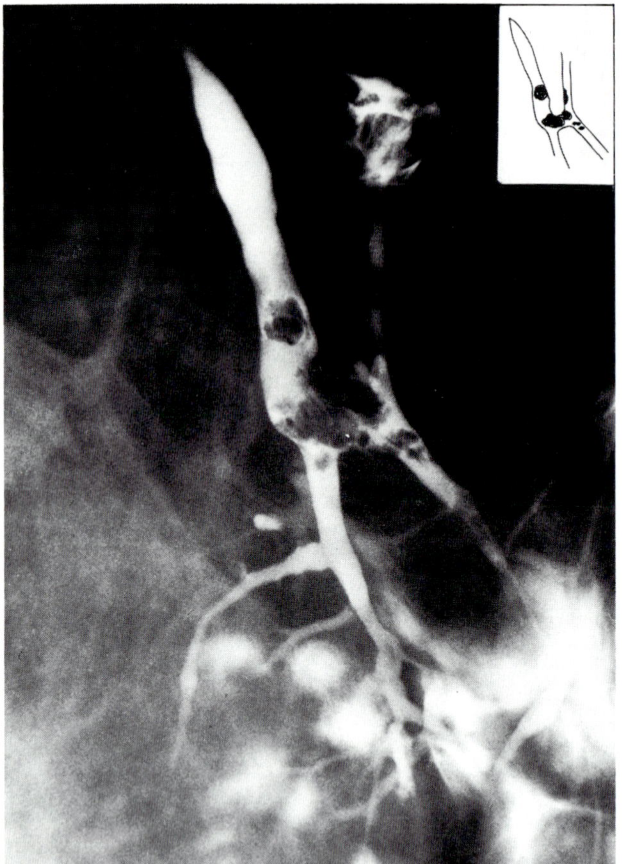

90 a

90 b

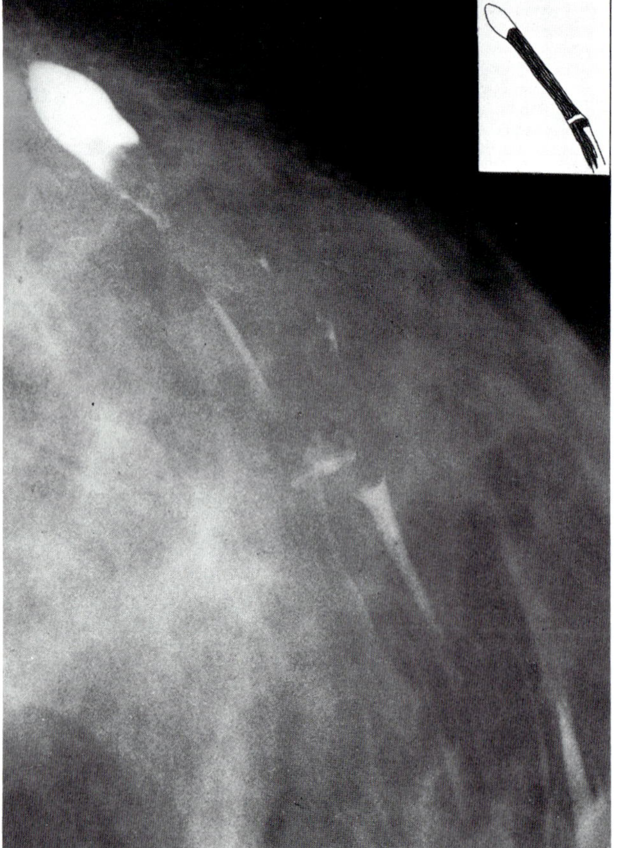

90 c

90 a–c. Localized, polycyclic, irregular filling defects in contrast medium within ectatic, lactiferous ducts. Varying extent of process. Histologically: benign papilloma or papillomatosis. Magnif 10×.

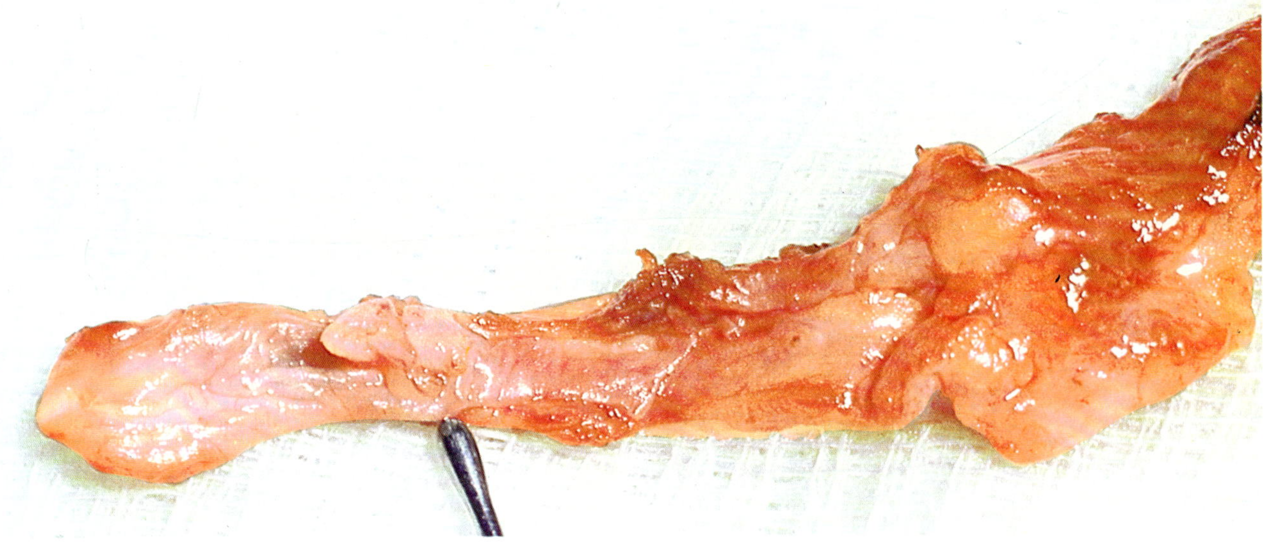

91

91 Extirpated and opened lactiferous duct showing cylinder-like tumor projecting into lumen.

92 a, b. *Histology and cytology.*

a) Histology. Intracanalicular papilloma of lactiferous duct. The plump, branched axes of the papillae consist of connective tissue and are covered by hyperplastic epithelium. With larger magnification no atypical epithelium.

b) Cytology. In secretion multiple small compact epithelial layers. The individual cells show broad cytoplasm, and partly eccentrically located nuclei can be recognized.

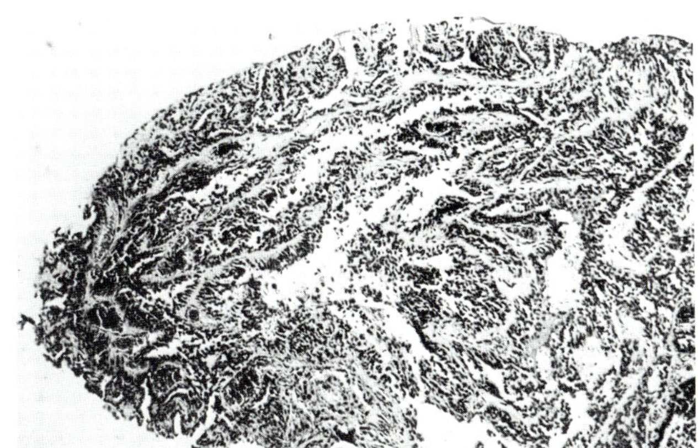

92a

92b

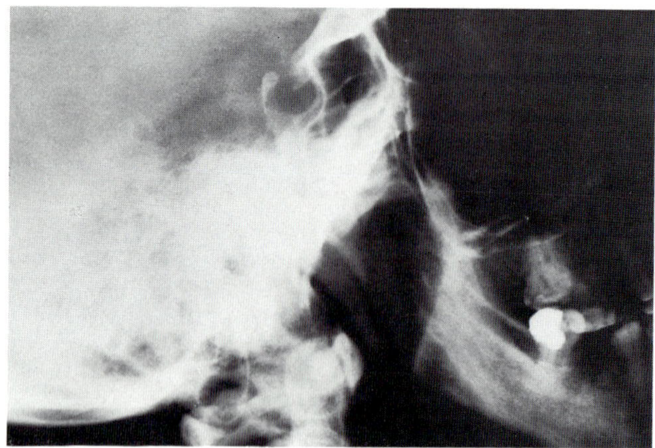

93a

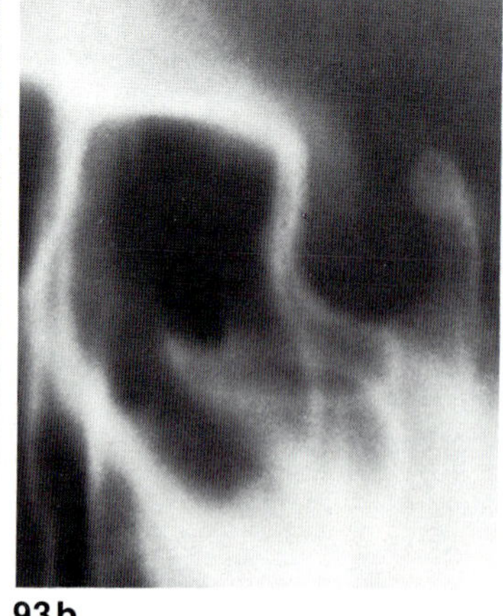

93b

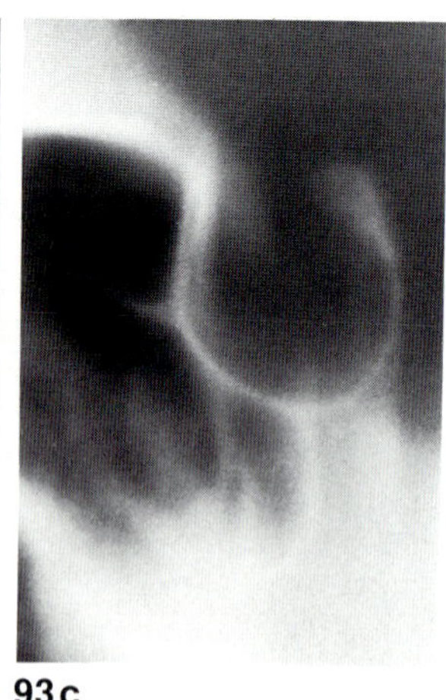

93c

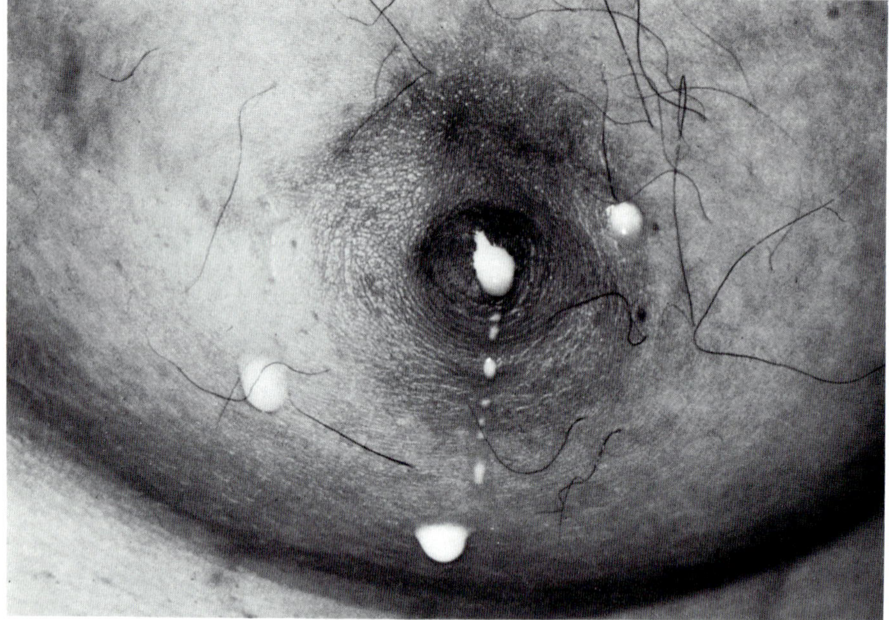

94

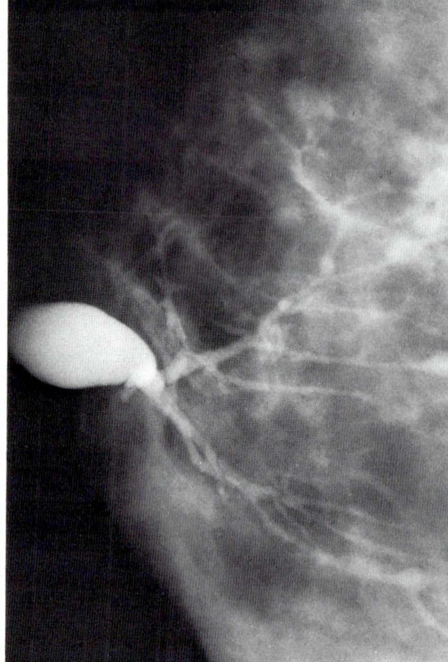

95a

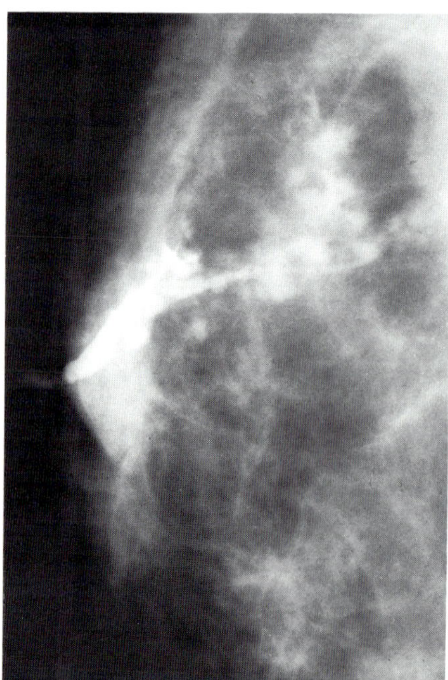

95b

43-year-old female. For 4 years marked milk secretion bilaterally, hirsutism. No headaches. Milk secretion induced by increased production of lactotropic hormone (prolactin) from pituitary tumor (Figs 93–95).

93 a–c. *Roentgenographic examination* of skull and tomograms of sella turcica.
a) Lateral view. Double contour of floor and dorsum sellae. Suspicion of unilateral excavation.
b) Left fossa of sella turcica normal. Dorsum sellae is not thinned.
c) Right fossa of sella turcica is enlarged. Dorsum sellae is markedly thinned. Unilateral pituitary tumor. Histology unknown.

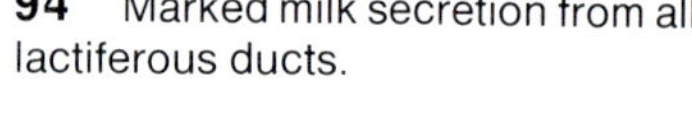

94 Marked milk secretion from all lactiferous ducts.

95 a, b. *Galactography* left (a) and right (b).
a) Markedly dilated lactiferous ampullae. Minimal cystic dilatation of lactiferous ducts in periphery.
b) Moderate retroareolar ductal ectasia. Contrasting lobuli. There are no proliferations of the ducts bilaterally.

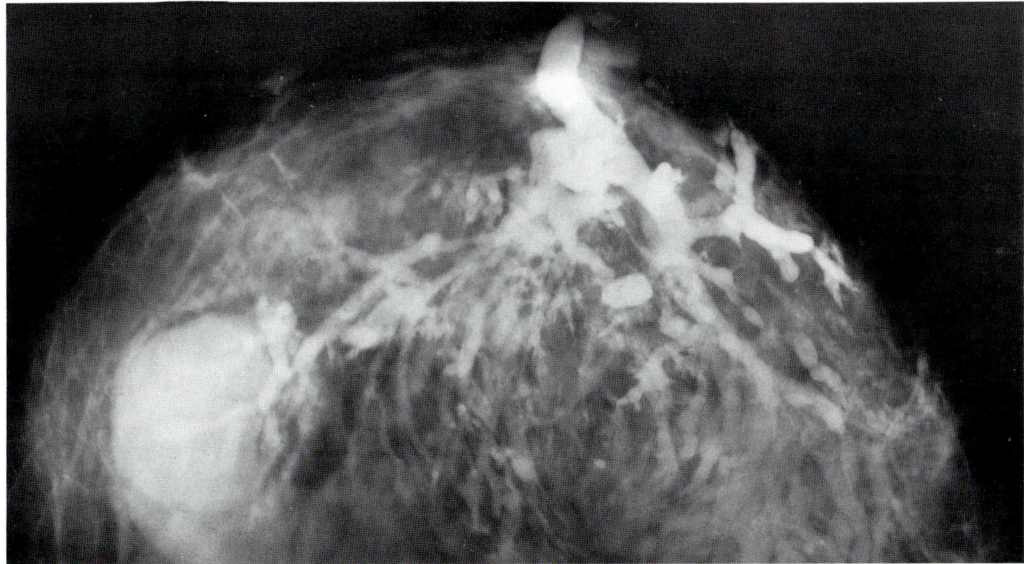

96

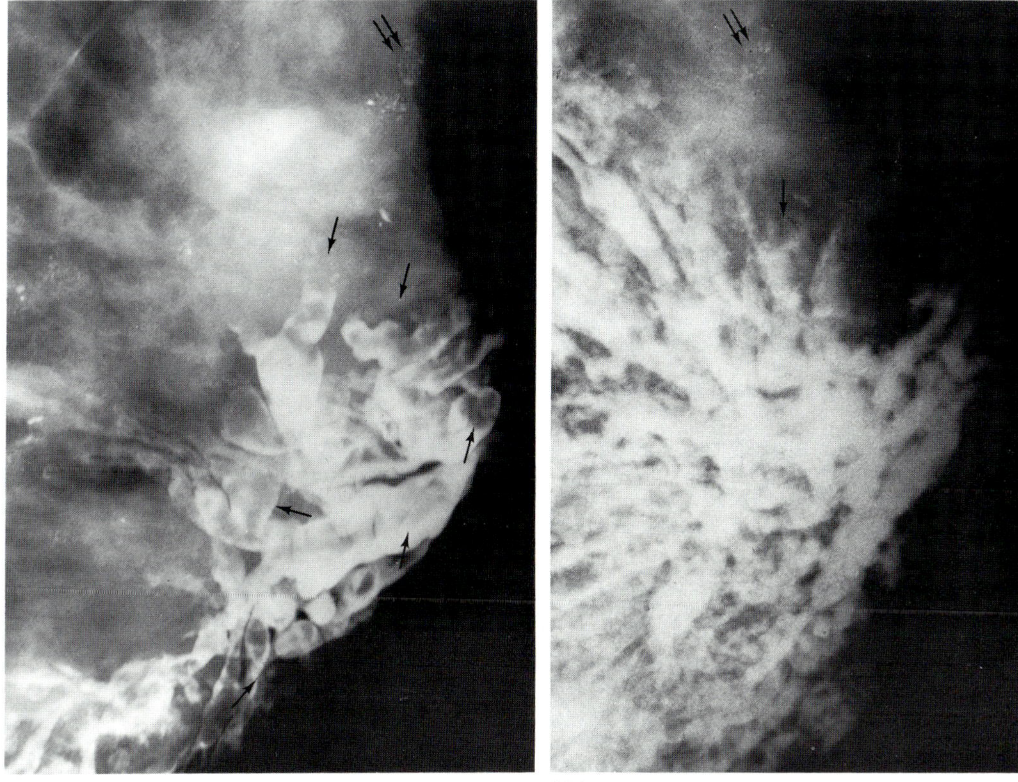

97a 97b

96 Right breast of a 57-year-old female. Markedly ectatic, retroareolar, lactiferous ducts in central and lateral quadrants. Histologically diffuse ductal carcinoma. Solitary cyst in medial quadrant. Severe mastitis after galactography.

97 a, b. Ductal ectasia and filling defect from cell debris.

a) Marked dilatation of contrast-filled lactiferous ducts with filling defects (arrow). Suspicion of epithelial proliferations. Microcalcifications at upper edge (double arrow).

b) Following flushing of ducts with saline solution and removal of a large amount of debris, repeat contrast filling of the ducts. Debris-produced filling defects seen in a) have now disappeared. Disruption of the contrast column in the upper area secondary to true proliferations with microcalcifications. Histology: ductal ectasia with benign epithelial proliferations and microcalcifications. No indication of carcinoma.

Calcifications in Benign Lesions of the Breast

Calcifications are common and may point to certain morphological changes.
The following types occur:

coarse,
circular and semicircular,
linear,
microcalcifications arranged in groups,
diffusely scattered microcalcifications.

KOEHL et al (1970) reviewed 238 cases of benign changes with calcifications and found the following distribution (Table **5**):

Table 5. Distribution of calcifications in benign lesions (from R.H. Koehl, R.E. Snyder, R.V.P. Hutter, F.W. Foote, Jr.: Am. J. Clin. Path. 53: 3, 1970).

Type of Lesion	Number of Specimens
Lobules and ducts	139
Sclerosing adenosis	45
Duct papilloma, duct hyperplasia	28
Apocrine metaplasia	20
Fibroadenoma	10
Scarring, fibrous tissue	10
Cysts	6
Arteriosclerotic vessels	5
Scarred ducts, duct ectasia	4
Fat necrosis	3
Lobular hyperplasia	3

Coarse calcifications are most common in *fibroadenomas*. These are calcified necrotic areas lying between strands of dense and hyalinized connective tissue (Figs **53** b, **76** c). In addition to coarse calcium particles, microcalcifications in the proliferating lactiferous ducts of the fibroadenoma may occur. In a breast rich in stroma, a fibroadenoma will be poorly defined in the mammogram so that such calcifications may be confused with the calcifications of a comedocarcinoma (Figs **82**, **83** a). Necrosis of the epithelium in carcinomas may cause both coarse and tiny calcifications (Figs **102**, **109**).
Ring and semicircular calcifications may be found in the cyst walls. In case of fatty degeneration of the cyst wall, calcium salts may be deposited within lipoid tissue (Fig **100** c). This causes a disc-like, ring-shaped or semicircular pattern of calcifications in the mammogram (Fig **99**). Cysts showing fatty degeneration with subsequent deposition of calcium are commonly solitary; multiple occurrence is quite rare (Fig **100**). Hypercholesterolemia of 340 mg/l was found in a patient with multiple fatty and secondarily calcified cysts with a fibrocystic mastopathy. Calcified cysts filled with oily fluid occur particularly following fat necrosis in surgical scars. Aspiration of these *oil cysts* reveals a gray-brown mass which may contain lipophages (Fig **100** d). Opening of the cyst reveals a thin, white layer of calcium lining the cyst wall. Pinpoint calcifications also occur in *surgical scars* and may be confused with a carcinoma if the calcium particles are not shown tangentially and are projected over the breast (Fig **106**). These calcifications lie in the subcutaneous lactiferous ducts. They consist of calcified debris and calcified microhematomas.
Linear calcifications are found with arteriosclerosis of the breast. They have a double contour and follow the course of the vessels. There is no problem in the differential diagnosis of these calcifications. Calcified thrombi (phleboliths) in the vessels of the breast are not well known. Organized and calcified thrombi lie in dilated veins and arteries and occlude the lumen of the vessel. These phleboliths are plump, homogeneous, and smoothly defined (Fig **107**). On occasion it may be difficult to differentiate these calcifications histologically from calcified debris in fibrosed ducts.
Needle-like calcium deposits are typical of plasma cell mastitis and are secondary to calcified debris filling the large ducts. These "calcium needles" may be localized but may also be distributed over the entire breast (Fig **98**).
The plasma-cell-mastitis calcifications must be differentiated from comedo-carcinoma calcifications which are shorter and stipple-like. Groups of microcalcifications indicative of carcinoma are discussed on page 96.
Coarse localized calcium particles are found with mastopathy. The individual calcium particles are of varying size. They may be distributed over the entire breast and are located anatomically in lobules and ducts (Fig **101** c). When they occur in groups, it is not possible to differentiate them from neoplastic epithelial growth. Surgical removal of the tissue with specimen radiography and histological examination must be done (Figs **101**, **102**).
Tiny *psammoma-like microcalcifications* are seen histologically with proliferating mastopathy. They lie in the epithelial layers but may also be located between the proliferating epithelium and the basal membrane. They are so small they can only be seen in a microradiograph or in an industrial film following electronic photographic enlargement.

A 60-year-old patient with previous removal of an intraductal carcinoma in the outer upper quadrant of the left breast showed a single microcalcification in a mammogram. Magnified radiographs of the removed breast with multiple sections showed duct-like calcifications in almost all parts of the breast (Figs **77–81**).

More than two types of calcifications are rarely found in one breast, but in the same mammogram one patient showed coarse calcium particles in a fibroadenoma, calcified cysts, microcalcifications of a carcinoma and calcified arterial walls (Fig **109**).

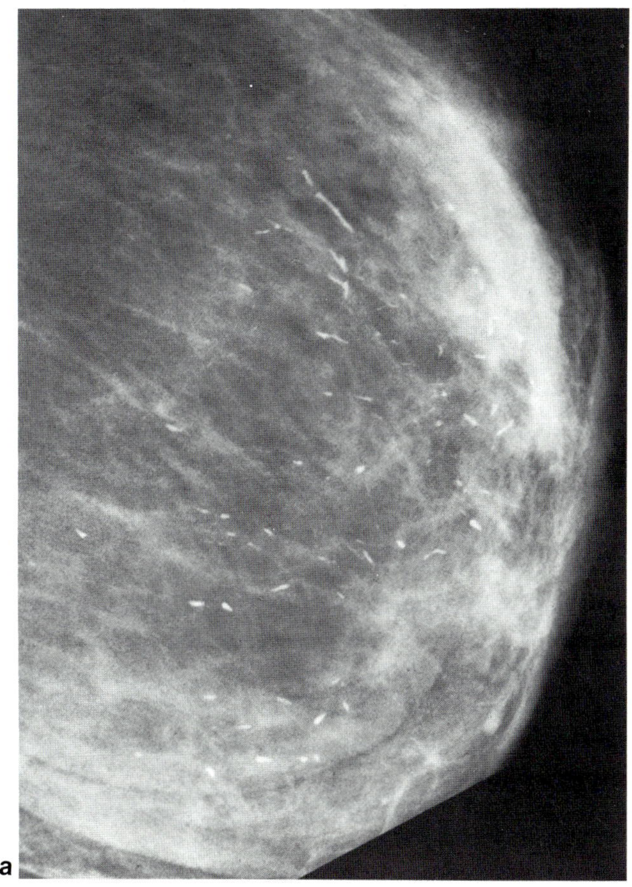

a

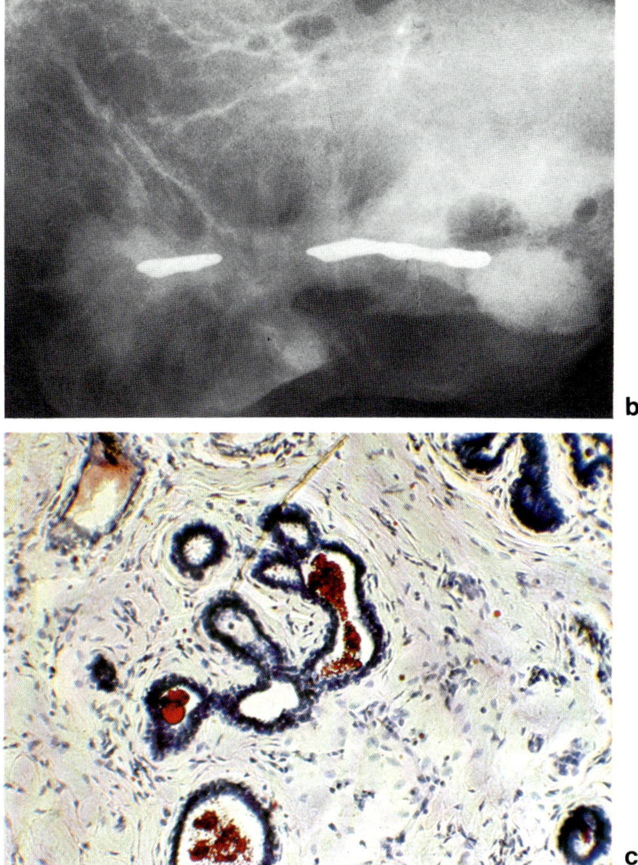

b

c

98

a) 73-year-old female, left breast. Multiple, needle-like calcifications located along the course of the ducts.

b) Magnif 20×, on industrial film. Calcium needles in a thickened, ill-defined duct.

c) *Histology.* Sudan stain (fatty tissue red). Dilated ducts, fatty debris deposits in the lumen. The deposition of calcium salts is possible.

(Also compare secretory disease and plasma cell mastitis, Figs 59–62.)

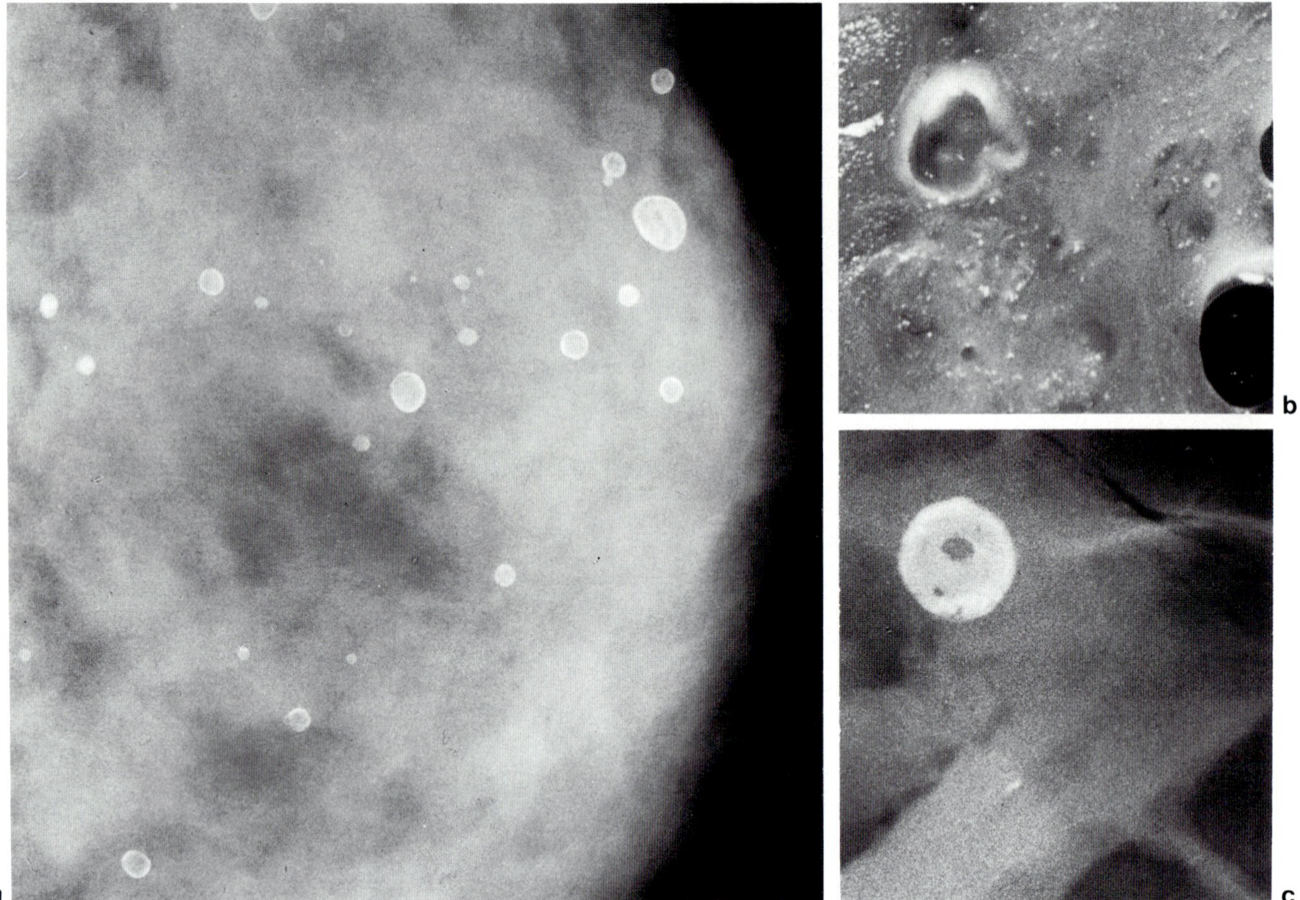

99
a) *Mammogram.* Several calcified cysts with disc-like calcifications. There is a ring-like thickening of the edge of the discs.

b) *Cut section of the anatomic specimen.* Opened cyst with markedly degenerated, fatty, gray-white wall. Histology: fatty degeneration and calcification.
c) *Specimen radiograph* of (b). Disc-like calcification with central lucency. Increased absorption of the x-ray beam traversing the cyst wall tangentially causes the ring-shaped thickening of the edge of the cyst wall.

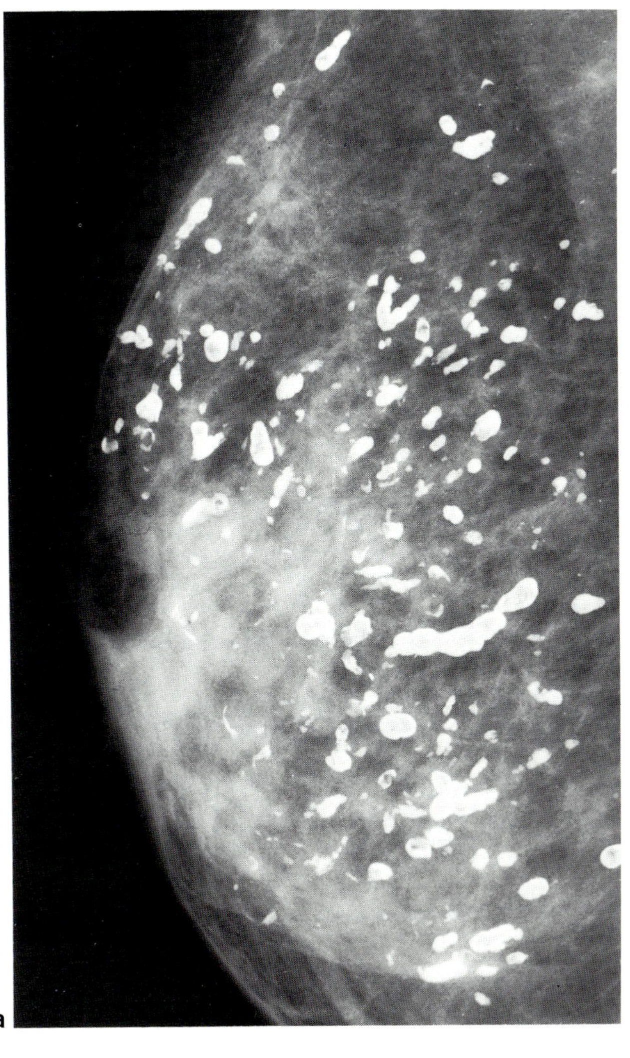

a

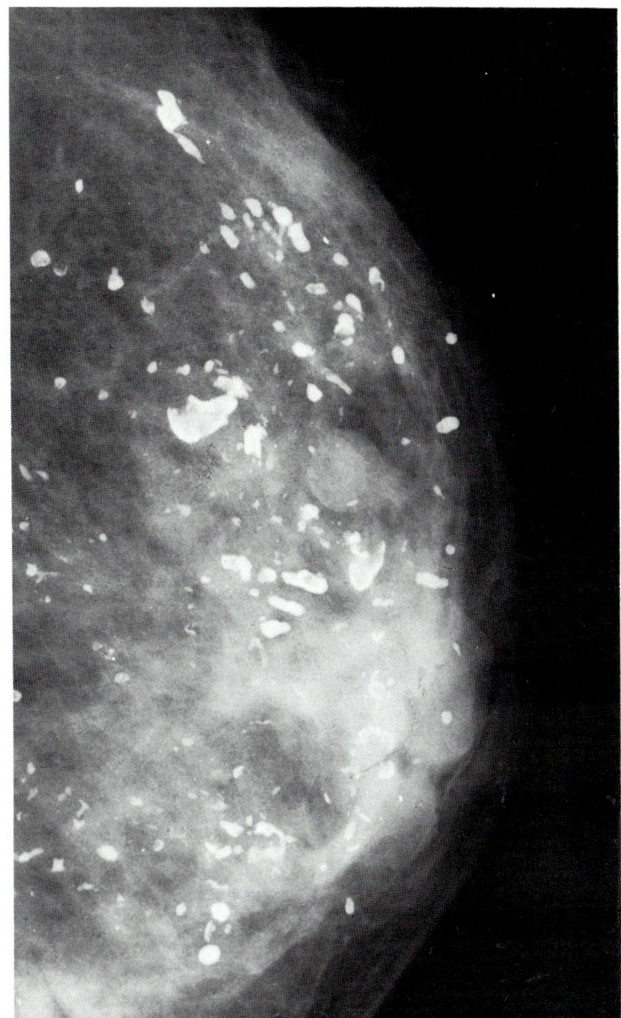

b

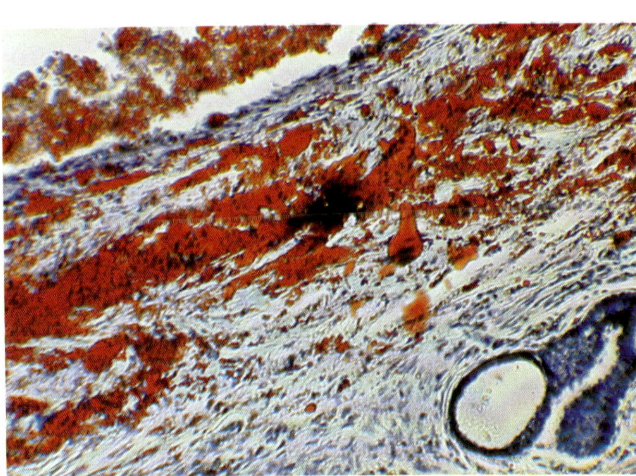

c

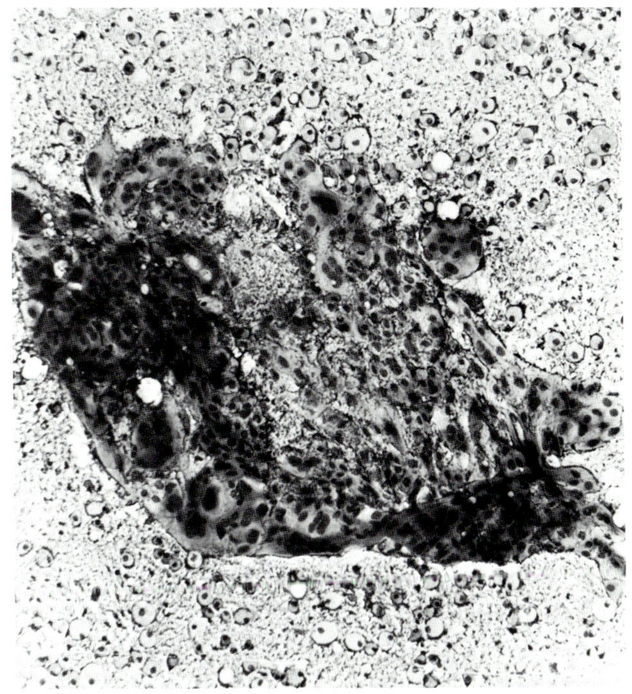

d

100 a–d. 57-year-old female. Hypercholesterolemia.

a, b) *Mammogram.* Multiple, markedly calcified cysts in both breasts. Next to them needle-like calcifications as in plasma cell mastitis.

c) *Histology* of cyst wall (Sudan stain: fat red, calcium black). Lipophages (foam cells) in cyst wall. Fatty debris on the inner surface (left above). Dilated lactiferous duct (lower right).

d) *Cytology* of aspirate of degenerated duct cyst. Large collection of lipophages with nuclei of varying sizes and multinucleated foreign-body giant cells as well as fatty debris (lipophage = fat-containing as well as fat-storing histiocyte).

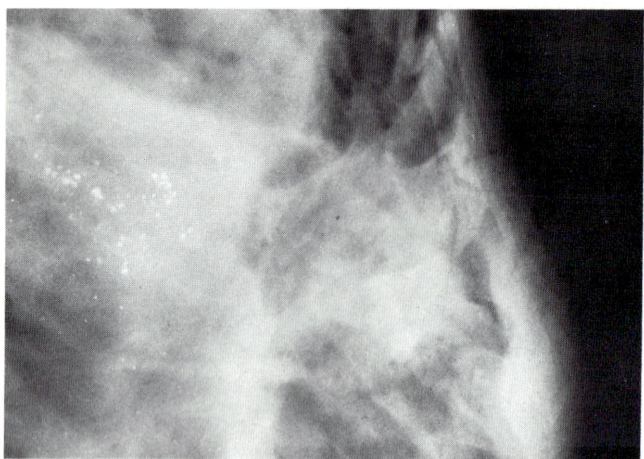

a

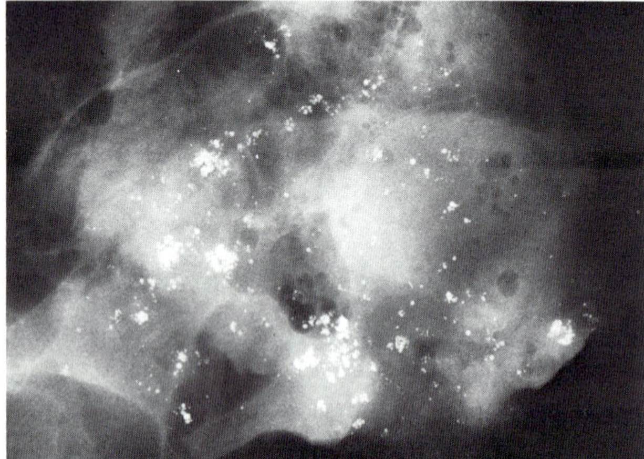

b

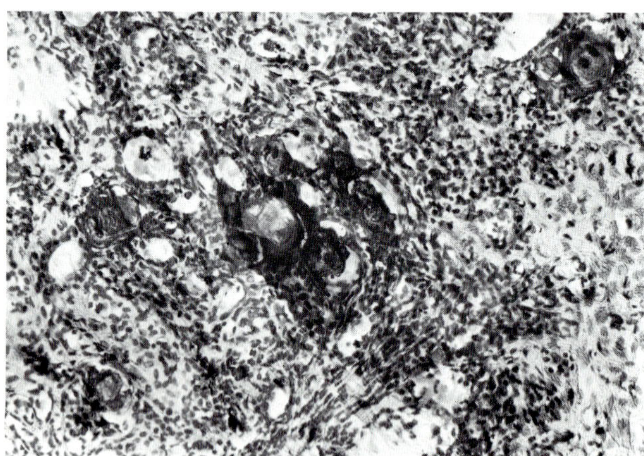

c

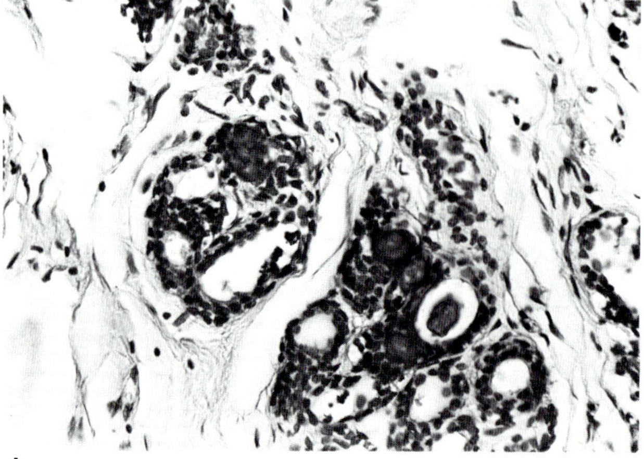

d

101 a–d. 24-year-old female, left breast.

a) *Portion of mammogram* (medio-lateral). Multiple groups of microcalcifications near chest wall. Suspicion of intraductal carcinoma.

b) *Specimen radiograph* of the surgically removed tissue: Multiple coarse groups of microcalcifications. Complete removal.

c) *Histology.* Focus of adenosis with marked calcium deposits in lobules and with perifocal round cell infiltration (reactive chronic mastitis).

d) *Histology* of lobule and duct. Calcium deposits between proliferating epithelium and basal membrane. Calcium particle in lumen of an acinus.

102 32-year-old female, right breast. Observation and routine examinations over 3 years of groups of microcalcifications in mammogram. For 1 year palpable nodule on right. Now fist-sized firm tumor. Retracted nipple. Peau d'orange skin (periareolar). Multiple, superficially-ulcerated skin metastases. Generalized bony metastases.

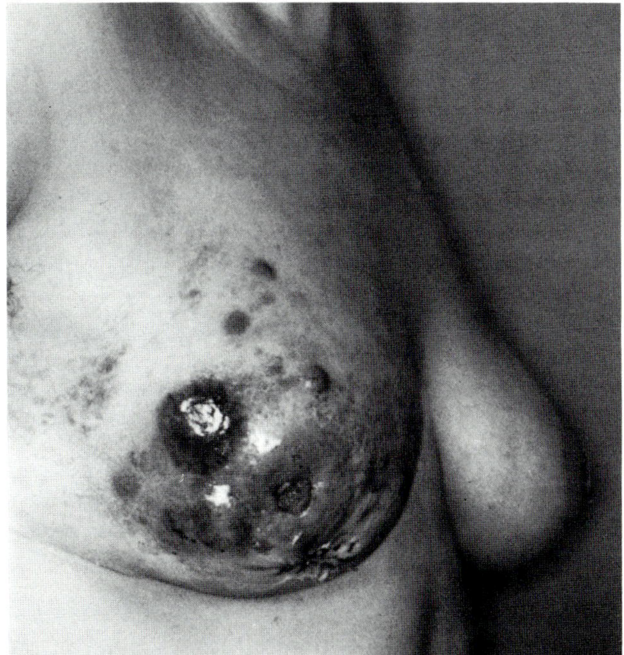

102

103 a, b. *Mammogram and histology.*

a) First mammogram 3 years ago. Group of microcalcifications suggestive of carcinoma. (Present mammogram cannot be evaluated. Homogeneous increased density not allowing differentiation of tissues.)

b) Histology of an intraductal carcinoma in another patient with similar mammographic changes as in a). Magnif 120×. Dilated lactiferous duct with proliferating atypical epithelium. Formation of acini. Central calcium particles. Basal membrane intact (intraductal carcinoma in situ). (In another area breakthrough of basal membrane with infiltration of surrounding tissue.)

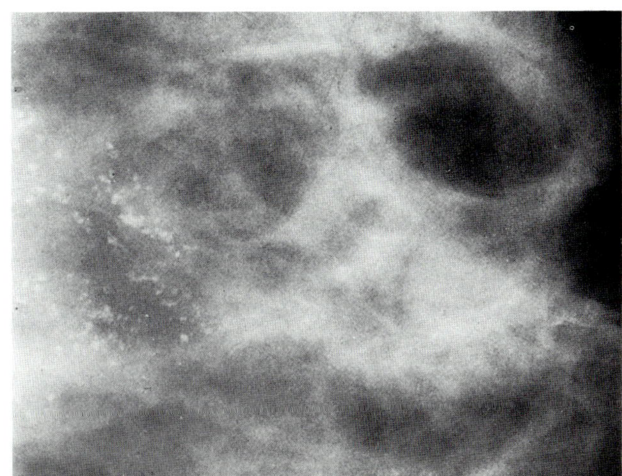

103a

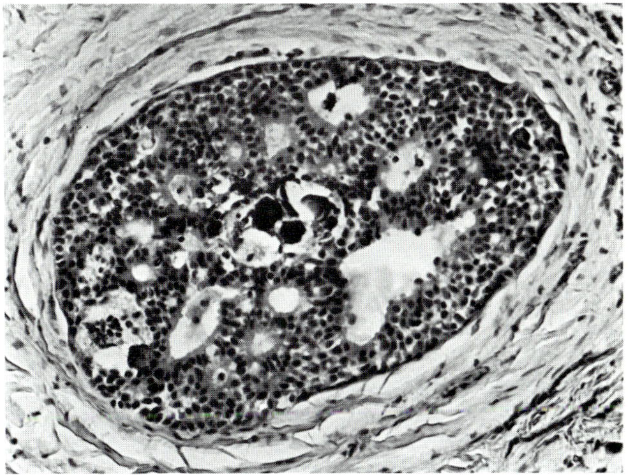

103b

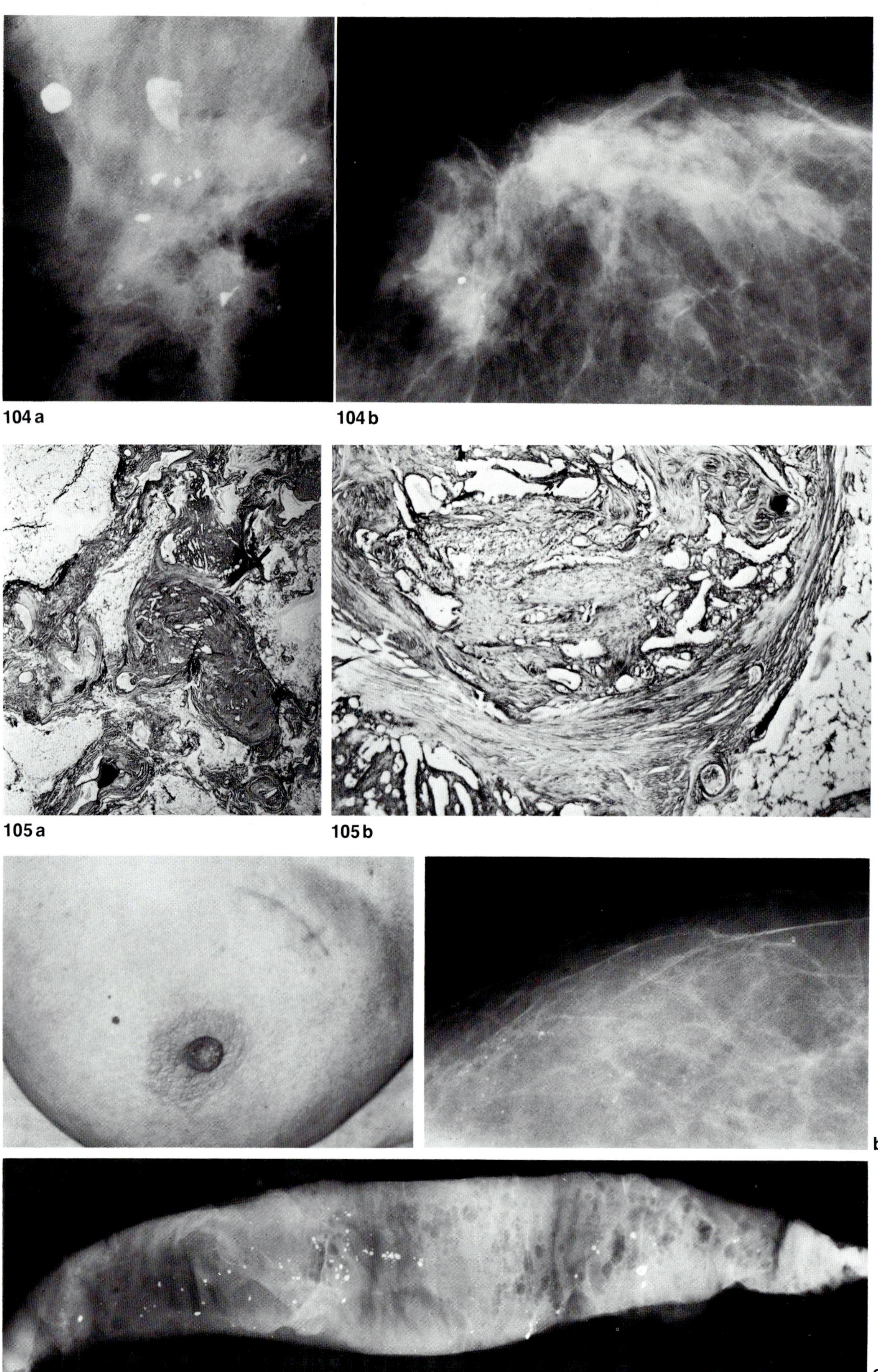
104 a
104 b
105 a
105 b
a
b
c
106

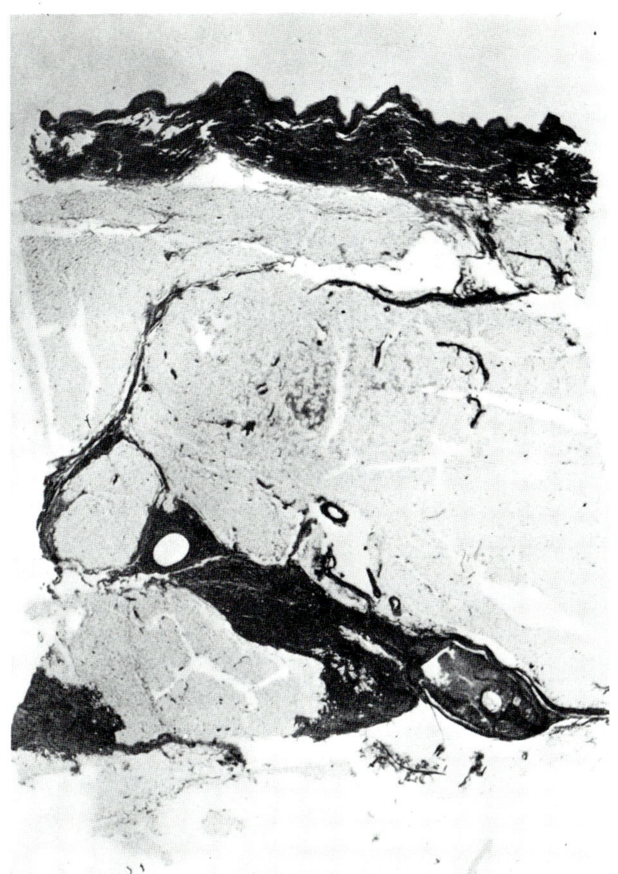

107 a

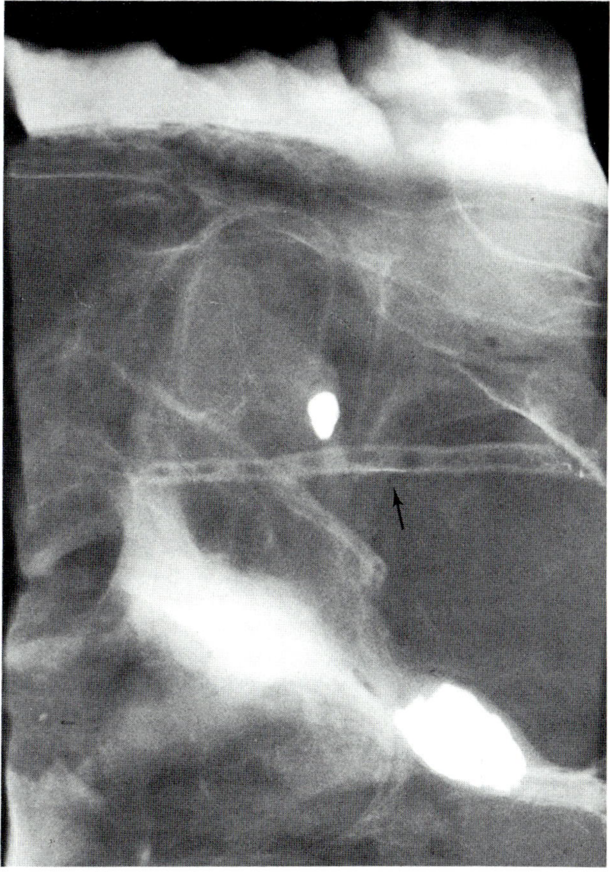

107 b

63-year-old female, left breast. Vascular calcifications and two coarse calcium deposits (Figs 107–108).

107 a, b. *Histological-radiological comparison.*
a) Histological macrosection, magnif 10×. Stroma septum with ectatic blood vessels. Calcified thrombus in a dilated artery.
b) Specimen radiograph, magnif 10×. Stroma island. To the right, coarse calcium deposit in a vessel; above, a second calcium deposit apparently also a thrombus. Between both calcium particles two arteries with calcified walls crossing each other (arrow).

108 *Histology following decalcification,* magnif 80×. Ectatic vascular lumen, sclerosed intima with calcification in the media of the wall of the vessel. The lumen is filled with an organized, centrally recanalized thrombus. Differential diagnosis: organized hematoma with secondary calcification in an ectatic duct.

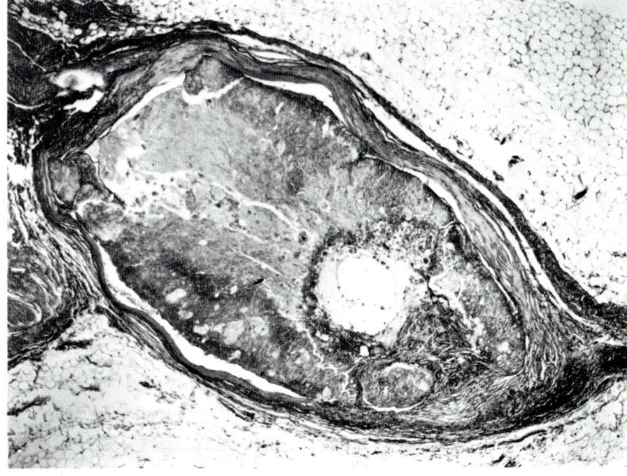

108

◁ **104** a, b. 43-year-old female, left breast. In mammogram nonhomogeneous opacity with radiating borders as well as coarse and fine calcifications.
a) Magnif 10× of *specimen radiograph.*
b) Original size in *mammogram.*

105 a, b. *Histology* of papilloma.
a) Intraductal sclerosing and hyalinized papilloma with circumscribed calcification of duct wall (right, above). At the lower left border, markedly sclerosed duct with calcified debris in the lumen. Magnif 60×.
b) Fibrosing duct wall, sclerosing and hyalinized papilloma in lumen. Calcium particles right. Magnif 160×.

106 a–c. Calcium in a scar.
a) Previous removal of benign nodule of inner upper quadrant of right breast.
b) *Mammogram.* Groups of microcalcifications in the inner upper quadrant.
c) *Specimen radiograph* of surgically removed scar. All calcium particles lie subcutaneously in the scar.

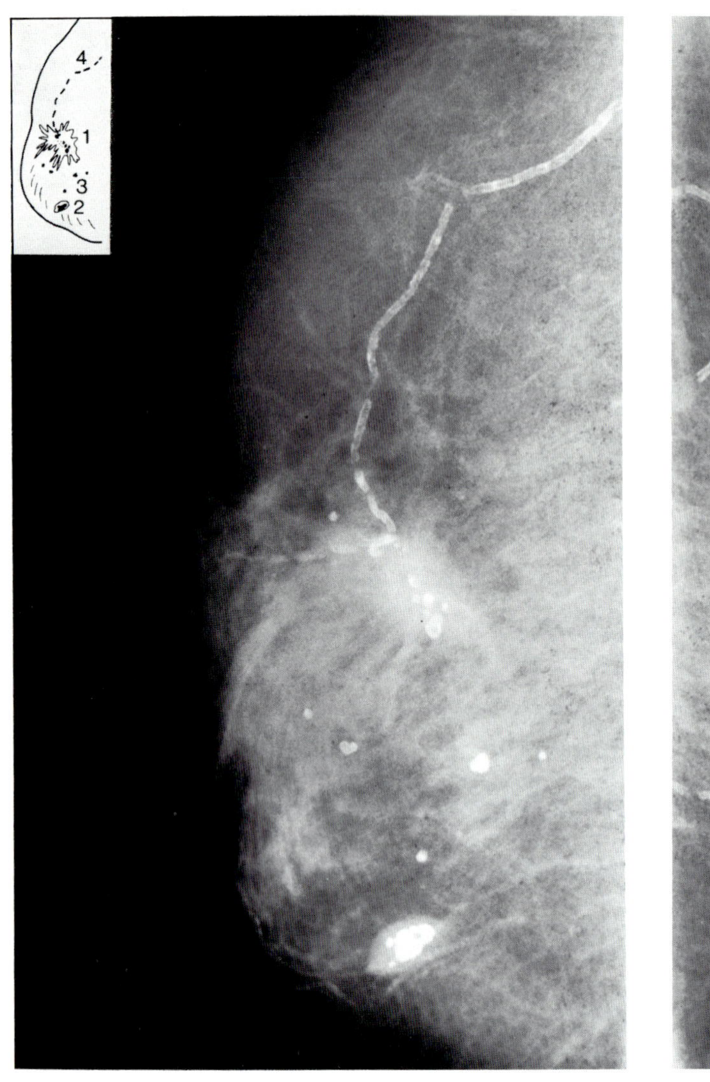

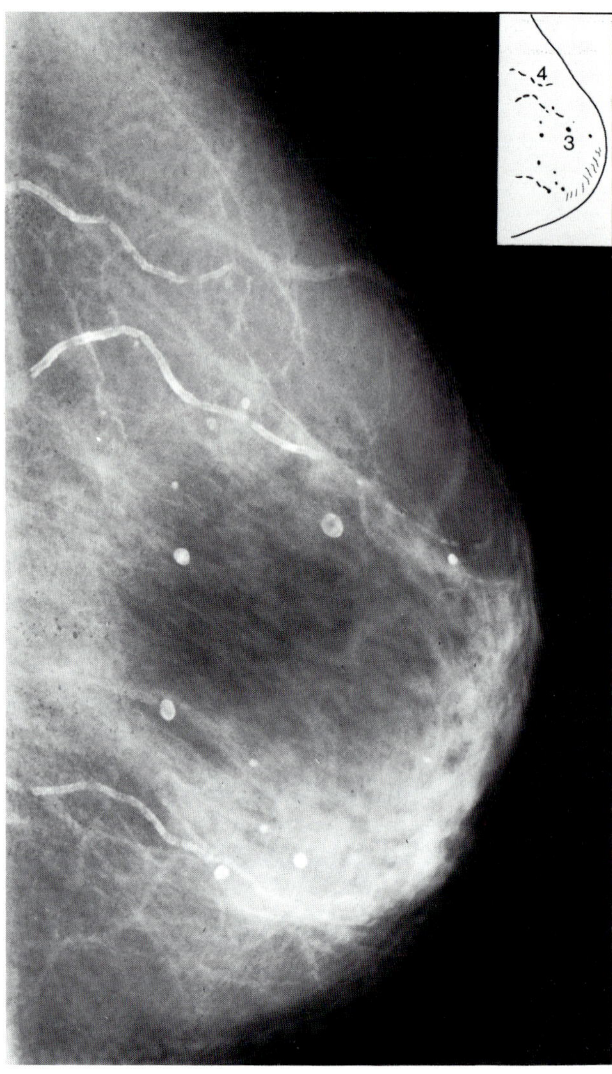

109 a **109 b**

72-year-old female, left and right breasts. A malignant tumor is palpable in the left inner upper quadrant.

109 a, b. *Mammogram* (medio-lateral).
a) Left.
b) Right.
On both sides marked vascular calcifications (4) and circular coarse calcium deposits in calcified cysts (3). In the left breast coarse, plump calcifications in a fibroadenoma (2). Microcalcifications are identifiable in the carcinomatous nodule on the left (1), in addition to calcium in vessels and cysts. Histology: solid carcinoma.

The Preinvasive Stage of Carcinoma of the Breast (Carcinoma in Situ) and the Clinically Occult Carcinoma

The tumor origin is in the lobule (lobular carcinoma in situ, Fig **110**; lobular neoplasia) and in the lactiferous duct (ductal carcinoma in situ, ductal neoplasia). The tumor has not yet broken through the basal membrane of lobule and duct. It does not infiltrate the surrounding tissue.

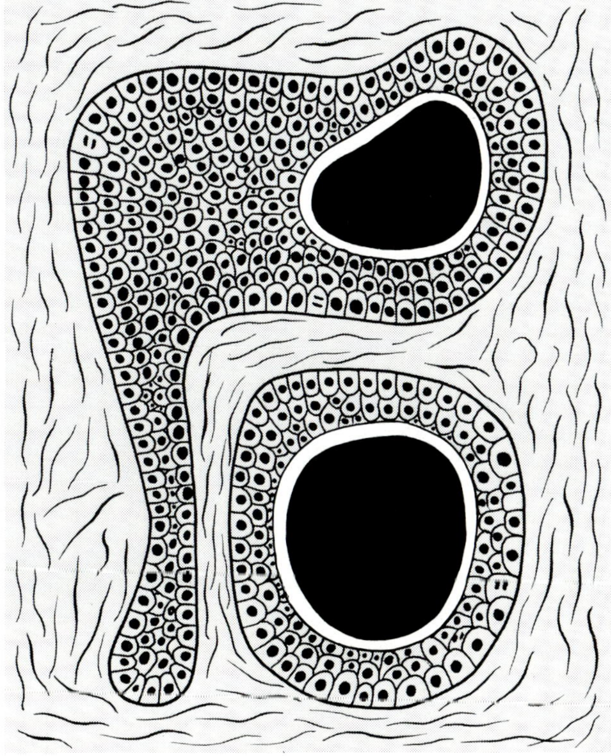

110 Lobular and ductal carcinoma in situ.

Lobular carcinoma in situ

Intraductal solid growths of the epithelium are called *epithelioses*. The lobules become enlarged and plump. According to BÄSSLER (1975), three morphologic types of intralobular solid epithelial growths can be differentiated:

a) Intralobular solid growths of the epithelium found at the *periphery of undifferentiated*, invasive, mostly *solid* and *scirrhous carcinomas*. In most cases, these are so-called concomitant intralobular epithelioses next to invasive carcinomas (Fig **197**).
b) Lobular epithelioses as manifestation of *an intraductal carcinoma which has grown beyond the ductal system*. This is *secondary lobular neoplasia* when tumor cells of a ductal carcinoma grow by way of the terminal ducts into the lobules (Figs **220**, **235**); 22% of all lobular neoplasias belong to this group.
c) *Primary lobular neoplasia of the breast.* Lobular carcinoma in situ tends to arise just prior to menopause and beyond age 60. Most tumors are found incidentally during the histological examination of papillomas, sclerosing adenosis or microcalcifications seen radiographically. There is no palpable tumor; 25% of lobular carcinomas in situ are bilateral. The epithelioses are found as a mirror image in the opposite breast in 40% (Figs **112–118**).

The time interval from the in-situ phase to invasive carcinoma may be from a few months to 23 years; 10% of primary lobular carcinomas in situ may become invasive within five years; 15% within ten (BÄSSLER et al, 1971).
Our own observations revealed that circumscribed, enlarged and confluent lobules in stroma-poor breasts may point to an epitheliosis (lobular neoplasia).

Histological examination of enlarged lobules in three patients revealed lobular carcinoma in situ. In one case histological examination revealed an infiltrating ductal carcinoma of the left breast and a lobular carcinoma in situ in the right. Specimen radiograph of left parenchyma showed additional multiple round opacities up to several millimeters in diameter, indicating epithelioses (Fig **115**).

The normal and the enlarged and confluent lobules have until now received relatively little attention mammographically. In the search for radiographic signs of preinvasive carcinoma enlarged and confluent lobules should be noted and included in the differential diagnosis. Not all enlarged lobule conglomerates can be surgically removed for histological examination. They should be examined regularly by mammography and *selectively* examined cytologically if necessary. Removal with histological examination should be done if

a) microcalcifications in the enlarged lobules appear or are already present,
b) the lobules increase in size,
c) the periphery of the lobules is indistinct and the surrounding ducts thickened, or the ducts seen in a galactogram are interrupted or displaced next to enlarged conglomerates of lobules (Fig **112**).

Specimen radiograph of the biopsy is absolutely necessary for selective examination of removed lobules. The enlarged lobules can thus be localized, properly stained, and subsequently examined in serial sections. This method also has proved successful in removal and histological examination of microcalcifications of breast parenchyma (see page 97).

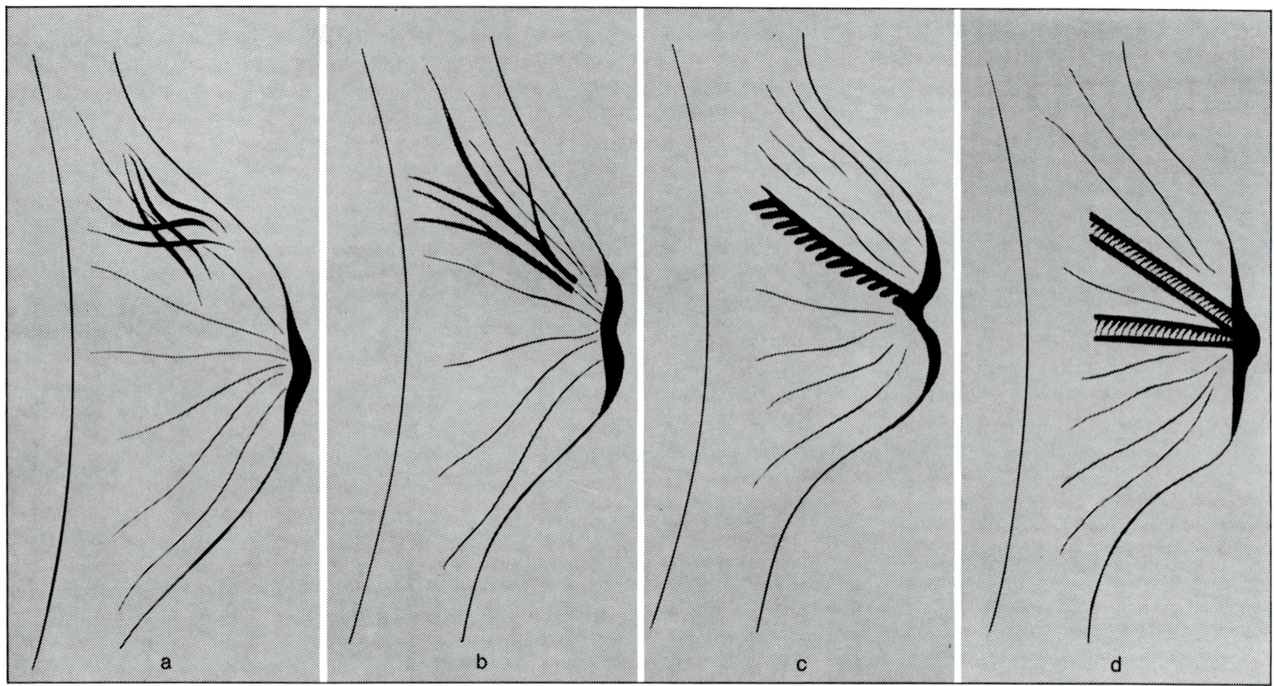

111 a–d. The radiographic-anatomic changes of infiltrated ducts.
a) Thickened lactiferous ducts in net-like arrangement.
b) Thickened and broadened but normally arranged lactiferous ducts, marked retraction of the nipple.
c) Band-like, partially ill-defined opacification with retraction of nipple.
d) Dilated, fibrotic, lactiferous ducts with thickened walls secondary to proliferating epithelium, double contour radiographically.

Ductal carcinoma in situ

Atypical, multilayered epithelium spreads continuously in lactiferous ducts. It may reach the *region of the areola* to cause *Paget's disease* or it may invade the lobules via terminal segments of lactiferous ducts producing a *secondary lobular* neoplasia (Baessler, 1975). These findings are shown schematically in Fig **235**.

Paget's disease of the nipple was proved histologically in a 53-year-old patient. For unknown reasons mammography was not done. There was no tumor palpable in the breast.
The Paget's disease was treated locally with a dose of 5000 rads (tumor dose) using the betatron. It regressed completely. After three months the nipple was scarred, there was no longer any secretion.
Eight months later the patient experienced discomfort in the same breast. Clinical examination showed a painful induration in the inner upper quadrant. Mammography demonstrated a suspicious density 2×4 cm in size in this region which proved to be cytologically a polymorphous carcinoma and histologically an infiltrating lobular carcinoma (Figs **232–234**).

Ductal carcinoma in situ has a different growth pattern than undifferentiated carcinoma; the tumor remains within normal boundaries of the ducts for a longer period of time during which it has a favorable prognosis. According to Bässler (1975), however, up to 95% of intraductal carcinomas are histologically no longer "in situ". They break through the basal membrane and infiltrate periductal stroma at right angles to the duct. Further growth is similar to that of undifferentiated carcinomas which do not remain in situ in the terminal ducts but grow as a small, invasive carcinoma into the stroma. Radiographic changes in the form of net-like enlarged and thickened ducts or enlarged lobules are then no longer present (Fig **119**).

In the *absence of microcalcifications* intraductal carcinoma in situ and the beginning infiltrating ductal carcinoma can be recognized radiographically in stroma-poor breasts by the thickened lactiferous ducts. The ducts also may show net-like branching. Marked ectasia of a duct made thick and fibrotic by proliferating epithelium will show double contour in mammogram (Fig **111**).

Wolfe (1966) reported the diagnostic significance of circumscribed, "torqued" and dilated ducts in intraductal carcinomas.

Thermography may show increased temperature of the nipple with intraductal epithelial proliferations. The temperature of the nipple is several 0.1 °C higher than the opposite nipple. Thermographically the nipple normally is cold. The sign of the *warm nipple* is not present in all duct carcinomas. Its presence is cause to suspect a retroareolar growth of intraductal epithelium.

Thin-needle biopsy of lobular and intraductal carcinoma in situ demonstrates cytologically dissociated individual cells and smaller epithelial groupings in most cases. The cells are very small; the nucleus is round or oval. The cell pattern may be uniform since the nuclei are not hyperchromatic. Mitoses are rarely seen in the smears. With this type of tumor, the danger of a "false negative" diagnosis is great. Contrary to benign processes in the breast, there are no bipolar naked nucleated cells in smears of ductal and lobular neoplasias. This finding may be a differential-diagnostic help.

According to ZAJICEK (1974) 21.4% of all intraductal carcinomas have small cells and show the picture described above in cytological smear. When lactiferous ducts have smooth contours, a preinvasive carcinoma as shown in Fig **111** is indicated. The duct will become unsharp with tumorous infiltration. A solid cancer nodule may develop at the site of broadened, ill-defined ducts seen radiographically. This typical evolution of breast cancer from preinvasive to clinically evident phase was found in a 36-year-old patient:

First mammogram was done 4 years earlier with normal clinical and radiographic findings.

The second a year later showed slight increase in density of both breasts. The ducts in the lower quadrant of the left breast were slightly thickened (seen only retrospectively).

A third mammogram showed a net-like, ill-defined opacity at the site of the thickened ducts. Palpation revealed induration of this area. Thin needle biopsy showed epithelial groupings with somewhat plump nuclei *cytologically*. A follow-up examination in three months was advised. Because of pregnancy, the follow-up examination was done 1¼ years later. The nonhomogeneous opacity noted in the previous mammogram had increased to a homogeneous partially smooth and partially spiculated tumor in the meantime (Fig **121**). Clinically there was retraction of the skin.

The *cytological picture* was consistent with a polymorphocellular carcinoma (Fig **122**).

Histologically a polymorphocellular, solid, infiltrating carcinoma was found.

The net-like opacities noted on the third mammogram apparently were no longer the preinvasive stage of the carcinoma; it had already progressed to the invasive stage as indicated by the ill-defined ducts.

Thermography was done only with the last mammogram. The involved breast was 2.5 °C warmer than the other.

Band- or net-like thickened ducts in the mammogram are particularly critical findings and require early follow-up examinations. Biopsy should be done at an early stage. In retrospect the parenchymal changes in the third mammogram are an absolute indication for biopsy with histologic examination, even in the presence of negative cytological findings.

Intraductal carcinoma in situ may be recognized early in the mammogram by the presence of microcalcifications. It will then be diagnosed and treated like an infiltrating comedo-carcinoma (see page 144).

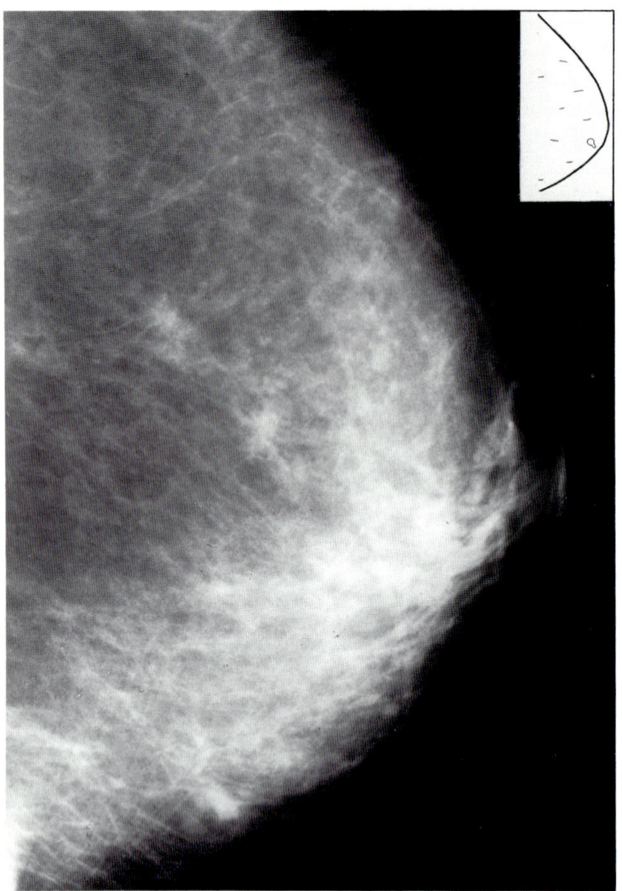
112a

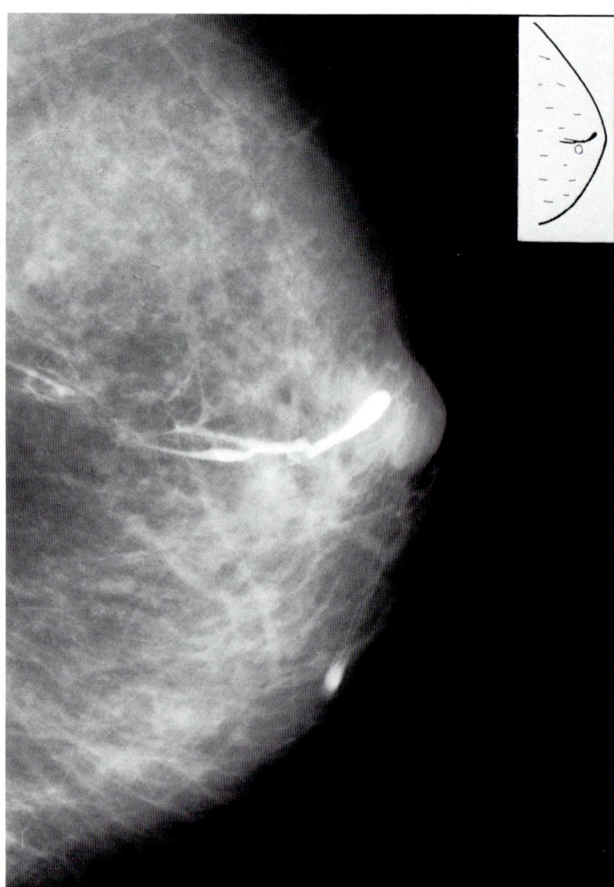
112b

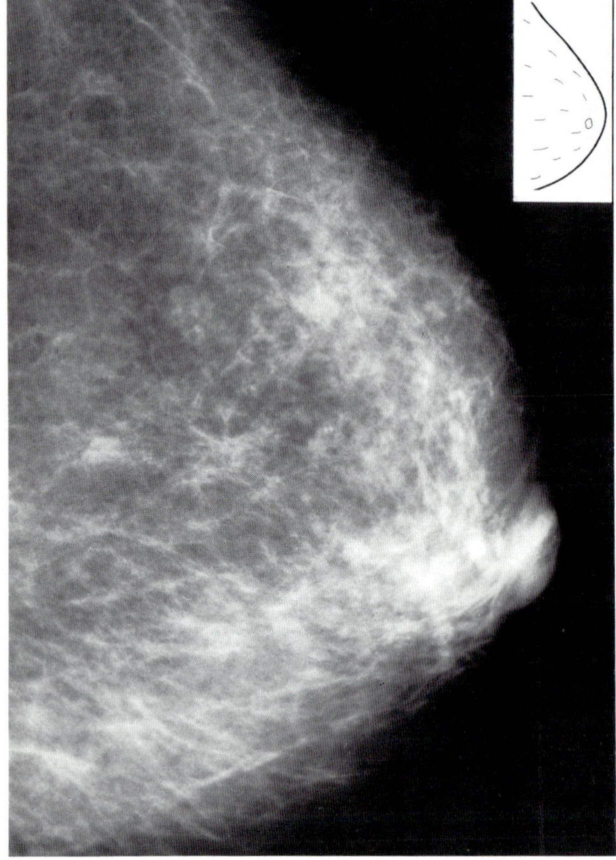
112c

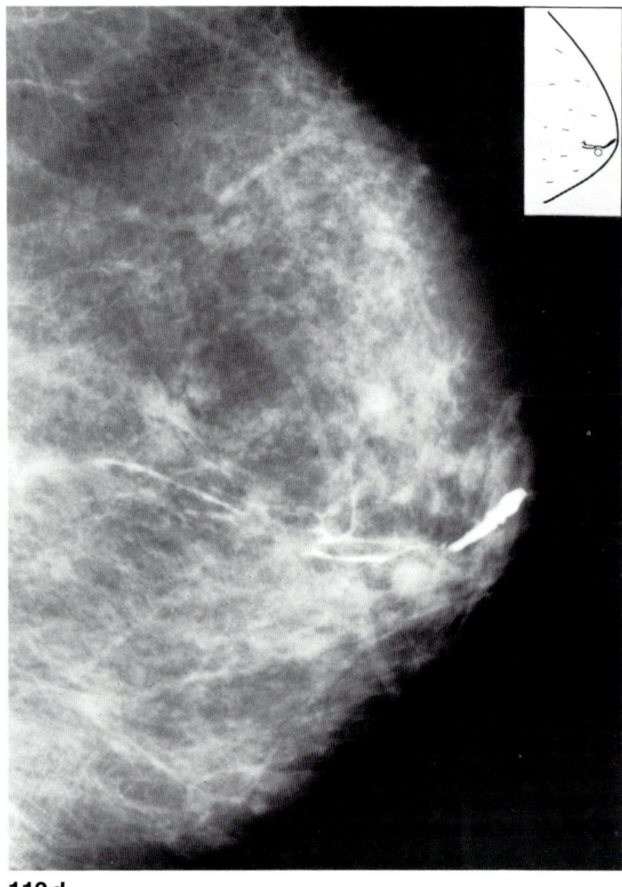
112d

56-year-old female, left and right breasts. Screening examination. Palpation normal. First examination 1 year ago, radiographic diagnosis: suspicion of malignant tumor left. Patient refuses treatment. Follow-up examination after one year: palpation still negative. Slight regression of secretion on the left (Fig 112–114).

◁ **112** a–d. *Mammogram and galactography* left (medio-lateral).
a) Mammogram 1 year ago. Unsharp, faintly radiopaque, small retroareolar nodule measuring a few mm (miliary).
b) Galactography 1 year ago. Retroareolar opacified duct, slight elevation of duct above nodule. No stenosis. Suspicion of lobular carcinoma.
c) Follow-up mammogram. Retroareolar nodule slightly larger and denser. Unsharp contour. Additional enlarged lobules in upper quadrants.
d) Follow-up galactography. Stenosis and elevation of opacified duct by the tumor. Suspicion of ductal carcinoma (invasion of duct system by lobular carcinoma). Histology: small ductal carcinoma with one axillary lymph node metastasis.

113 a, b. *Cytological examination* of breast secretion (follow-up examination).
a) Milky secretion from a duct.
b) Solid epithelial layer with marked polymorphous nuclei. Increased number of plump nuclei. Suspicion of malignancy.

114 a–d. *Electronic thermovision,* examination 1 year ago.
a) Right breast normally vascularized.
b) Left breast with diffuse hyperthermia and striking periareolar vascularization.
c) Right. Follow-up examination after 1 year.
d) Left. Increase in periareolar hyperthermia with warm nipple. Otherwise unchanged vascularization bilaterally.

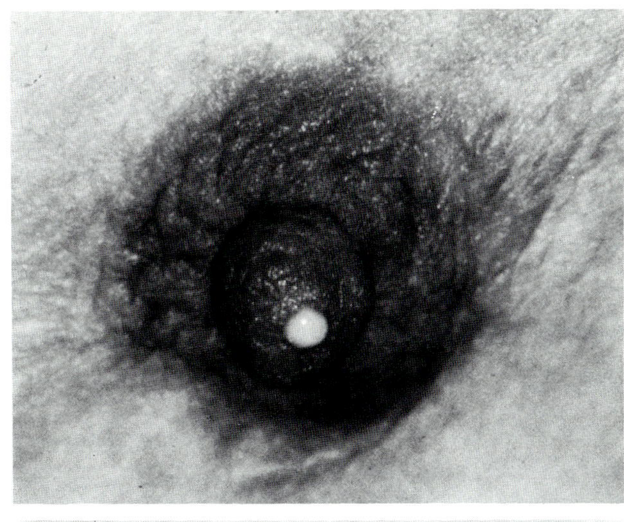
a

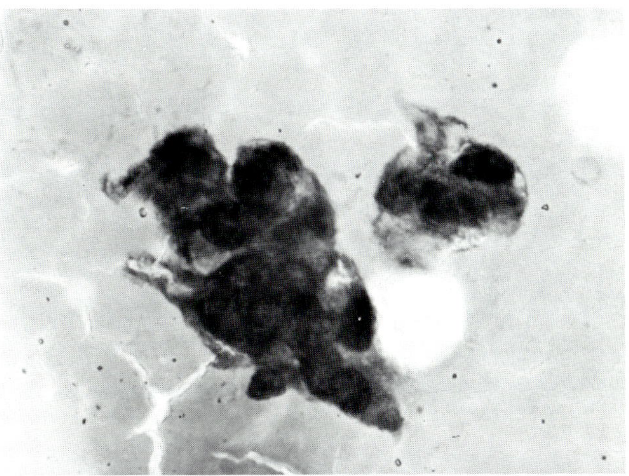
b

113

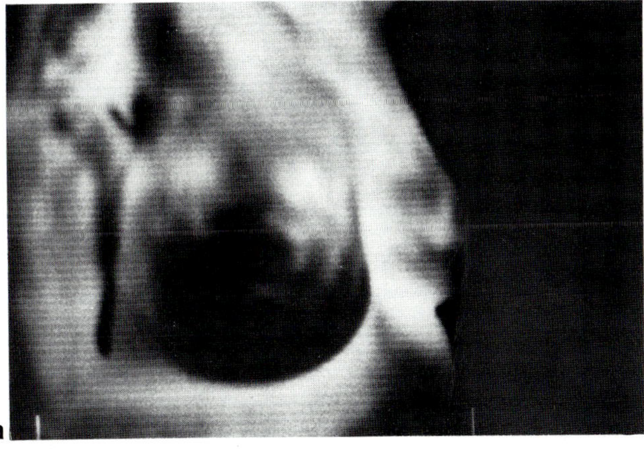
a

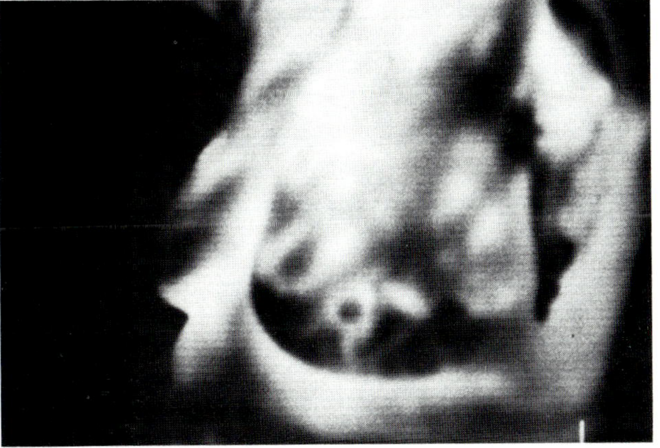
b

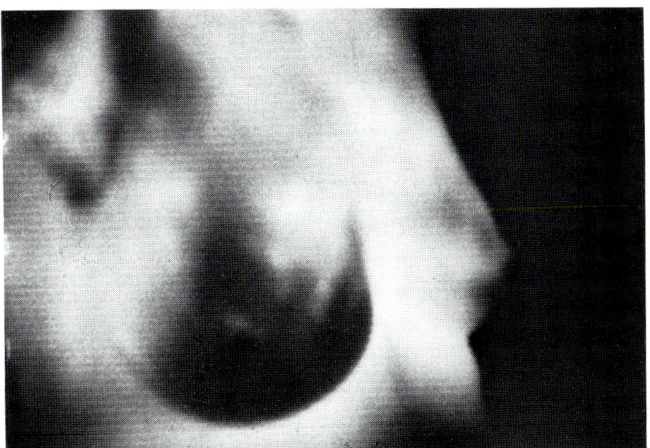
c

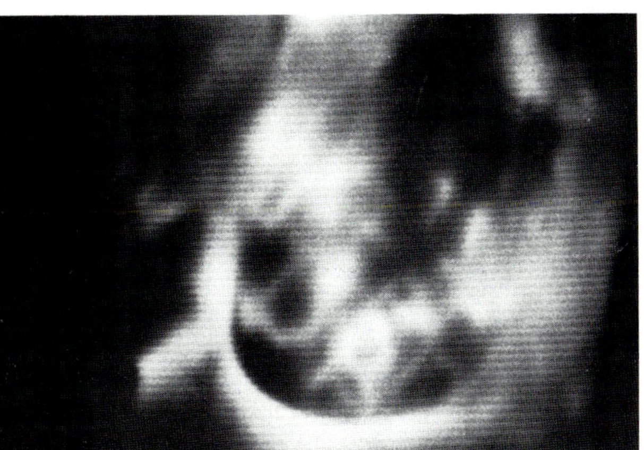
d

114

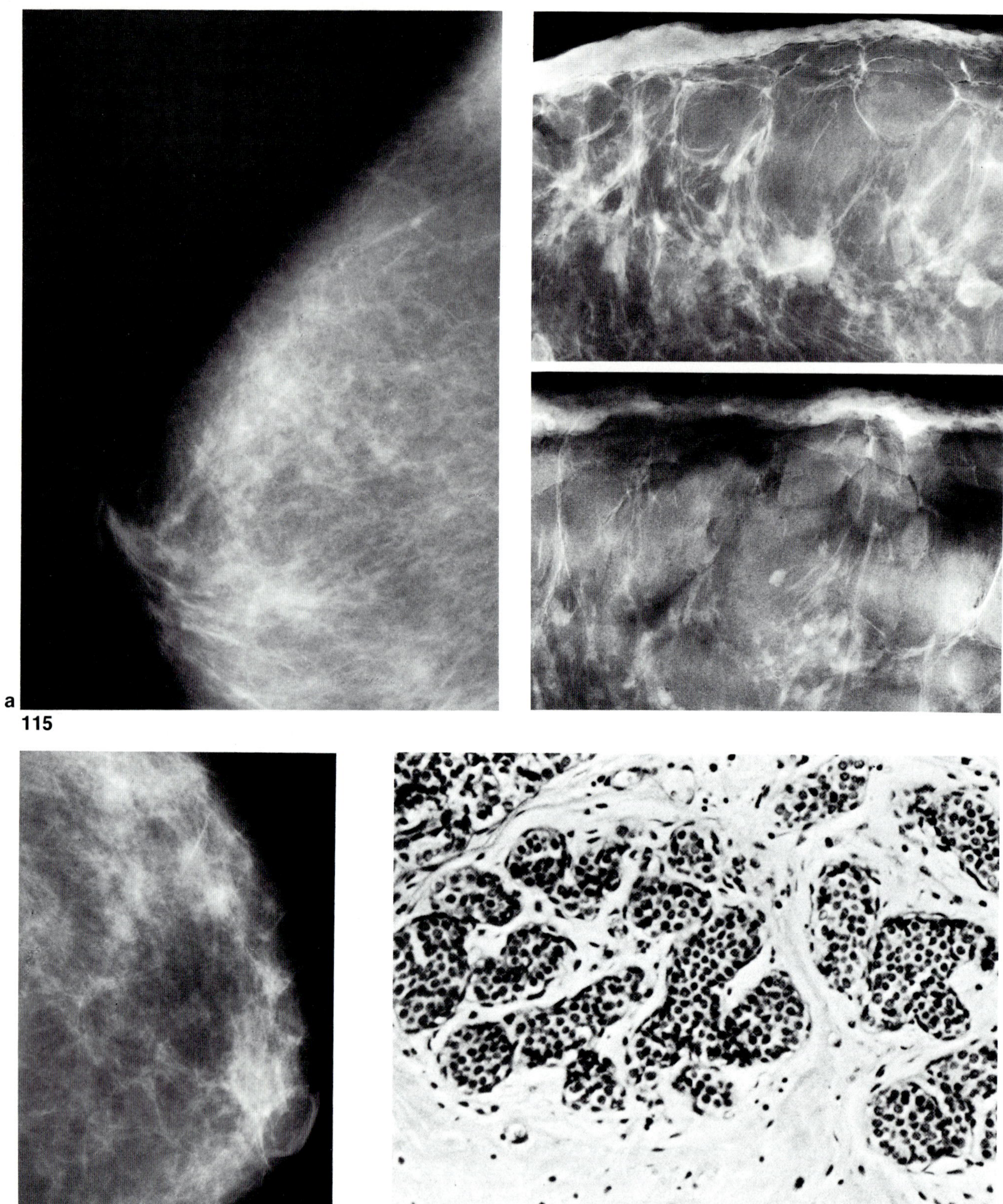

115 a–c. Enlarged lobules with lobular carcinoma in situ. **a)** *Mammogram* of right (left in Fig 112). Multiple enlarged lobules and a group of microcalcifications in upper quadrants. **b, c)** *Specimen radiography* of breast shown in Fig 112. There are additional enlarged and confluent lobules in two different cuts. Lactiferous duct and its corresponding lobules identifiable in (c). Histology: lobular carcinoma in situ in all areas. The patient has multifocal tumor growth in both breasts.

116 53-year-old female, left breast. Several enlarged and confluent lobules in upper quadrants. Histology: lobular carcinoma in situ.

117 *Histology* of radiographically enlarged lobule. Proliferation of tumor cells in lobule with preservation of its basic structure. Lobular carcinoma in situ.

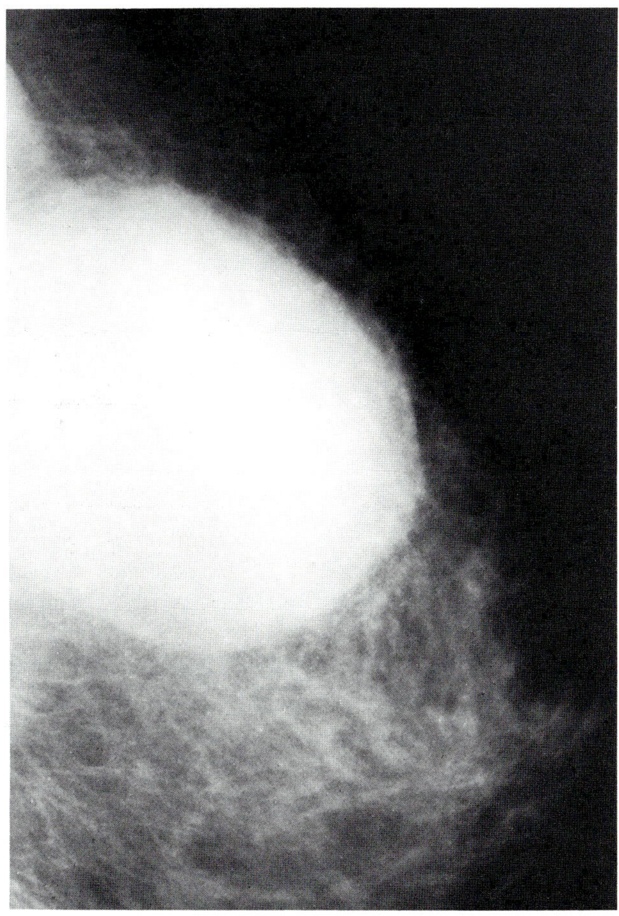
a

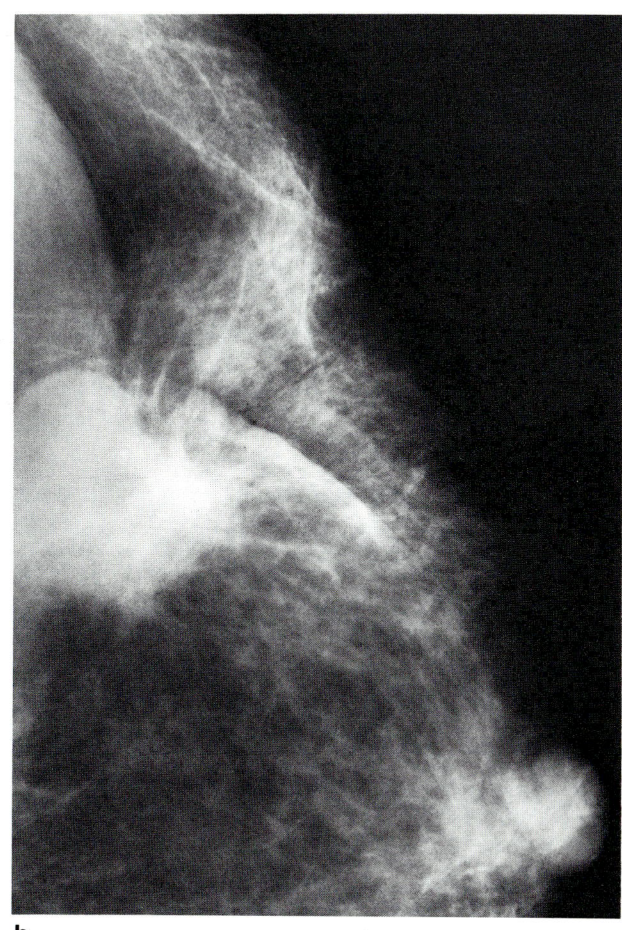
b

After biopsy of breast shown in Fig 115, a tangerine-sized tumor developed in the other (right) breast of this patient (Fig 118).

118 a, b. Original findings and follow-up examination.
a) *Mammogram* (medio-lateral) 14 days after biopsy. Smooth, round, sharply-defined tumor, benign. Clinically and cytologically hematoma following biopsy.

b) *Follow-up examination* (medio-lateral) after 4 months. Regression and marked decrease in size of the hematoma, radiating scar and skin retraction. No palpable tumor. No tumor cells in cytologic smear.

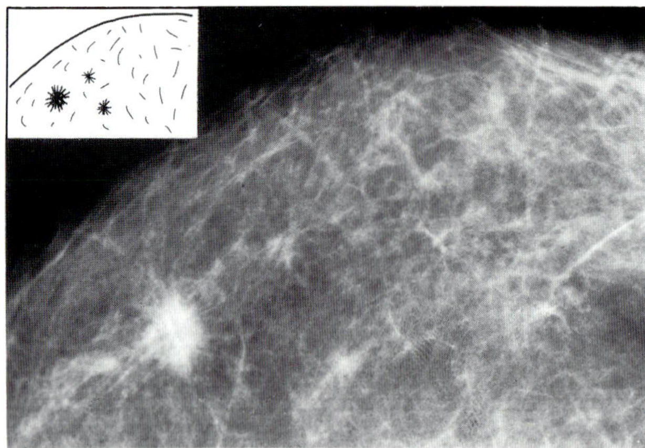

119

Survey examination. Normal palpation. On thermography bilateral normal vascularization (Figs 119, 120).

119 *Mammogram* left (cranio-caudal). Radiograph of 62-year-old female. Involuted breast. Lentil-sized stellate carcinoma in upper-lateral quadrant. Two tiny radiating opacities medially. Histology of large nodule: solid carcinoma. The additional two opacities were not found histologically.

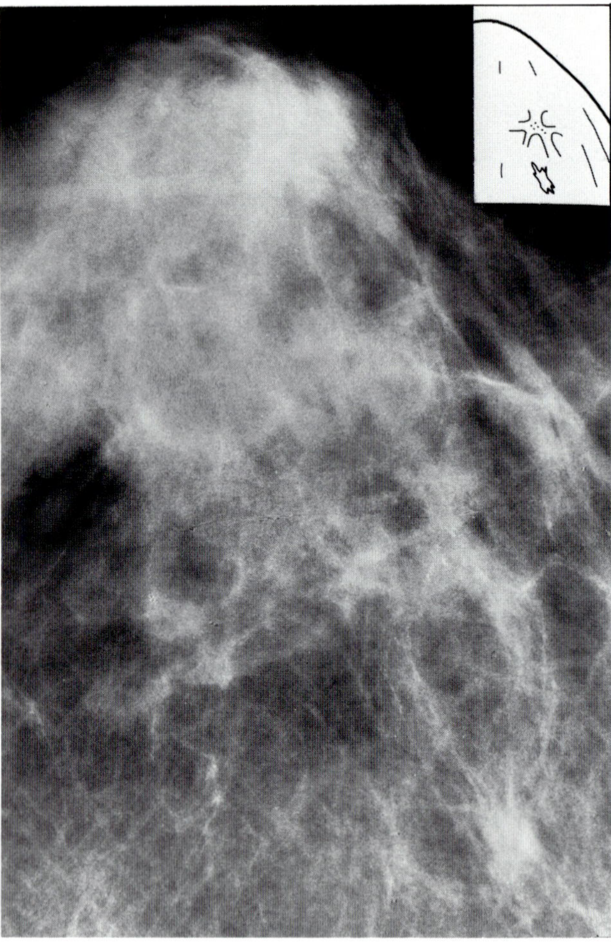

120

120 *Mammogram* left (cranio-caudal). 41-year-old female with partially homogeneous, partially focal opacities consistent with fibrosis. Distorted trabecular architecture with stellate opacities in inner-quadrant region. Comedo-calcifications recognizable. Removal of abnormalities and examination with specimen radiography. Histology: multilocular ductal carcinoma.

36-year-old female, left breast. First examination 4 years ago. Clinically and radiologically normal. Second examination one year later showed bilateral, increased density and retrospectively somewhat thickened ducts. Third examination 1 year later showed net-like, unsharp opacities in lower quadrants. Increased resistance (induration) to palpation. Since thin-needle biopsy was negative a follow-up examination in 3 months was suggested and not done until $1^1/_4$ years later because of pregnancy. At that time, clinical examination showed a definite carcinoma. ▷

121 a–d. *Serial mammograms.*
a) First mammogram (7/15/72). Normal breast structures. No evidence of malignancy.

b) Second mammogram (8/26/73). Diffuse increased density. Slightly broadened and thickened ducts in lower quadrants. Otherwise negative.

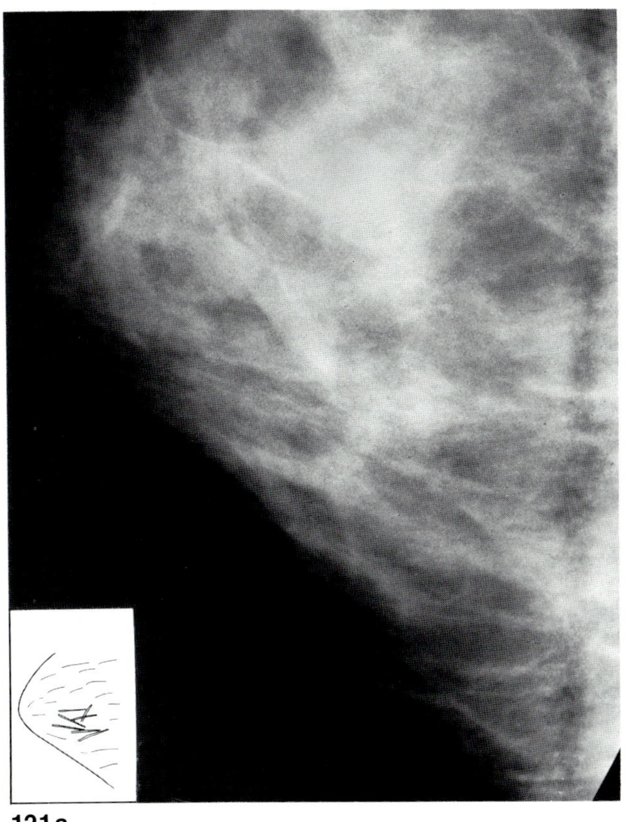

121a

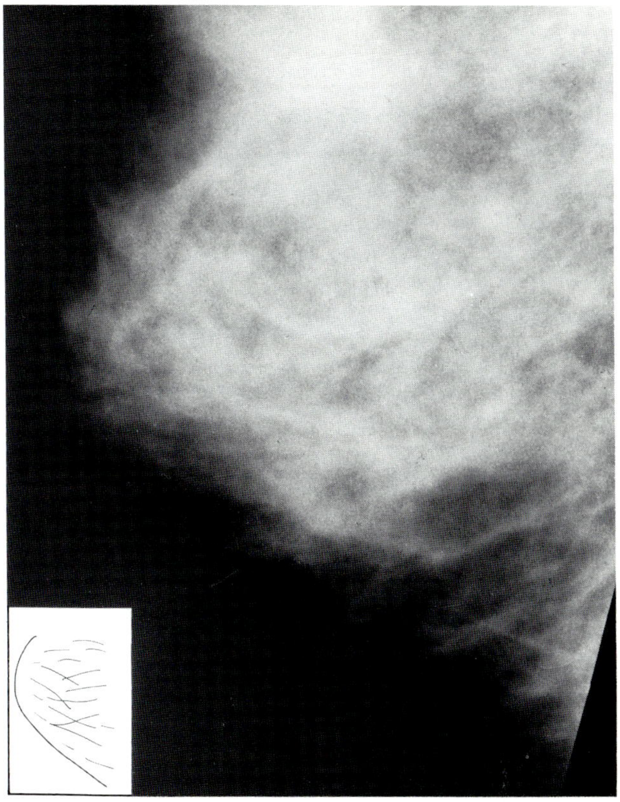

121b

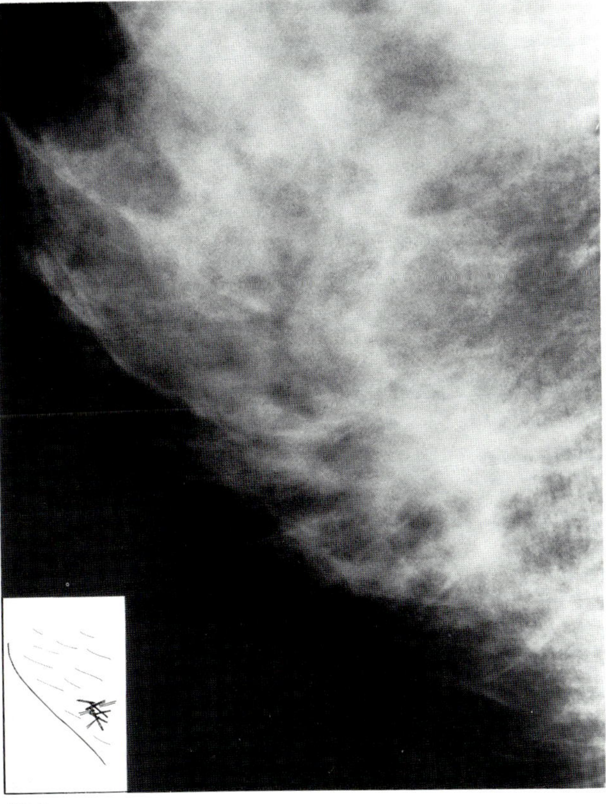

121c

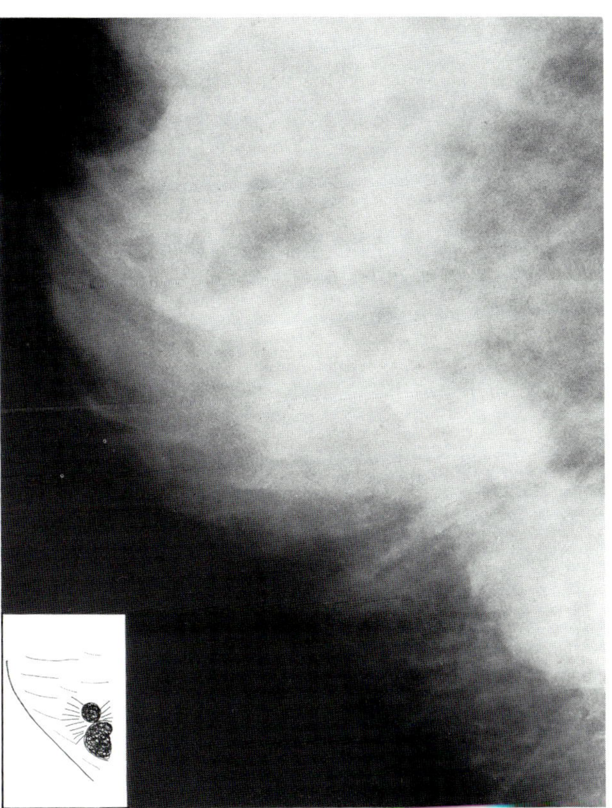

121d

121 **c)** Third mammogram (9/25/74). Retroareolar portion of breast is again more radiolucent. In inframammary fold partially net-like, partially spiculated opacities with thickened ill-defined ducts can be seen. Atypical induration on palpation. Thin-needle biopsy reveals abundant epithelium (Fig 122a). Follow-up examination in 3 months advised.

d) Fourth mammogram (11/25/75). The suggested follow-up examination was delayed because of pregnancy. Palpable nodule in lower outer quadrant toward end of pregnancy. Several smoothly defined tumor nodules on mammography. Radiating strands of tumor between these with retraction of skin.

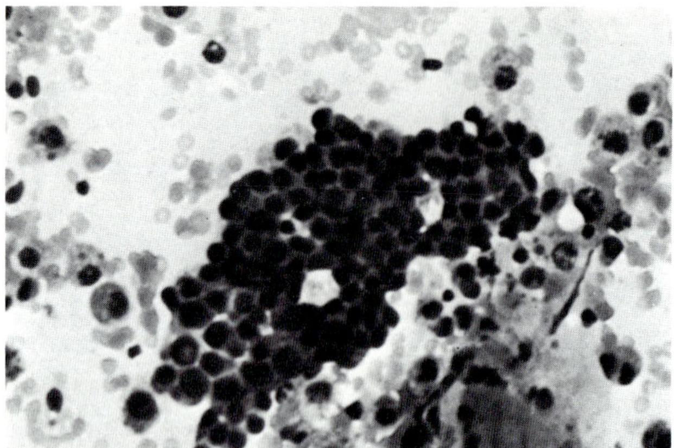

122a

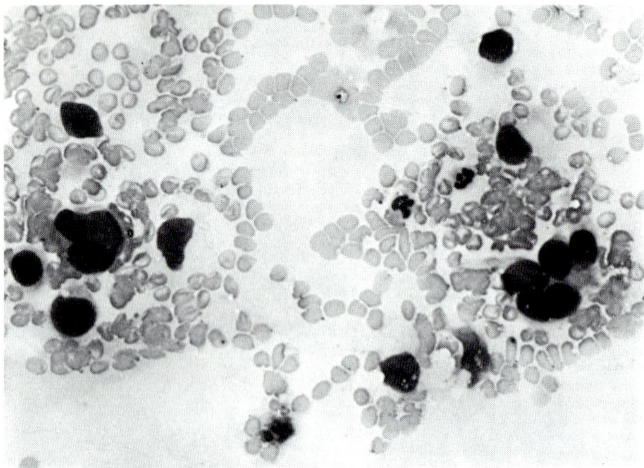

122b

122 a, b. *Cytology* (same case as Fig 121)

a) Thin-needle biopsy on 9/25/74. Epithelial layer with uniform nuclei and small rim of cytoplasm of epithelial cells. In lower portion of epithelial layer are enlarged and hyperchromatic nuclei. Next to them are individual cells with broad rim of cytoplasm. Slightly hyperchromatic nuclei. Diagnosis: cell architecture similar to mastopathy with epithelial changes. Follow-up in a short period of time advisable.

b) Thin-needle biopsy on 11/25/75. Tumor cells in small groups and plump, polymorphous and polychromatic nuclei. Partially naked nucleated cells. Diagnosis: polymorphocellular carcinoma.

56-year-old female. Repeated radiographic examinations over past 6 months. No abnormal findings. Patient worries with apparently psychosomatic symptoms centering on left breast (Figs 123–124). ▷

123 a, b. *Bilateral mammogram* (medio-lateral).

a) Left breast. Fibrous mastopathy. Periductal thickening (compare Figs 75, 77–81). In upper quadrant fibroadenoma with coarse calcifications. Elongated stellate opacity with some microcalcifications hidden in breast structure. High suspicion of malignancy.

b) Right breast. Fibrous mastopathy. No evidence of malignancy.

124 a, b. *Specimen radiography.*

a) Radiograph of specimen. Stellate opacity with tongue-like tumor projections in the dense breast. Some microcalcifications in the center.

b) Central calcification, magnif 20×, using fine grain industrial film. Extensive microcalcifications in small groups, partially confluent. The extent of this calcification is not recognizable in mammogram nor in specimen radiograph.

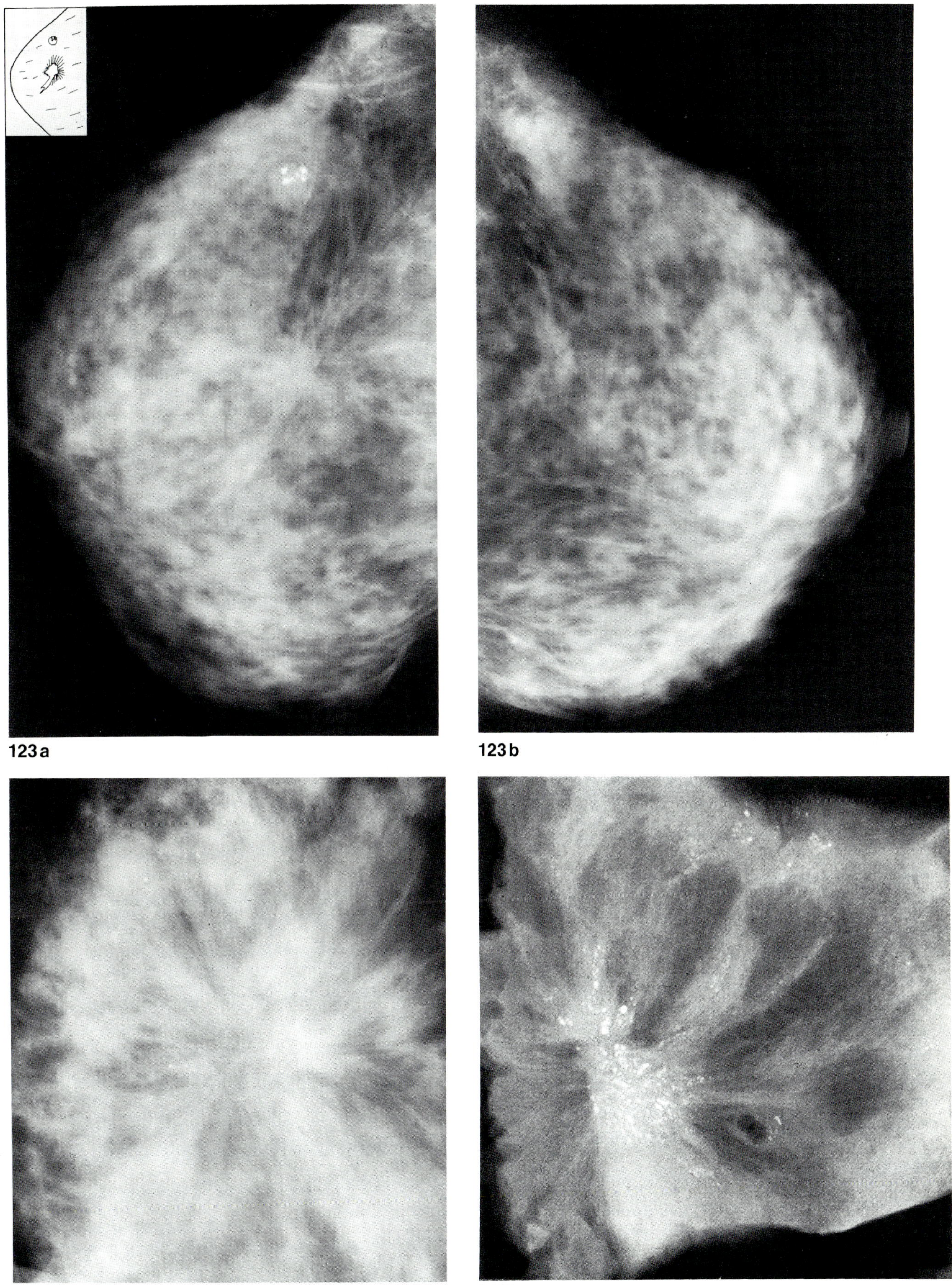

123 a

123 b

124 a

124 b

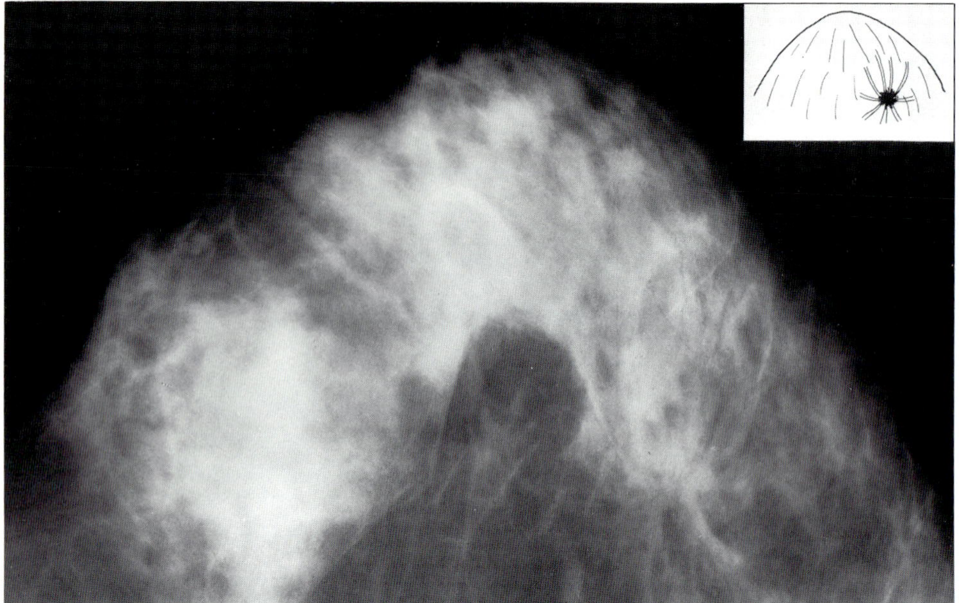

125a

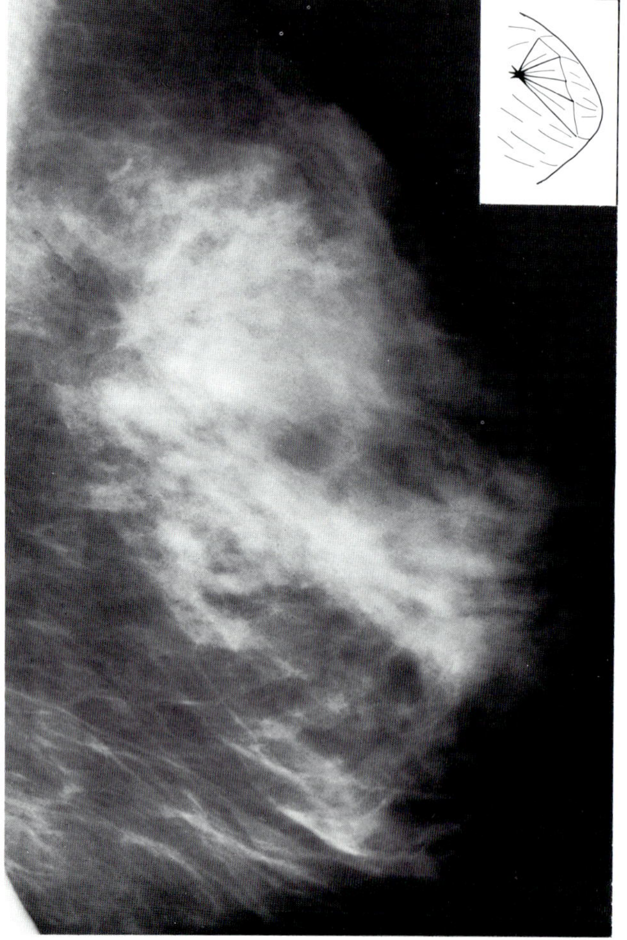

125b

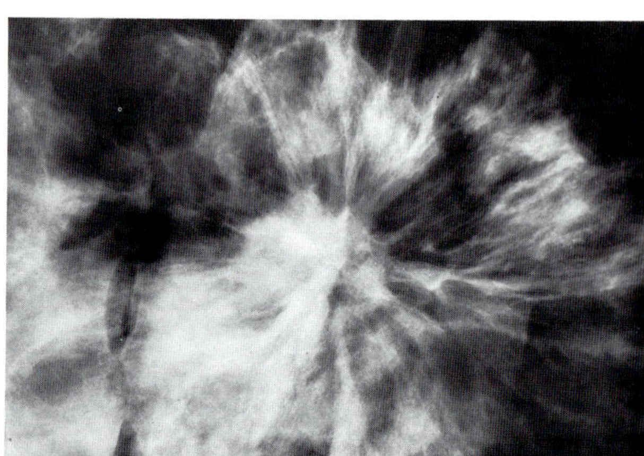

126

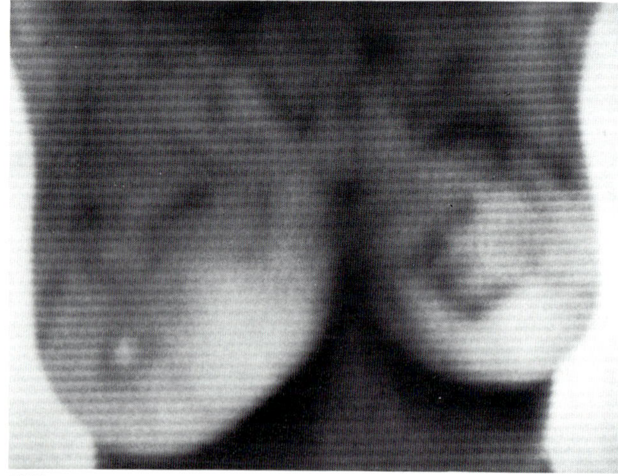

127

53-year-old female, left breast. Survey examination. Normal palpation. Left breast smaller than right since puberty (Figs 125–127).

125 a, b. *Mammogram.*
a) Cranio-caudal.
b) Medio-lateral.
Retroareolar thickened ducts. Homogeneous opacity in outer upper quadrant. Curved, stellate opacities in inner upper quadrant. Suspicion of malignancy.

126 *Specimen radiograph.* Tumor nodule with long projections into surrounding breast.

127 *Thermovision.* Right breast of normal size, left breast hypoplastic. Left breast, inner quadrant, atypical vessel with hyperthermia of 0.5 °C.

Malignant Invasive Tumors

Malignant breast tumors are new growths predominantly originating from the epithelium of lobules or lactiferous ducts *(carcinomas)*. Malignant transformation of breast connective tissue is very rare *(sarcomas)*. *Systemic diseases* may involve the breast (leukemias, lymphosarcoma, lymphogranulomatosis, reticulum cell sarcoma and others). *Metastases* to the breast from other organs are possible (hypernephroma, thyroid carcinoma, melanoma and others).

Cell-stroma relationship

Every tumor consists of a basic connective tissue framework (stroma) and of cells. The proportion of both components varies from tumor to tumor and causes its characteristic morphological appearance.

Stroma predominates in *acellular tumors*. These new formations grow in stellate forms and separate themselves from the surrounding tissue in a radiating fashion. Calcifications are common.

In *cellular tumors* there is little stroma present. They grow in a nodular form and separate themselves from the surrounding parenchyma in a smooth or polycyclic fashion. Calcifications are rare or absent. Cellular tumors grow more rapidly than acellular.

Morphometric tumor analyses reveal an average of 21.5% tumor epithelium in stellate growing malignancies. Cell content increases in the parenchyma-rich nodular tumors to an average of 64.5% (UNDERWOOD, 1972). Of all breast carcinomas, about 0.7% are completely smooth, 15% partially smooth, partially radiating, 84% completely radiating with radiograph corresponding to anatomic findings (HAMPERL 1968, GALLAGER and MARTIN 1969, CASTANO-ALMENDRAL et al 1971).

Cellular malignancies show a tendency toward hemorrhagic necrosis, producing spontaneous hematomas in the breast which, on occasion, may be the first hint of a malignant process (Figs **188**, **190**, **282**). Cellular malignancies have increased metabolism resulting in their increased vascularization and greater-than-normal parenchyma, so they may be recognized by electronic and/or plate thermography by unilateral, localized or diffuse hyperthermia, by atypical vascular patterns or by a warm nipple (TRICOIRE et al 1970, MÜLLER et al 1974) (Fig **185**). However, cellular, nodular, growing tumors retract the surrounding parenchyma only minimally or not at all. In contradistinction, depending on their elastic fiber content, stellate growing tumors show more or less marked retraction of the surrounding tissues. Strands of tumor growing toward the skin (associated with thickening and retraction of the skin, 52%), nipple retraction (55%), deranged architecture surrounding the tumor and peritumoral lucency in the mammogram are manifestations of this process (BUCHWALD and HYLSE 1971). The stimulus regulating the stroma content of a tumor is unknown. According to VON ALBERTINI (1974), the stroma originates not from tumor parenchyma but from the invaded tissue. It consists of connective tissue with vessels. The reaction of the connective tissue normally present is initiated by unknown stimuli acting from the tumor parenchyma on the connective tissue.

While BUSCH and MERKER (1968) and LUNDMARK (1972) believe that the production of new connective tissue is a defense reaction of the organism toward the tumor cells, GULLINO and GROMTHAM (1963), UNDERWOOD (1972) and DOUGLAS and SHIVAS (1974) believe that the fibroblastic reaction is biologically specific for the individual tumor and not a reaction of the organism to the tumor. Apparently, local and endocrine immunological factors play an important part (OZZELLO 1970), since primary tumors and metastases have a differing morphologic appearance. The production of connective tissue secondary to lymphangitic skin cancers is very impressive (Fig **293**). Concentric layers of loose connective tissue are formed to surround the growing tumor cells within the lymph channels of the skin.

Elastic and fibrous tissue content

The growing stellate carcinomas show a remarkable amount of elastic tissue (DOUGLAS and SHIVAS 1974); normal connective tissue has only relatively few elastic fibers. The elastic tissue of the cut section of a cancer appears as net-like, yellow spots and strands (JACKSON and ORR 1957, LEVITAN et al 1964) (Fig **291**).

There is an apparent relationship between elastic fiber content of a tumor and the survival of the patient. SHIVAS and DOUGLAS (1972) examined elastic content of carcinomas and length of survival of 103 patients. Those with tumors without elastic fibers had an average survival time of 33.5 months while the survival time of patients whose tumors had extensive elastic tissue was 93.7 months.

The reverse is true for the *connective tissue* content of a tumor. According to ANASTASSIADES and PRYCE (1974) the higher the content of connective tissue in a tumor, the poorer the prognosis. The connective tissue portion is remarkably high in the undifferentiated carcinomas (scirrhous carcinoma, solid carcinoma). According to DOERR and ULE (1970) the cell-stroma relationship is 1:3 to 1:2 depending on the histological type of the tumor. According to VON ALBERTINI (1974) undifferentiated carcinomas have an equally poor prognosis. Only medullary carcinoma has a somewhat better prognosis. Mucoid carcinoma and comedo-carcinoma have the best survival rate; it is poorer for adenocarcinoma. This is reflected radiographically as follows.

Poorest prognosis: stellate growing tumors (scirrhus, solid carcinoma, adeno-scirrhus). *Relatively good prognosis:* predominantly smooth or multilobular nodular tumors (medullary carcinoma, mucoid carcinoma). *Very good prognosis*: pure duct carcinomas (comedo-carcinoma).

Tumor cells

The stroma of a tumor plays only an unimportant role in the tumor diagnosis of the pathologist (VON ALBERTINI 1974). In contradistinction, it may be the earliest sign of a malignancy radiographically. There is no significant difference between the stroma and the remaining interlobular connective tissue (BLACK and YOUNG, 1965). Physically denser than normal interlobular connective tissue, tumor stroma absorbs a larger percentage of the x-ray beam.

To this date there is no *absolute* morphological sign of tumor cells under the light microscope. According to BUSCH (1968) and VON ALBERTINI (1974), there are also no specific neoplastic changes of breast cancer in distinction from normal breast epithelium to be seen with electron microscopy. The tumor cell has a number of characteristics differentiating it distinctly from the normal cell; each *individual* characteristic, however, is not conclusive of malignancy while in toto they indicate a very high probability of malignancy. One particular characteristic of a tumor cell is its variations in size and form (polymorphism). It varies from microelements to giant cells. The nucleus is polymorphic; it varies in size, is often irregular in shape and may have a bizarre form and plump lobulation.

The tumor cell frequently contains several nuclei. The structure of the chromatin of the nuclei may be markedly different on one slide. Fine granulation and coarse septum formation may be noted. Abnormal nucleoli are characteristic. They are always enlarged in tumor cells. Not all cells with enlarged nucleoli, however, are tumor cells. In carcinoma cells the nucleoli may become so large that the remaining cell nucleus is only a small rim surrounding the nucleolus. Mitoses are common in tumor epithelium and are noted more commonly in the histological section than in the cytological smear (Fig **181** b). Atypical mitoses of cells are common.

Tumor cells commonly have naked nuclei. It is also notable that the appearance of tumor cells in the primary tumor and in the metastasis may be different. Tubular collections in the cytological carcinoma smear are prognostically favorable. In contradistinction, absent or deficient coherence of cells with many free epithelial cells outside the cell collections indicates a less favorable prognosis (STEGNER and PAPE 1972).

Tumor calcifications

In addition to stroma and epithelium, calcifications play an important part in the diagnosis of cancer. Carcinomas rich in stroma and growing in a stellate pattern calcify more extensively than carcinomas poor in stroma (Figs **156**, **157**). Coarse calcium particles usually lie in the center of the tumor. In carcinoma of the duct they are secondary to necrosis of duct epithelium and lie within the duct (LEVITAN et al 1964, BLACK and YOUNG 1965, HAMPERL 1968, HASSLER 1969, KOEHL et al 1970, BARTH and DEININGER 1971, STEGNER and PAPE 1972, HOEFFKEN and LANYI 1977). Delicate and very tiny, in part dust-like calcifications tend to lie more in the periphery of the tumor (Fig **140**), usually interstitially. According to STEGNER and PAPE (1972) interstitial calcifications originate in tumor cells and migrate into the interstitium. He was unable to demonstrate early interstitial calcifications by electro-optical means. In lobular carcinoma the calcifications are commonly found outside the tumor. KOEHL et al (1970) found such calcifications in the tumor itself only in six of 32 such tumors. In the remaining malignancies they were outside in normal tissue. Medullary and mucoid carcinomas, as a rule, show no calcifications (LEVITAN et al 1964, KOEHL et al 1970, HOEFFKEN and LANYI 1977) (Figs **184**, **186**, **196**, **200**).

Incidence of microcalcifications is quoted differently and varies between 29 and 63%: EGAN (1963) 35 to 45%, LEVITAN et al (1964) 29%, ZUCKERMANN (1965) 63%, HAMPERL (1968) 50%, KOEHL et al (1970) 62%, GERSHON-COHEN (1970) up to 40%. The number of proved calcifications is only the minimal incidence; where no calcifications were found in histological sections examined, they may have been present in other sections. More calcium can be shown in the radiograph than in the histological section (particularly after phototechnical and electronic enlargement), because the radiograph includes the entire tumor parenchyma. Not all microcalcifications are recognizable on large grain mammography film. The calcifications are identifiable in thin specimen sections (5 mm thick) as well as microradiographs (40 to 50 μm thick) using high resolution industrial film (Figs **77**, **114**, **115**, **123**, **124**).

According to HASSLER (1969) a group of microcalcifications of more than ten particles is typical of carcinoma. A smaller number of particles does not exclude a carcinoma but neither can it be differentiated from a benign lesion. We came to the conclusion that the nature of a process cannot be determined either by the number of calcium particles or by their relation to themselves. KOEHL et al (1970) found calcifications to be identical in 62% of all carcinomas and 23% of all benign diseases. The genesis of tumor calcification is still unclear. OZZELLO (1970) explains the process as follows. The ducts and lobuli are coupled with an avascular stroma. This stroma together with the basal membrane, the intercellular spaces, the plasma membrane of the epithelial cells and the myoepithelium forms an electronic-optically identifiable morphological unit called "epithelial-stroma-junction" (ESJ). The ESJ forms a functional unit transporting substances to and from the epithelium. The ESJ is rich in acid mucopolysaccharides which in turn may cause calcifications. The nature of the disorder of this control function is unknown.

Specimen radiography

Surgical removal of microcalcifications of the breast may create problems. The cooperation of surgeon, radiologist and pathologist is necessary to detect, remove and histologically define the nature of the calcifications. The exact location of the calcifications in the breast must be described preoperatively. The distances from the nipple, from the adjoining quadrants and from the skin surface are important. The surgeon removes a larger specimen from the area which is either opacified or marked by a small steel ball (implanted near the calcification through a cannula with a 2 mm lumen). This specimen should be subsequently examined radiographically. Without palpable findings, specimen radiography of microcalcifications is an absolute necessity. It shows whether the calcium has been completely removed from the breast and also marks the location of the calcium in the tissue for the pathologist. The method is important since it is difficult for the pathologist to recognize a group of five, ten or fifteen microcalcifications in a larger tissue specimen. From this point of view the installation of a small, low-voltage x-ray unit in the pathology department merits consideration.
A particularly time-saving method in the removal of microcalcifications was proposed by KOEHL et al (1970). The calcium particles in the specimen are marked with a needle. The pathologist attempts to dissect the microcalcifications from the designated portion of the specimen. A frozen section is then made from the suspicious area. Should a carcinoma be found in this region, any additional examination of the tissue specimen is unnecessary. The remaining specimen will be prepared under radiographic control in case no tumor (and in particular no calcium) can be found. The tissue containing calcium is embedded and serially sectioned and examined. KOEHL et al (1970) state that out of 515 selectively removed calcifications, $^2/_3$ were found in the frozen section and $^1/_3$ following selective preparation under radiographic control.

Round cell infiltrate

Opinions vary regarding the prognostic significance of the infiltration of a tumor by lymphocytes and plasma cells. The round cells either penetrate the tumor diffusely or lie in its immediate vicinity; this occurs commonly in medullary carcinomas (Fig **193** c). While many authors consider the penetration of the tumor by lymphocytes and plasma cells an immunological defense reaction to tumor parenchyma (BERNDT and LANDMANN 1969, CUTLER et al 1969), WALLACE (1971) found no correlation between infiltration of the tumor by round cells and prognosis, based on observations over a period of five years.

A patient with a locally metastasizing breast carcinoma has been treated for several years. The tumor is radiosensitive, tends to have recurrences which occasionally regress spontaneously. Prior to each spontaneous regression there was increased penetration of the tumor epithelium with round cells as seen in cytological smear (Fig **288** d, e).

Age distribution

From the table (Fig **128**) based on 4000 tissue biopsies, it becomes apparent that in the age group *up to 20 years* one half of all breast tumors are adenofibromas. The other half are adenofibromatoses, breast fibroses, adenomas and mastopathies.
In the age group *40 to 49*, every third histological examination will reveal a carcinoma, but only 10% have fibroadenomas. Mastopathies occur in 40%.
In the age group *60 to 79*, carcinomas are much more common than benign diseases and are found in 80% of all examinations.

Histological classification

KRAUS (1973) classifies three main groups histologically:
a) *non-infiltrating tumors*—intralobular and intraductal carcinoma in situ (see page 83);
b) *infiltrating carcinoma*—undifferentiated carcinoma—scirrhous, solid and medullary carcinoma; carcinoma with little structural differentiation—adenocarcinoma;
c) *carcinomas with specific histological differentiation*—papillary, cribriform, duct, mucin producing or mucinous (mucoid, colloid), lobular and squamous-cell carcinoma, Paget's disease.

This classification is of prognostic importance since better therapeutic results can be expected with carcinoma which has not yet infiltrated than with infiltrating carcinoma.

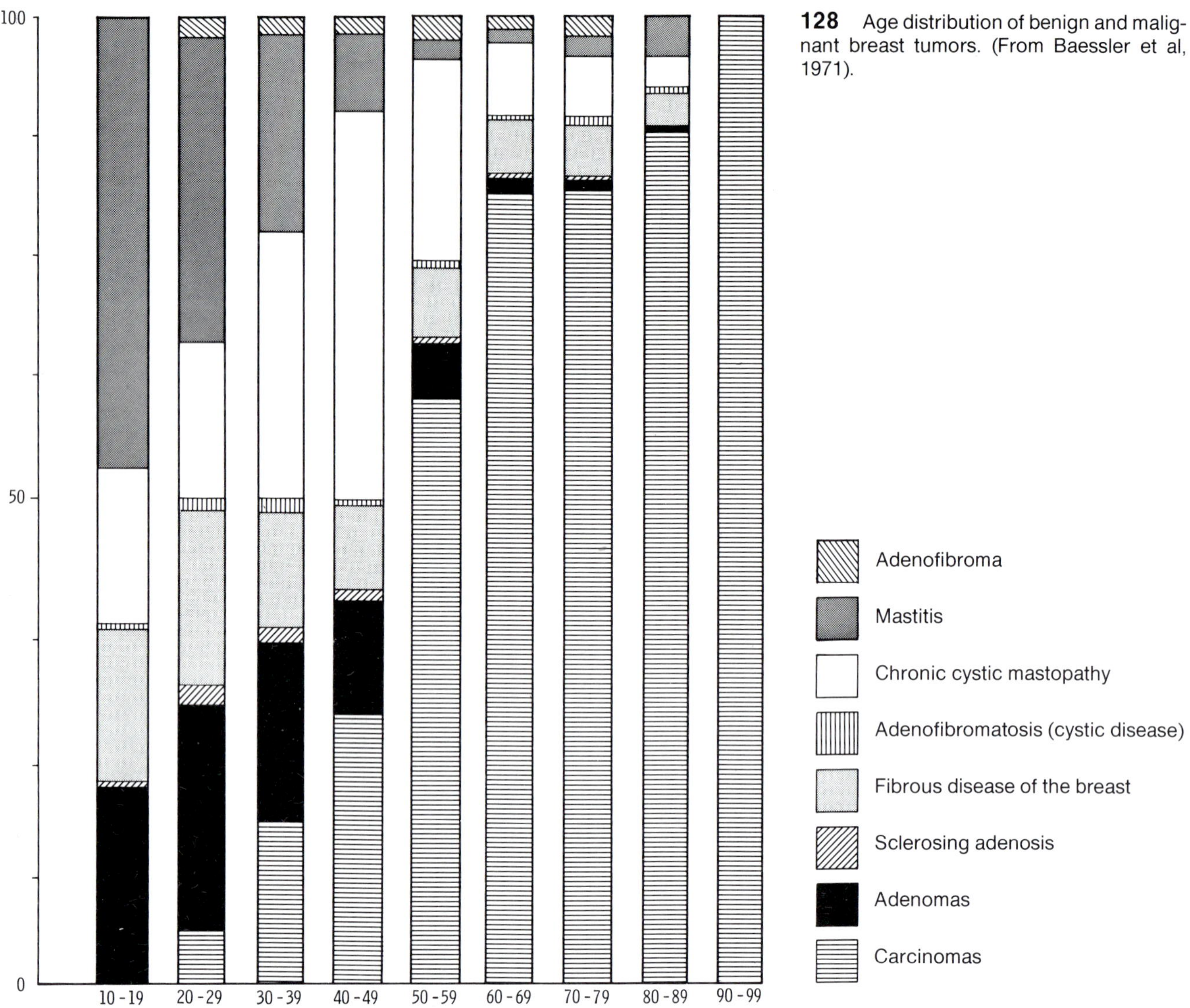

128 Age distribution of benign and malignant breast tumors. (From Baessler et al, 1971).

Carcinoma in situ

For description see page 83.

Infiltrating carcinoma

Most carcinomas seen in daily routine of the pathologist belong to this group. The tumor epithelium has broken through the basal membrane of duct and lobule and infiltrates surrounding tissues.

The most common form is the *scirrhous carcinoma* (Figs **129**, **147** a). It consists of small collections of tumor cells in one to three layers with abundant connective tissue in between. Fibrosis and hyalinization predominate. According to DOERR and ULE (1970) the cell-stroma relation is 1:3. The tumor tends to have central and peripheral interstitial calcium deposits. In addition to the anaplastic carcinomatous tissue, there may be a tendency to differentiate into adenoid structures and hence a histological picture of an adenocarcinoma growing in scirrhous form (adeno-scirrhus), having lost its distinctive character.

Macroscopically the scirrhous portion is characterized by irregular, poorly demarcated, radiating, whitish, coarsely fibered tissue extending into the breast parenchyma (Fig **142**).

The *simple solid* (uncomplicated, circumscribed) carcinoma (Figs **130**, **148** a) shows about a 1:1 ratio of tumor cells to connective tissue. The solid epithelial layers consist of three to six rows of cells. There may be more- or less-cellular types. The less-cellular types have a radiating contour; the more-cellular types are uniform and smooth (Figs **154**–**157**). Microcalcifications are more common in the less-cellular types.

In the surroundings of the carcinoma, there are occasional coarse calcifications following fat necrosis.

Adenocarcinoma (Figs **131**, **149** a) is rarely found in pure form in the breast. It occurs more often in older women and has an irregular radiating contour.

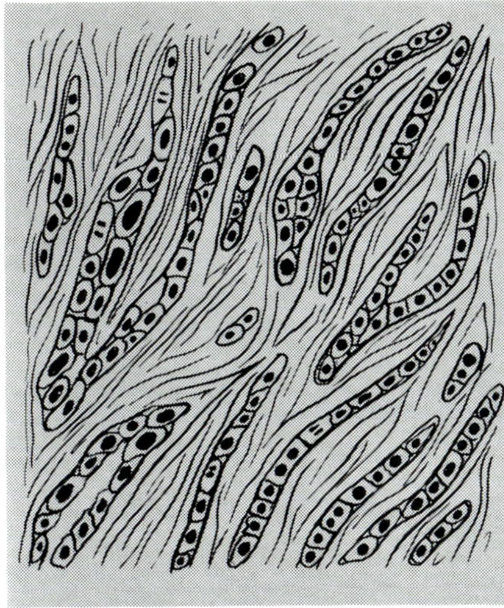

129 Scirrhous carcinoma.

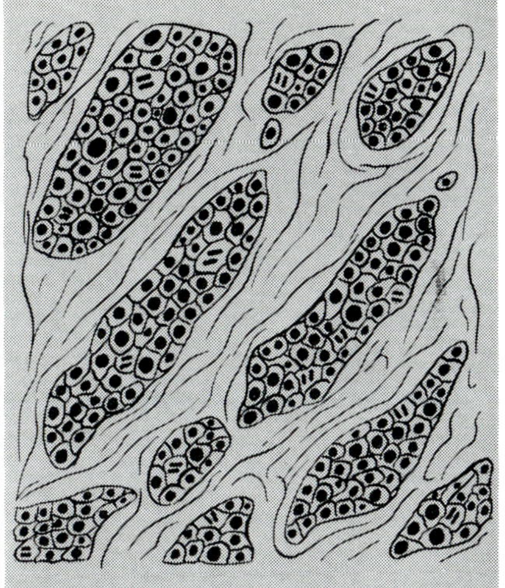

130 Uncomplicated circumscribed carcinoma.

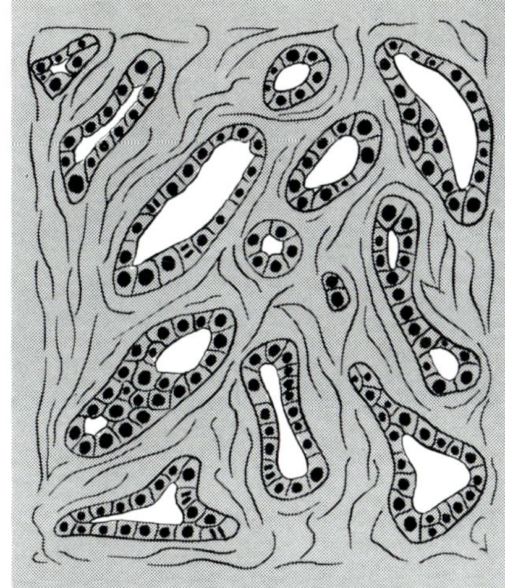

131 Adenocarcinoma.

Differentiation of the above-mentioned tumor types is not possible either macroscopically, clinically, mammographically or cytologically.

Mammographically the contour of these carcinomas is stellate and poorly demarcated. In accordance with cell-stroma relationship, the projections vary in length from short to several centimeters long. They grow in radiating fashion for varying distances into surrounding tissue (Figs **141**, **145**, **146**).

Medullary carcinoma (Fig **132**) grows predominantly by production of cells from the center of the tumor toward the surrounding tissue. The tumor commonly shows histologically and cytologically only a minimal number of atypical cells and nuclei. There is very little stroma. The tumor grows in an expansive as well as infiltrating fashion, so it may be smooth or polycyclic or poorly demarcated.

Macroscopically the carcinoma is so sharply defined that it almost appears to be "encapsulated" even in the advanced stage. Microscopically this encapsulation is a zone of peritumoral fibrosis with infiltration by lymphocytes and plasma cells (Fig **193** c). There may be central necrosis and hemorrhage resulting in rapid enlargement of the tumor. There may be spontaneous hemorrhages into the surrounding breast tissue (Figs **188–190**).

The tumor can be distinguished from its surrounding tissue by palpation and also radiographically. As a rule, the size of the palpable tumor corresponds to the size of the tumor in the mammogram because there is little infiltration into the surrounding tissues. Because of its shape, a medullary carcinoma may be mistaken for a cyst or a fibroadenoma. In breasts rich in stroma it may be overlooked because of its low density, particularly since microcalcifications are usually absent (Fig **198**).

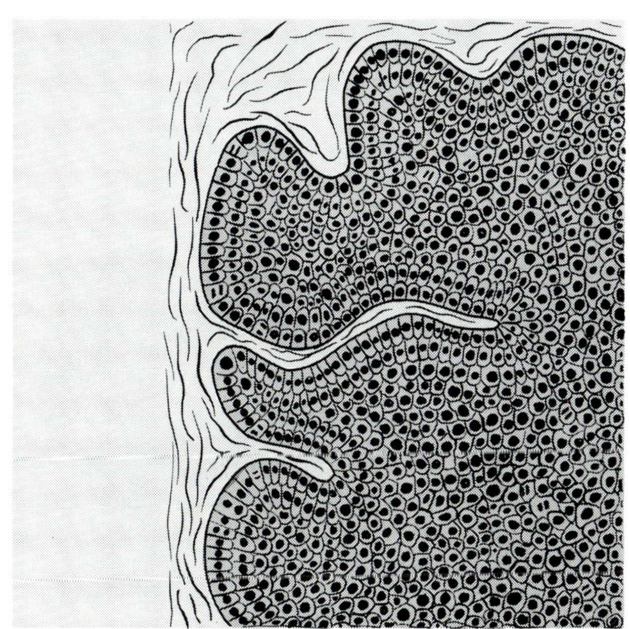

132 Medullary carcinoma.

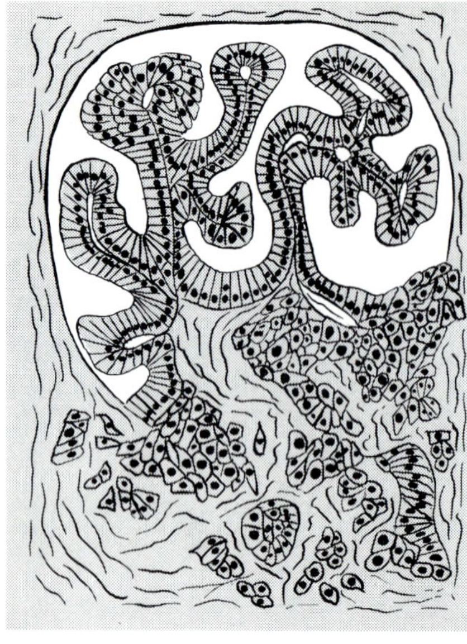

133 Papillary carcinoma.

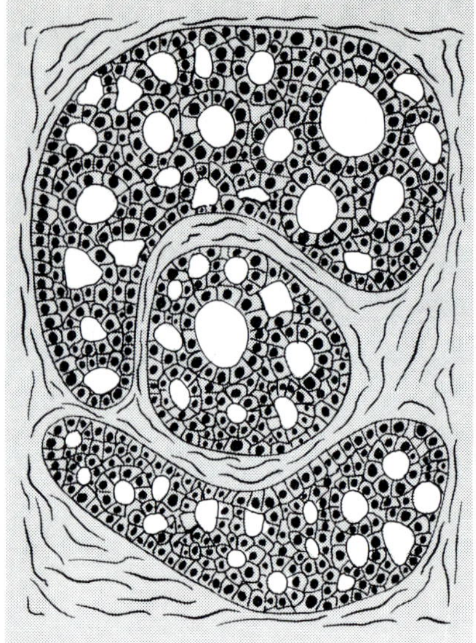

134 Cribriform carcinoma.

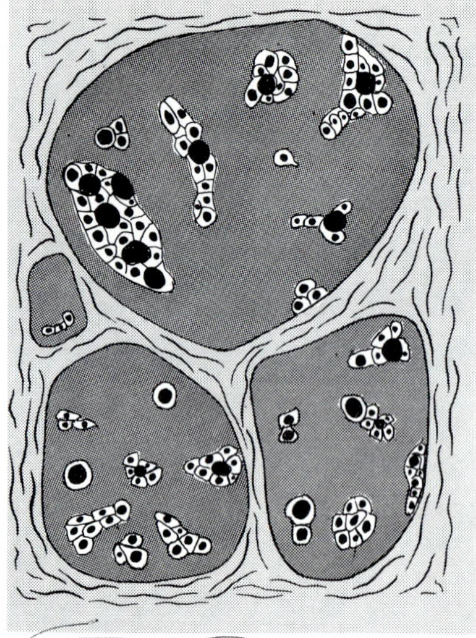

135 Mucinous carcinoma.

Specific histological variants of breast carcinoma

Papillary carcinoma (Fig **133**) may arise in a cyst or a lactiferous duct. It may develop by malignant degeneration of a benign papilloma or may occur as a primary papillary carcinoma. The tumor is nodular and "cauliflower-like" (Fig **202**) and infiltrates the surrounding breast parenchyma from its base.

Lactiferous duct carcinoma (see Fig **138**) is (according to von Albertini 1974) morphologically as well as prognostically in a separate category. It demonstrates primarily diffuse growth without formation of nodules, is limited to the ducts and appears porous and grey-yellow on the cut surface. Running the knife over the cut surface makes a scratchy noise because of the calcified necrosis within the dilated ducts (Fig **212**). The comedos can be squeezed out of the tumor and consist of grayish-yellow, thickened, tenacious, crumbly material. Histologically this type of tumor shows *cell proliferation in the ducts*. Normal duct epithelium is replaced by atypical cells. Loosely arranged, they are polygonal or round. Mitoses are absent most of the time. In the ducts epithelial tumors show progressive cell necrosis appearing macroscopically as comedos.

According to Walther (1948) this type of carcinoma represents 0.3% of all breast carcinomas. According to von Albertini (1974) it has a very good prognosis. Tumor occasionally penetrates ducts and infiltrates parenchyma but does not produce metastases.

Cribriform carcinoma (Fig **134**) originally grows intraductally but later penetrates the ducts and infiltrates surrounding tissue. The infiltrating growth occurs relatively late, however, so such tumors have a very good prognosis. Sieve-like perforation of intraductal epithelial proliferations is characteristic (Fig **144** b). Differentiation from intraductal epithelial proliferations found in mastopathy is difficult and cytologically often impossible (Finsterer and Prechtel 1971, Barth 1972).

The *mucus-producing or mucoid (colloid) carcinoma* (Fig **135**) is rare, occurs in older females and has a good prognosis. The tumor produces a large amount of mucus containing floating epithelial clusters. According to von Albertini (1974) and Barth (1979), it is a specific type of carcinoma characterized histologically as a solid undifferentiated carcinoma with marked epithelial mucoid degeneration. Solid and mucoid carcinomas have similar stroma as shown on microradiographic examination (Fig **201**). Mucus production results in the mucoid portion of the solid carcinoma.

The tumor grows and expands slowly; there is little infiltration, a sharp separation from surrounding tissue. It has a good prognosis and metastasizes late. Radiographic contrast is satisfactory (because of the liquid content of the tumor nodule) but less than that of the stroma of a solid carcinoma or of breast parenchyma (Fig **201**).

Lobular carcinoma (Fig **136**) is characterized by proliferation of epithelium of lobules and terminal ducts. It occurs in 0.6 to 10.2% of all diagnosed carcinomas (according to the author). According to Baessler et al (1971), 3.5% of all carcinomas are of this type. Microscopic findings are characteristic: lobules and terminal ducts filled with plump, loosely arranged epithelial cells (Fig **220**), no polarization, little variation in nuclear size. Mitoses are rare.

In most cases, lobular carcinoma is multifocal, as shown

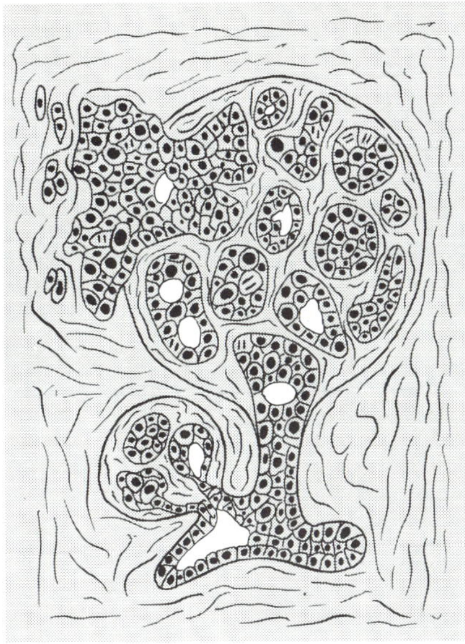
136 Lobular carcinoma.

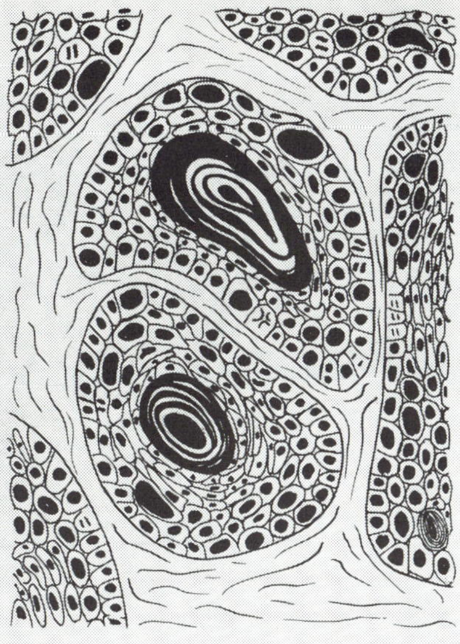
137 Squamous cell carcinoma.

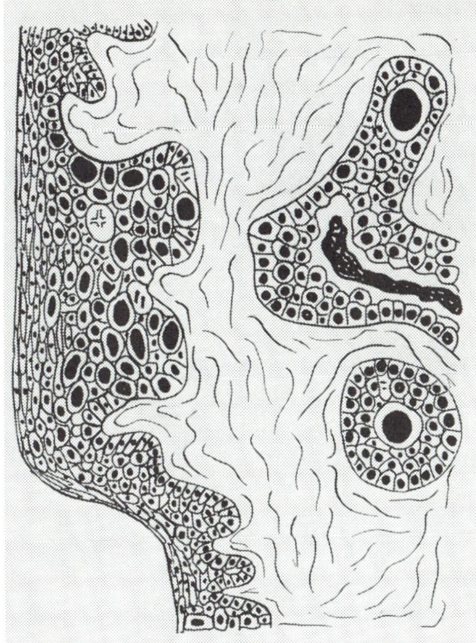
138 Paget's disease of the nipple with duct carcinoma below.

by biopsy examinations of breast specimens. In 70% of those examined, there were many foci. It is assumed that lobular carcinoma occurs bilaterally in more than 20% of the patients (HAAGENSEN 1971, VON ALBERTINI 1974). In 40% the localization in the contralateral breast is a mirror image.

Squamous cell carcinoma (Fig **137**) occurs rarely in the breast. It may develop in skin and nipple and infiltrate the breast. Histologically it shows the typical formation of prickle cells with keratin pearl formation.

Paget's disease is primarily an *intraductal* carcinoma (Fig **138**). It originates in the ducts next to the nipple and from there grows into the nipple. Tumor cells penetrate lower epithelial layers of nipple and areola and typically appear as large, clear, glycogen-rich cells (Fig **225**). The Paget carcinoma grows very slowly, displaces but does not invade surrounding tissue and is nondestructive. It causes eczema-like changes of the nipple (Figs **229–231**). Following penetration of ducts, the tumor grows in invasive fashion into the breast and may appear as a solid or scirrhous carcinoma. It then takes the same unfavorable course as do these tumors (Figs **229–231**). Any eczema of the nipple which does not respond to treatment within two weeks is possibly Paget's disease. In case of weeping eczema, typical clear cells may be seen on a smear of secretion (Fig **226** a). Mammographic changes are found only in later stages (retroareolar tumor, thickening of nipple, sub- or retroareolar microcalcifications and others) (Figs **228**, **232**, **233**).

The above-mentioned histological types of breast carcinoma only rarely show a single pattern. Most of the time the carcinomas demonstrate varying degrees of differentiation. It is therefore practical to classify such tumors histologically by the predominant growth pattern (i.e., partially solid, partially scirrhous carcinomas). Malignant epithelium is not present exclusively in the carcinomatous nodule. In addition to clusters of carcinoma cells, adenoses and epithelioses also can be seen. Thin-needle biopsy of a carcinomatous nodule will therefore not demonstrate carcinoma cells alone, but also normal and proliferating epithelium (Figs **143**, **144**).

Clinical and radiological aspects of breast carcinomas

The histology of a tumor determines its morphology, clinical course, and radiological appearance (GALLAGER and MARTIN 1969, BARTH 1979). Malignancies with few cells grow predominantly in a radiating fashion, multicelled tumors in nodular form. The following clinical and radiological classification is found after exclusion of the specific group of the ductal carcinomas and the characteristic growth pattern of certain tumors (Fig **139**).

a) *Predominantly radiating tumors with spicule-like contour* (see page 102):
   microcalcifications, retraction of surrounding tissue, slow growth, unfavorable prognosis.
b) *Predominantly nodular, smoothly defined tumors* (see page 126):
   minimal or no microcalcifications, spontaneous hematoma, no retraction of surrounding tissue, rapid growth, more favorable prognosis.

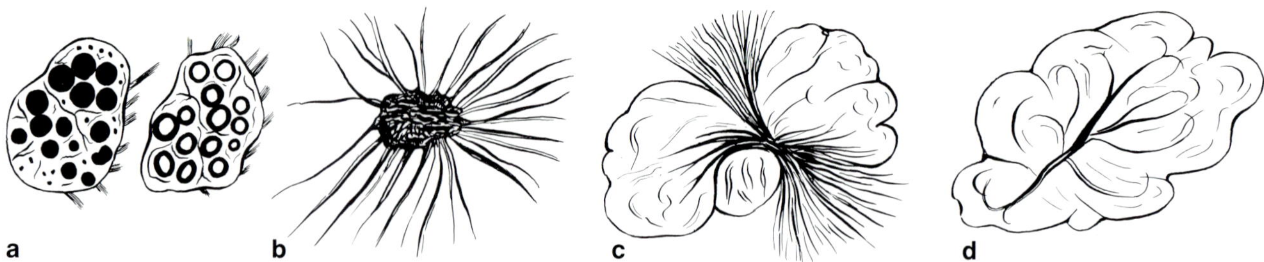

139 a–d. The radiological anatomy of breast carcinoma in correlation with the histological type of tumor.
a) Ductal carcinoma with and without comedo-calcification.
b) Stellate growth (scirrhus, adenocarcinoma, solid carcinoma).
c) Stellate and nodular growth (solid carcinoma, mixed types).
d) Nodular and polycyclic growth (medullary carcinoma, mucinous carcinoma, cellular metastases, sarcoma).

c) *Predominantly ductal growth* (see page 144): with calcifications or without, nipple retraction, favorable prognosis.
d) *Specific growth pattern* (see page 151): Paget's disease and others.

Predominantly stellate growth

Scirrhous, solid and adenocarcinoma show predominantly stellate growth; radiograph reflects the morphological findings. Tumor extensions of varying size infiltrate the surrounding tissue. Depending on the degree of fibrosis and the number of elastic fibers, there is varying traction by the tumor on the surrounding structure. At first the parenchyma of the breast is retracted resulting in a disrupted architecture. A broad, relatively radiolucent halo surrounds the tumor radiographically. More forceful traction leads to retraction of skin and nipple. In more advanced stages, increasing infiltration makes the breast smaller. Without treatment it may shrink markedly over a period of months or years (Figs **236**, **290**). Of all stellate carcinomas 90% have groups of microcalcifications which tend to be more numerous in slow growing tumors and tumors rich in connective tissue. The calcifications do not follow the course of the ducts and occur very commonly in the tumor periphery (Fig **140**).
The tumor epithelium occurs predominantly at the periphery of the carcinoma and in extensions from its borders. The tumor appears smaller radiographically than by palpation since the radiograph essentially shows only the stromal portion of the tumor (Fig **145**).
In addition, palpation depends upon the degree of concomitant epitheliosis in ducts and lobules surrounding the carcinoma (Fig **154**). Invasion of the tumor into lymph channels may block the flow of lymph and cause first localized and subsequently diffuse lymphedema. In the mammogram the broadened lymph channels appear as net-like increased reticular structures in the breast and subcutaneous tissues. Clinically there is swelling of breast and skin and resultant deep retraction of pores (so-called orange-peel effect). The nipple appears retracted because of the thickened skin of the areola.
The *clinical signs* of stellate tumors (particularly by palpation) depend on content of cells and stroma in the tumor. With *minimal fibrosis* palpation reveals an irregularly bulging nodule retracting the skin or causing formation of a flat plateau. With *marked fibrosis* the tumor is very firm and relatively immobile. Skin and nipple show early retraction. The tumor appears larger on palpation than on the radiograph (Figs **145**, **146**, **150**, **155**).

The radiographic findings in stellate carcinomas may be grouped as follows:

a) Nonhomogeneous tumor opacity.
b) Ill-defined, radiating contour with delicate short and long projections into surrounding breast.
c) Band-like, increased density of tissue between tumor and nipple, thickened and retracted nipple, infiltrated subcutaneous fat, plateau formation of skin in neighborhood of carcinoma (so-called thumb tack phenomenon), shrinking of breast.
d) Microcalcifications and/or coarse irregularly arranged calcium particles.
e) Discrepancy between palpation and radiograph; essentially only the stroma component of the tumor is shown in mammogram.

With *diffusely growing* scirrhous carcinomas, breast structures do not necessarily exhibit radiographic changes. There is no tumor-specific opacity. In general the breast appears smaller and denser (Figs **251** b, **252** c). Usually the cell material obtained with *thin-needle biopsy* of a stellate carcinoma is sufficient for diagnosis even in cell-poor, scirrhous carcinoma. If the tumor is not palpable, it may be possible in breasts with a large amount of fat to "palpate" it with a longer aspiration needle.

Vascularization varies depending on metabolism of the tumor and may result in an altered *thermographic picture*. While the cellular, stellate carcinoma may be well vascularized and show a 0.5 to 1 °C rise in temperature above that of normal parenchyma, the cell-poor, scirrhous tumor usually shows a normal thermogram even in advanced stages and, on occasion, even shows a so-called "cold spot" secondary to disruption of vascular supply by the tumor. In one observation, however, thermography was the only examination pointing to diffusely growing scirrhous carcinoma (Fig **248**).

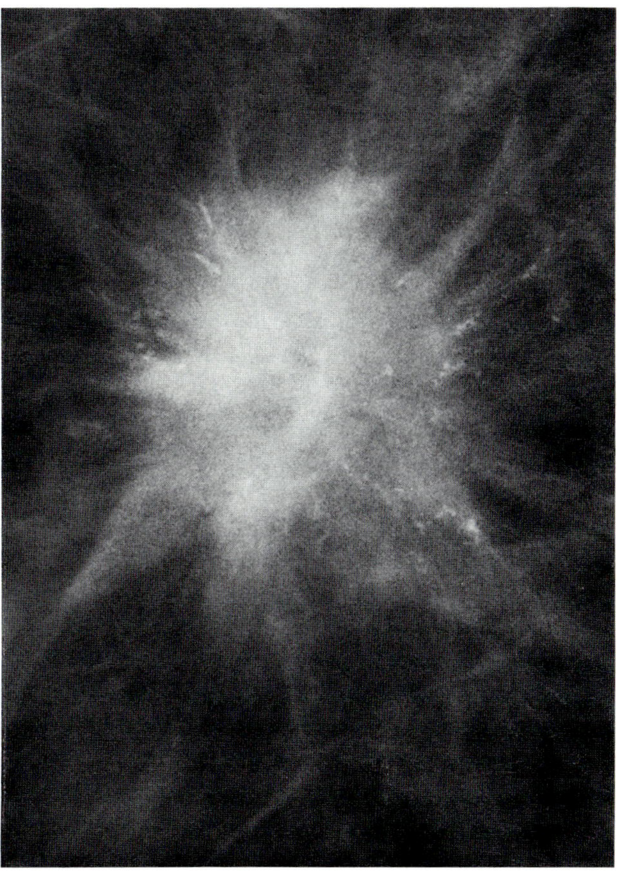

140 Star-shaped radiating carcinoma (histologically: adenoscirrhus). Multiple microcalcifications in tumor periphery and projections.

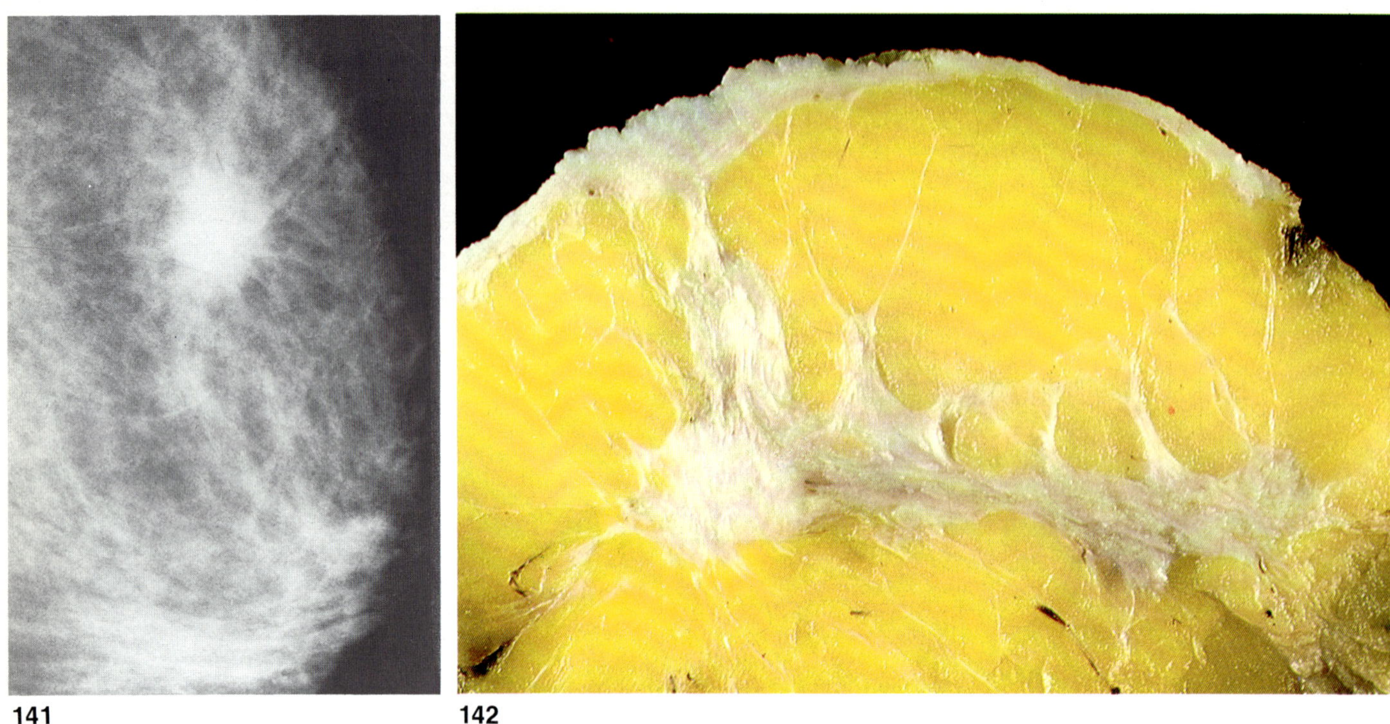

141 142

63-year-old female, left breast. Malignant tumor palpable in outer upper quadrant. Slight nipple retraction (Figs 141–144).

141 *Mammogram* (medio-lateral). Carcinoma growing in stellate fashion. Short radiating projections from the tumor. A few microcalcifications. In remaining parenchyma, band-like, duct-like opacities arranged predominantly behind the nipple.

142 *Macroanatomy.* White-gray ill-defined tumor nodule. Tissue bridges of varying widths between tumor and nipple with nipple thickening and retraction. Breast parenchyma (right of tumor) light brown with projections into fatty tissue (yellow).

143 a, b. *Radiological-histological comparison.* ▷

a) Specimen radiograph. Tumor in left portion of breast. Radiating contour with short and long projections into surrounding fat. Nonhomogeneous, dense tumor center. Right below the nodule a group of microcalcifications. Nipple is thickened and slightly retracted. Behind the nipple ground glass-like nonhomogeneous opacities. Breast parenchyma right of tumor shows band-like and small nonhomogeneous opacities with radiating contours. Increased radio-opacity at right edge of breast. Fat traversed by vessels.

b) *Histological macrosection.* Carcinoma nodule on left with nonhomogeneous center. Short tumor extensions of varying widths. Infiltrated by a small amount of fat. (Fig 144b shows greater enlargement of tumor.) Further enlargement shows thickened and retracted nipple and retroareolar space diffusely infiltrated by scirrhous tumor. Greater enlargement shows ducts cut longitudinally in breast parenchyma with marked periductal fibrosis. Enlarged lobules with marked proliferation of acini consistent with adenosis lie between. At the right side of the breast, there is fibrosis with adenosis and scattered atypical intraductal epithelial proliferations. In the fatty tissue delicate septa of stromal tissue with vessels.

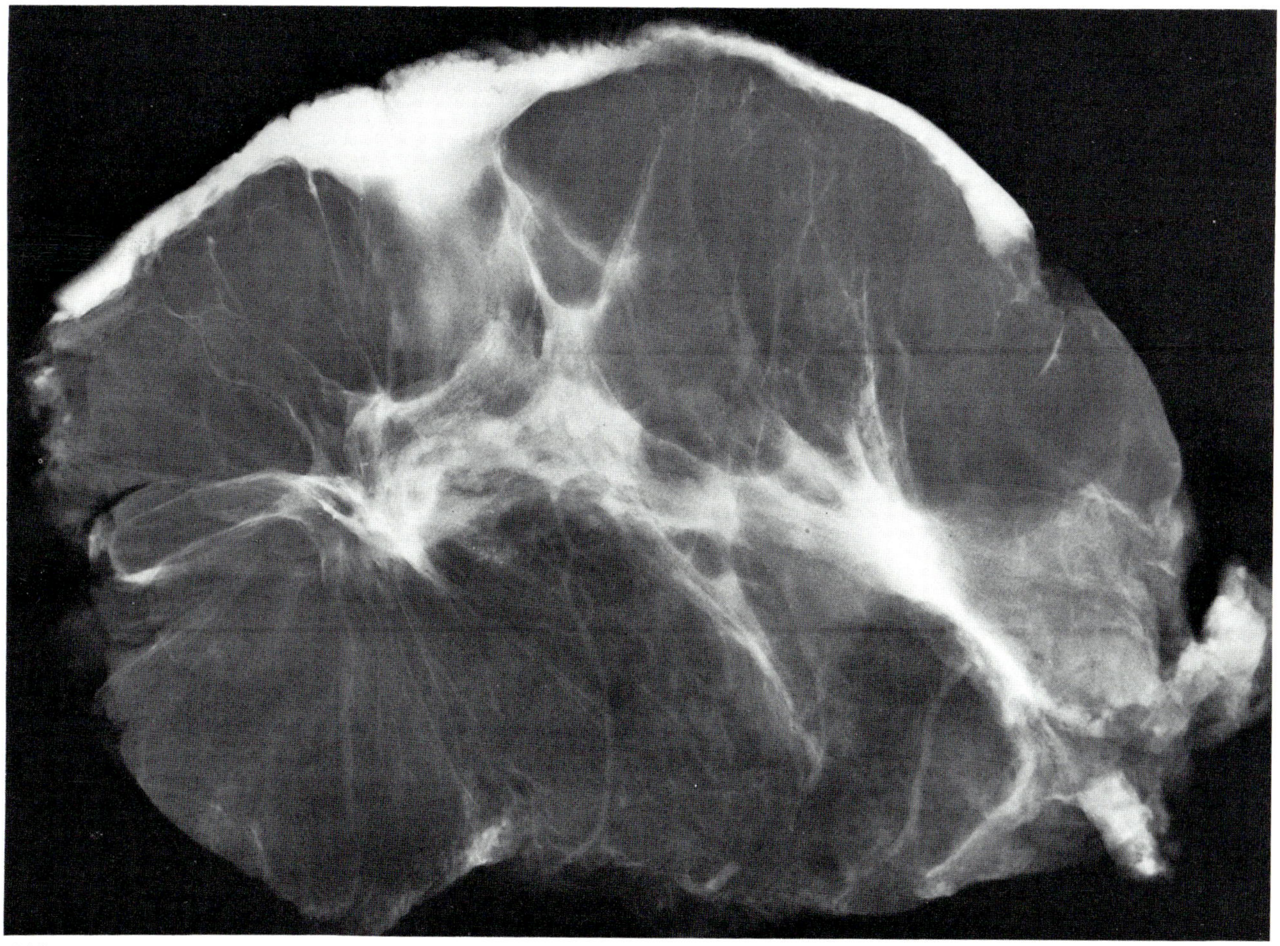

143 a

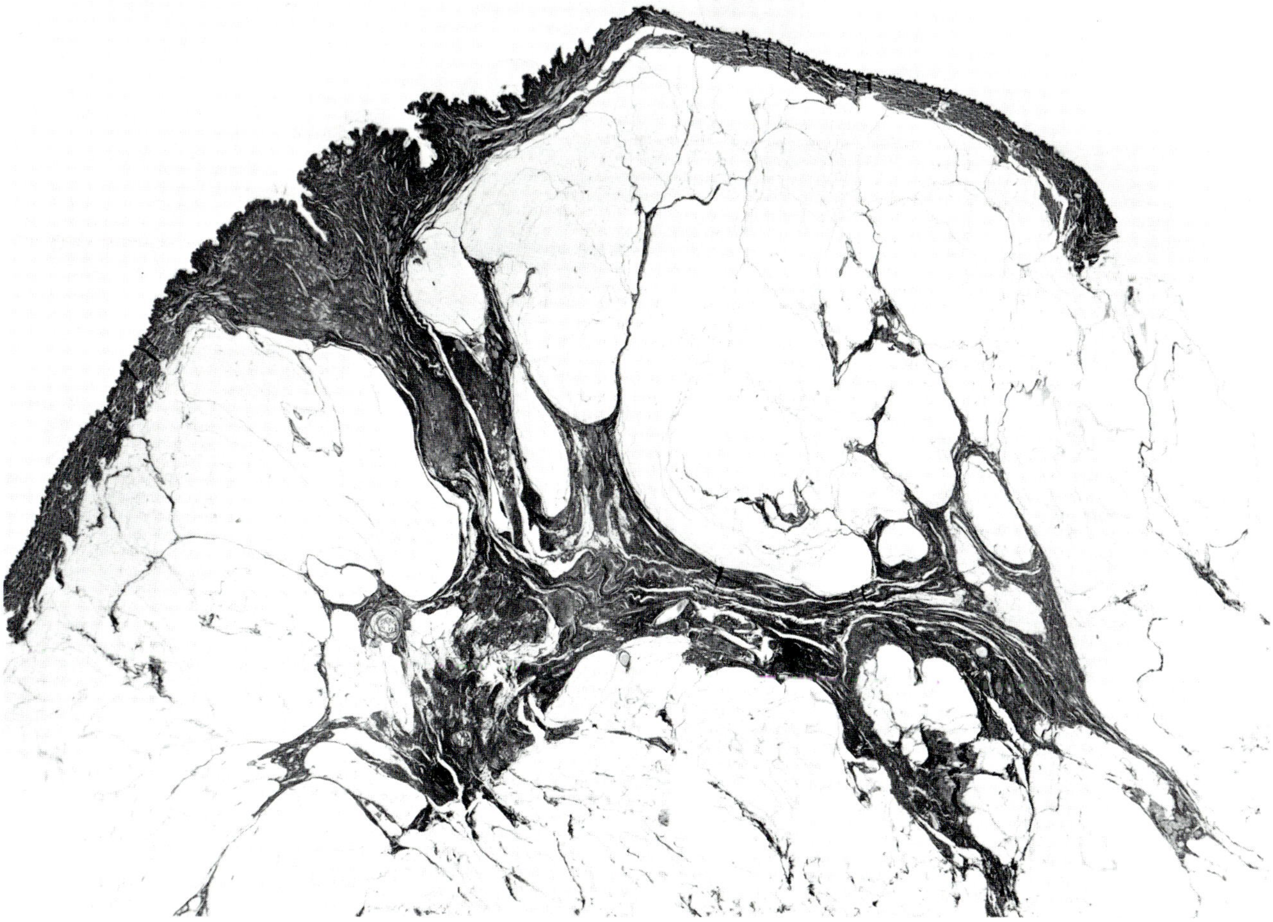

143 b

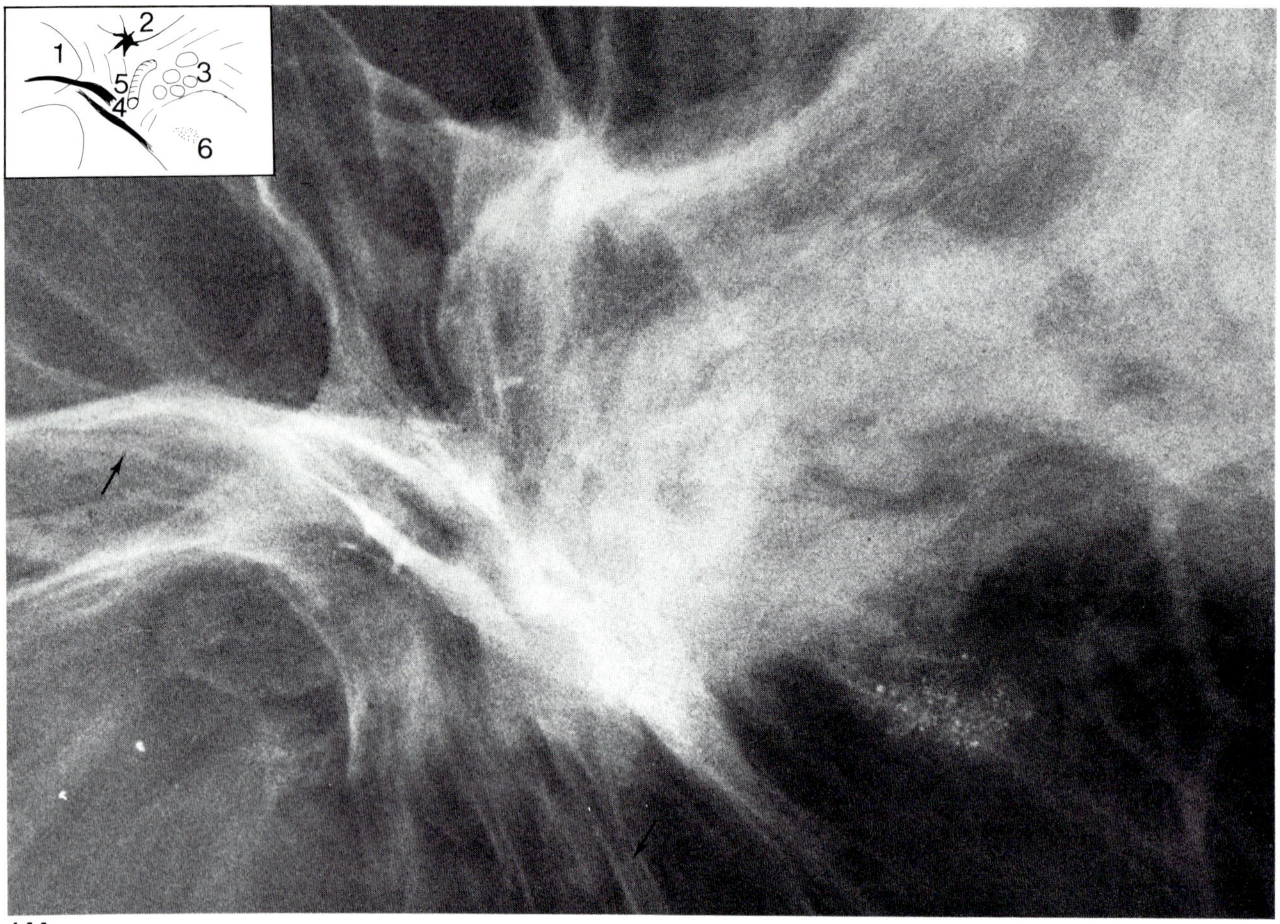

144 a

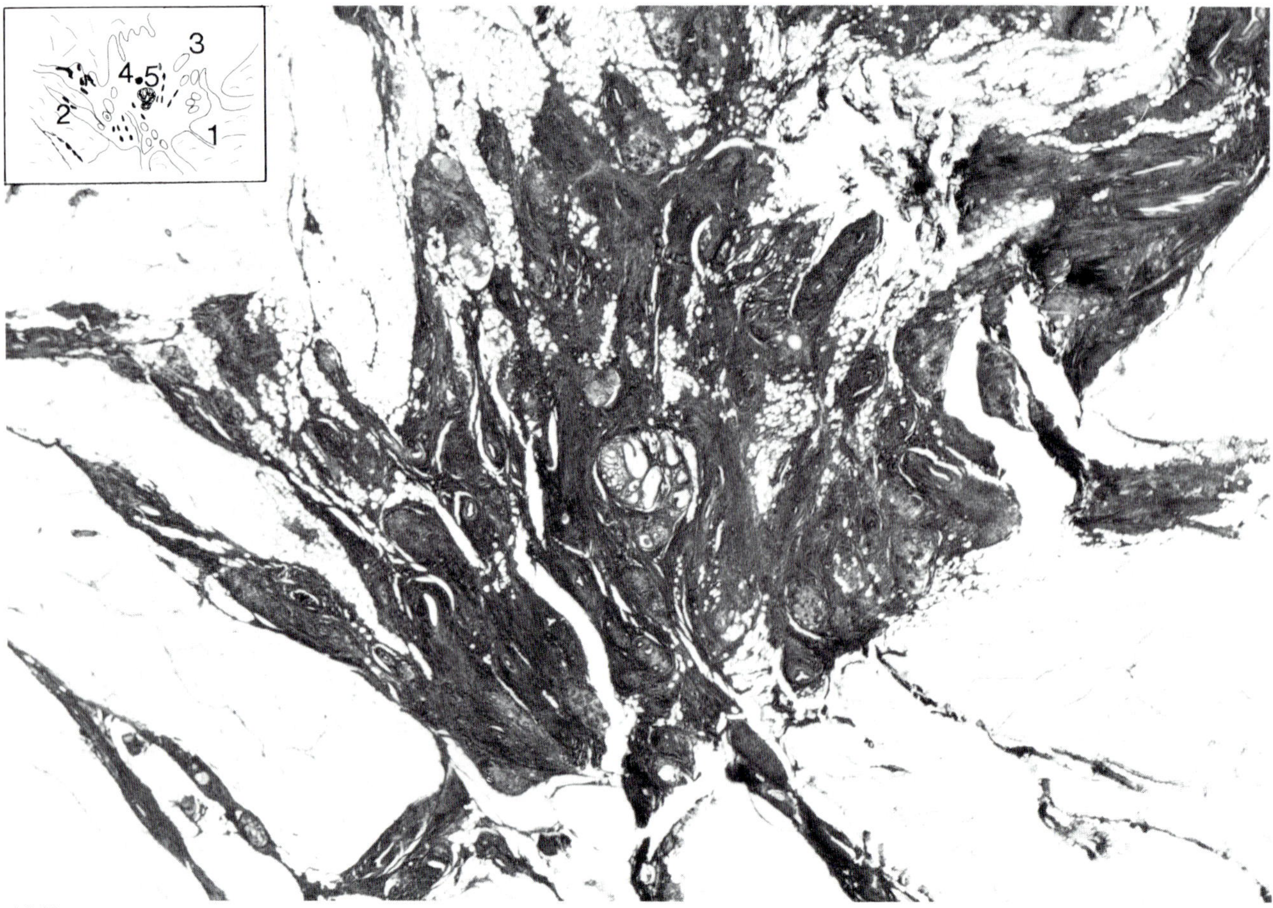

144 b

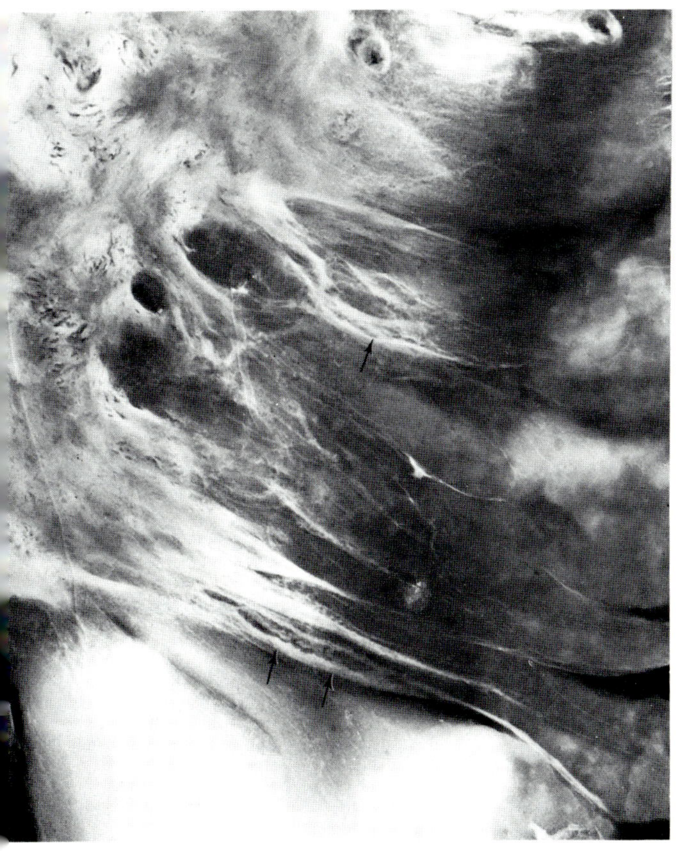

5a

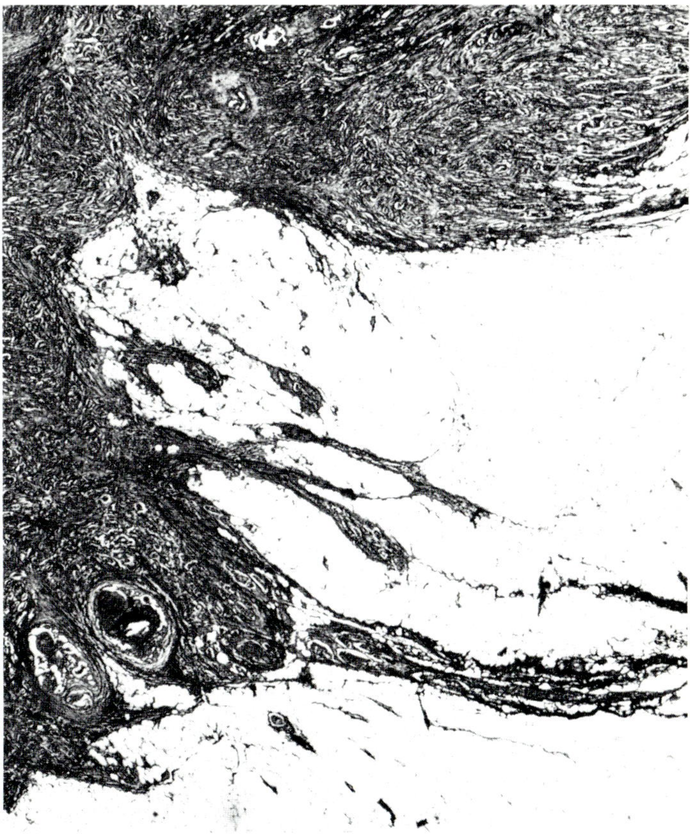

145b

145 a, b. Radiating contour of a scirrhous carcinoma.
a) *Microradiograph,* magnif 120×. Delicate tumor projections; the tumor cells are less radiopaque and can be delineated from the stroma (arrow). So the tumor appears smaller radiographically than on palpation. Fat immediately surrounding the tumor is more radiolucent than fat farther away (retractive effect of the tumor?). Oblique to the tumor projection is a small vessel shown with a double contour.

b) *Histology,* magnif 120×. Scirrhous carcinoma. Septa of stromal tissue with clusters of tumor epithelium in carcinoma projections.

◁ **144** a, b. *Radiological-histological comparison,* magnif 120× (same case as in Fig 143).
a) Specimen radiograph. In a specimen 0.5 cm in thickness, there are 500 morphological structural changes in comparison with a histological section 10 μm in thickness (as shown in b). The tumor projections are seen in radiograph as radiating densities and extend for great distance into surrounding fatty tissue. Filling defects are recognizable at the sites of epithelial layers (arrow). Right next to the tumor a group of microcalcifications appear (6), but there is no morphological correlation in the histological section (b). In the center of the nodule there are two tissue areas of different densities. In addition to radiopaque scirrhous carcinoma (2) there is an opacity of lesser density; in the latter there are oval shadows (mastion) (3) and adenoses. The duct noted on histologic section (b) is identifiable over a longer section as a band-like opacity (5) in the tumor center.

b) Histology. Tumor surrounded by fat (1) which also lies between the plump short tumor projections. In these projections are clusters of scirrhous carcinoma (2), enlarged acini with marked acini proliferation (adenoses) (3). The tumor contains a large amount of connective tissue; within the connective tissue there are sections of scirrhous carcinoma (2), adenosis (3), and epitheliosis (4). In the center of the nodule are dilated ducts with sieve-like proliferations of atypical epithelium (5). This section of 10 μm thickness represents one of 1000 morphological variants of a 1 cm cancer nodule. The tumor consists of fat and connective tissue, benign (adenosis) changes, semimalignant (atypical epithelial proliferations in ducts and ductule) and malignant changes (scirrhus). This explains why in aspirates of stellate malignancies normal proliferating epithelium may be found in addition to clusters of tumor cells.

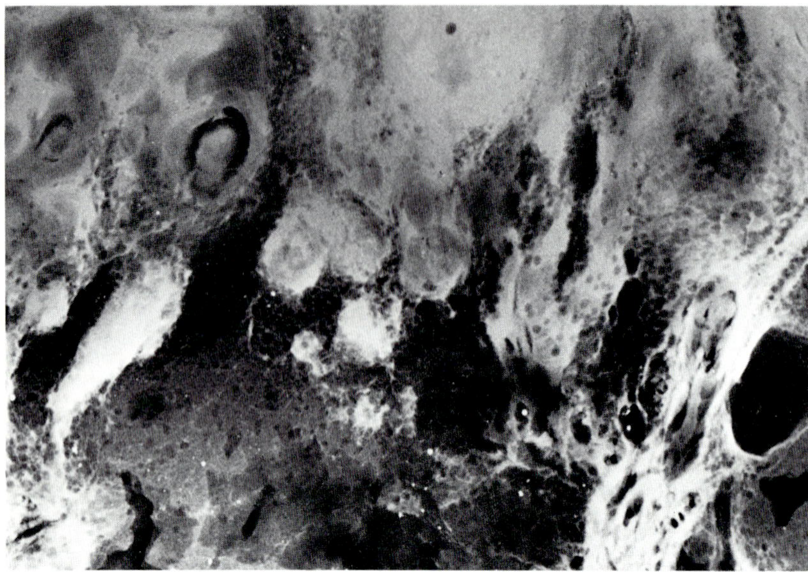

146a

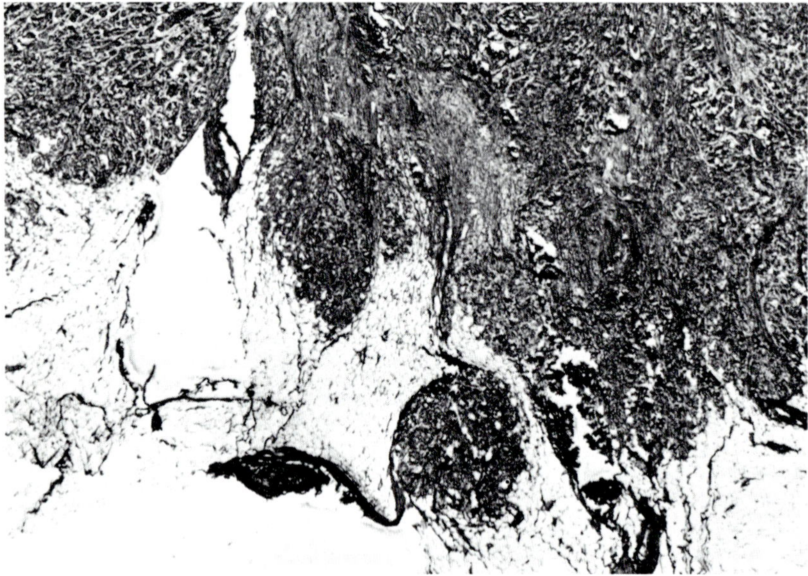

146b

146 a, b. Irregular contour of a cellular solid carcinoma.

a) *Microradiography.* Round and oval opacities at the edge of the tumor (light). Infiltration of fatty tissue (dark). Stroma with little septa (right below). In mammogram this type of spread shows smooth tumor contour (summation effect). Little discrepancy between radiograph and palpation.

b) *Histology.* At edge of solid carcinoma broad and plump cell layers of tumor epithelium infiltrating fatty tissue. Little variation in width of septa.

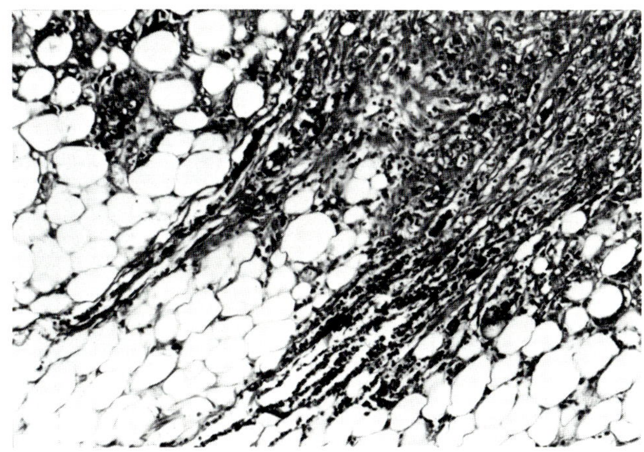

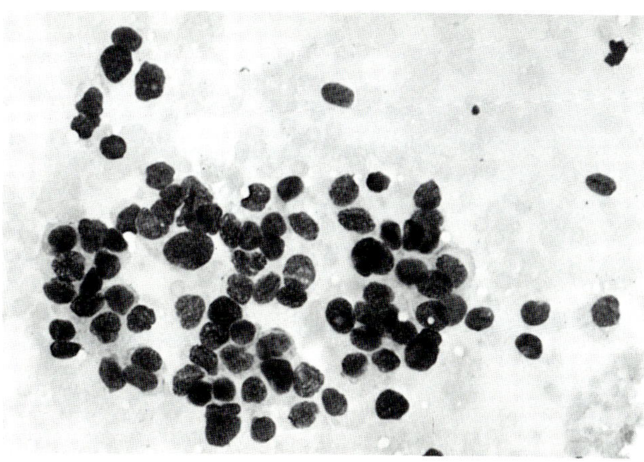

147 a, b. Scirrhous carcinoma.
a) *Histology,* magnif 80×. Atypical single rows of epithelial strands between abundant stroma; tumor extensions infiltrate bordering fat (unsharp contour).

b) *Cytology,* magnif 105×. Clusters of tumor cells with moderately polymorphous, loosely arranged cells with naked nuclei (absent coherence).

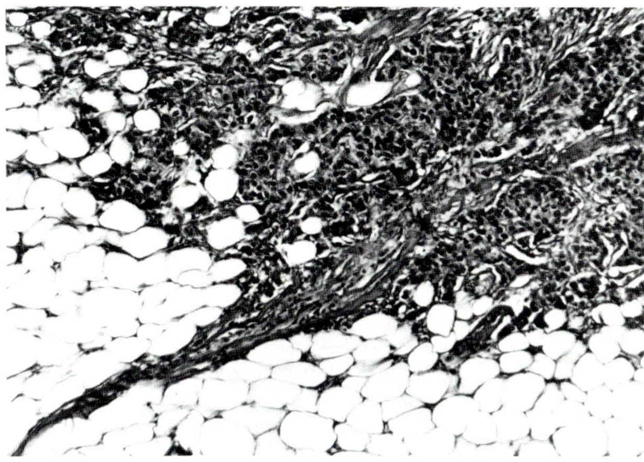

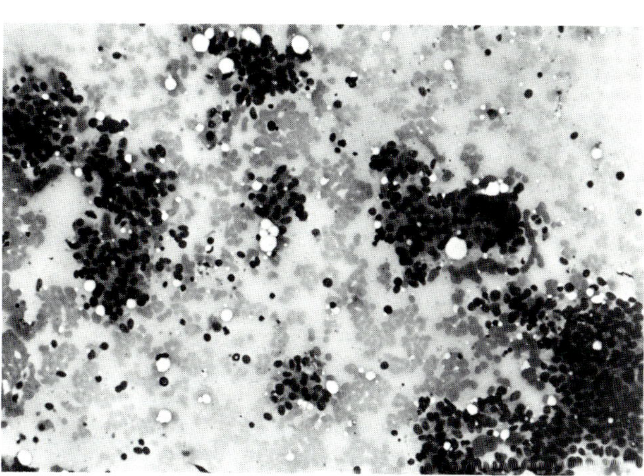

148 a, b. Solid carcinoma.
a) *Histology,* magnif 80×. Four to six rows of tumor cells between broad strands of stroma; infiltration of fatty tissue.

b) *Cytology,* magnif 80×. Clusters of tumor cells with plump nuclei and a small rim of cytoplasm. Little polymorphism of nuclei.

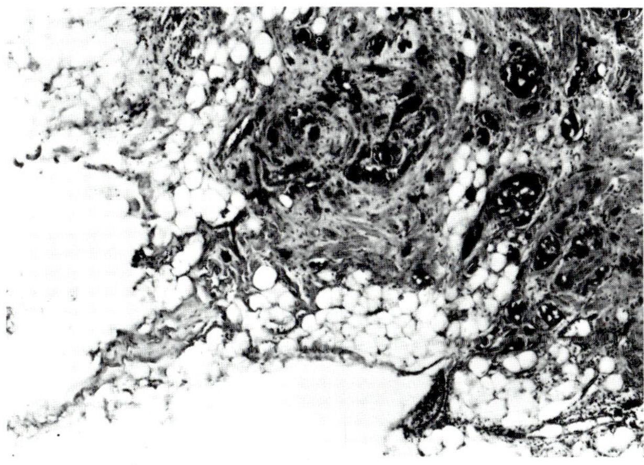

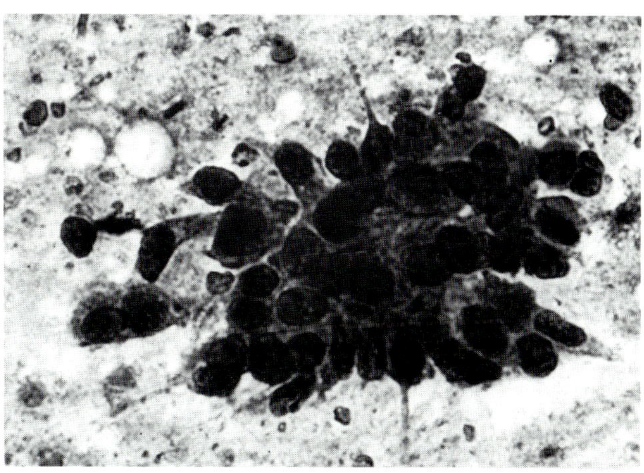

149 a, b. Adenocarcinoma.
a) *Histology,* magnif 80×. Atypical epithelium (suggestion of tubular arrangement), plenty of stroma (adeno-scirrhus). Infiltration of fatty tissue.

b) *Cytology,* magnif 140×. Tumor cells in gland formations with plump, moderately polymorphous, hyperchromatic nuclei. Shift of nucleus-plasma ratio in favor of nuclei.

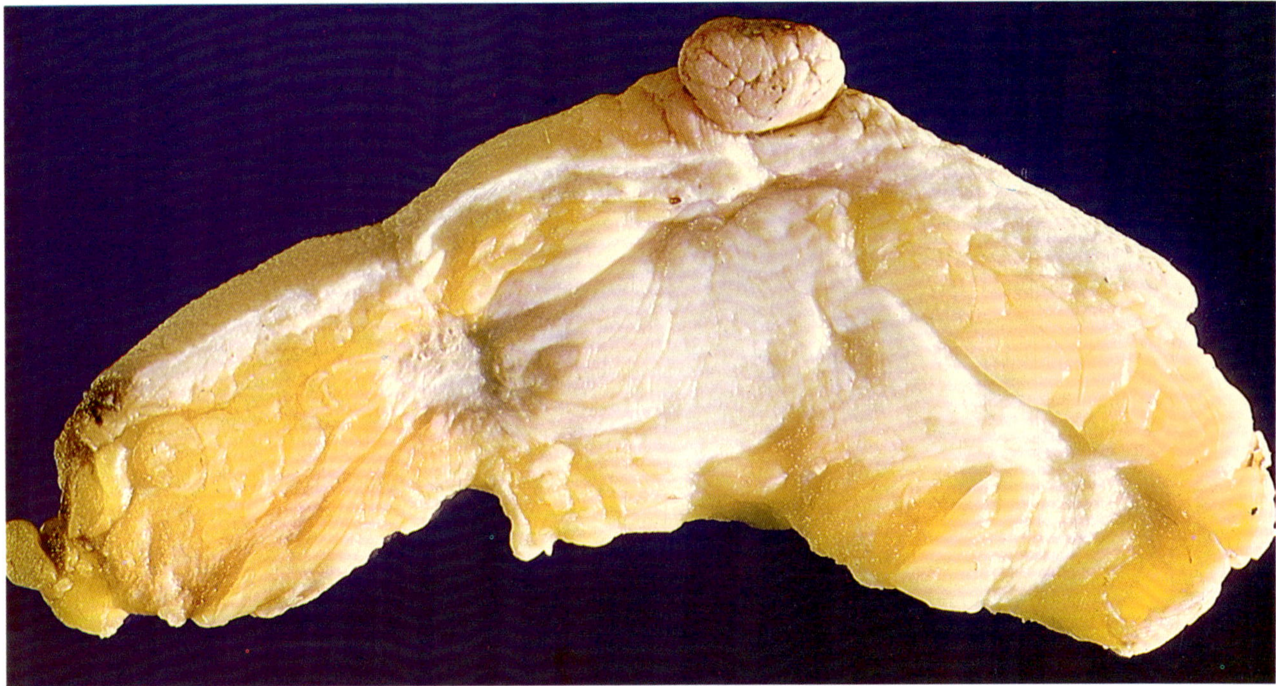

△

150 *Cut section of anatomic specimen.* Tumor of 1 cm size (scirrhus) at lateral edge of breast. Skin retraction. Surface of tumor sunken because of shrinking of malignancy. Plenty of perilobular connective tissue in remaining breast.

151 *Microradiograph,* magnif 40×. Nonhomogeneous tumor opacity. Increased density of tumor stroma. Tumor component less radiopaque than stroma (comma-shaped radiolucencies in tumor: artifacts secondary to shrinkage of tumor cells during fixation). Tumor cells are considerably less radiopaque than stroma in tumor projections (tumor larger on palpation than on the radiograph). Retraction and infiltration of skin (upper edge of illustration).

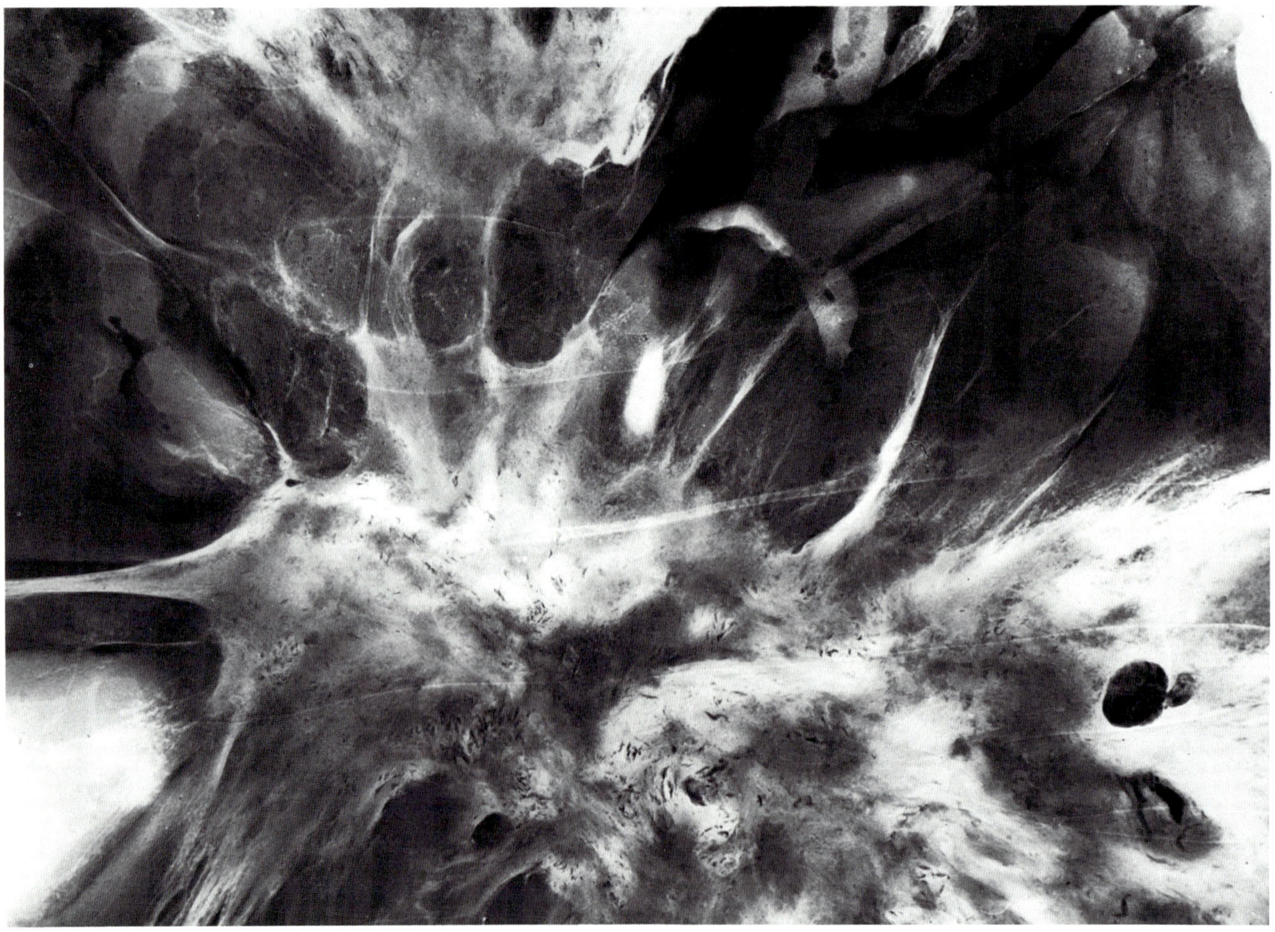

151

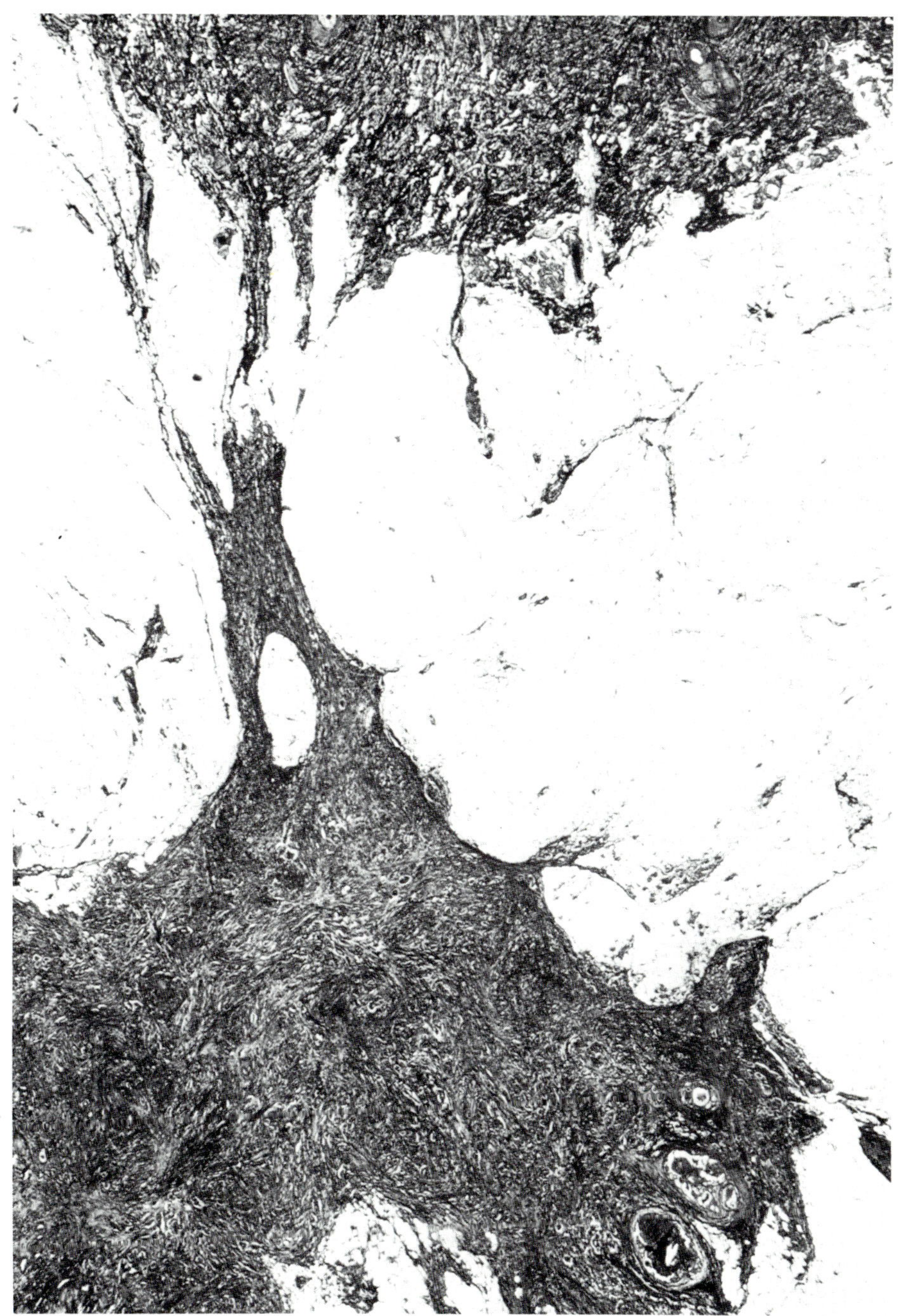

152 *Histology* of section shown in Fig 151. Scirrhous carcinoma with tumor extensions to infiltrated nipple.

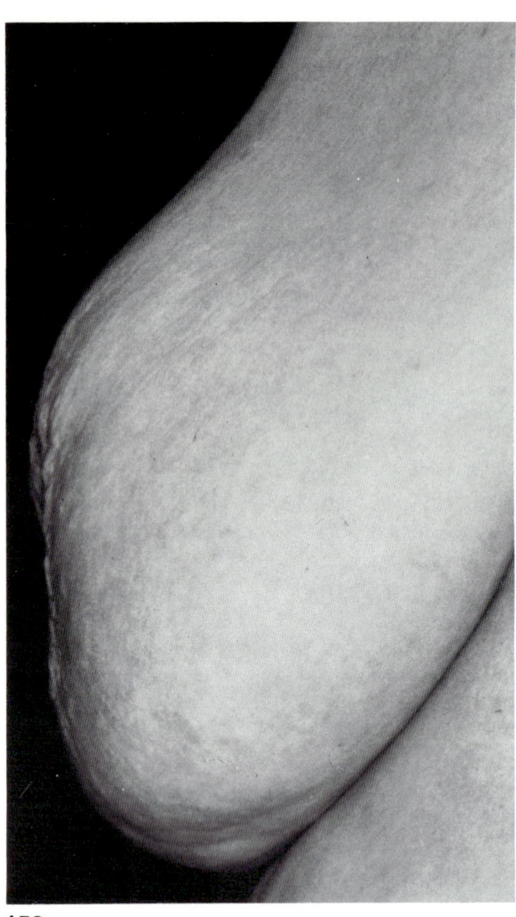

153

153 59-year-old female. For 4 weeks tangerine-sized node in right-upper-outer quadrant near chest wall following weight reduction. Flattening of nipple.

154 a, b. Infiltrating lactiferous ducts.
a) *Mammogram* (medio-lateral). Double carcinoma. Smooth, lobulated nodule near chest wall. No microcalcifications. Radiating second tumor near the nipple with microcalcifications.
b) *Galactography* (medio-lateral). Filling of lactiferous duct up to 3 cm prior to the stellate tumor. At this point disruption of column of contrast medium and obstruction of duct by tumor tissue (upper arrows). In one duct in the outer inferior quadrant, further proliferations of epithelial tissue have led to multiple defects in the contrast image (lower arrows). This shows the multilocular character of the tumor. Extensive extravasation of contrast medium in surrounding fat (right below).

155 *Macroanatomy.* ▷

156 *Specimen radiography.* Nodule left, little stroma, cellular, lobulated contour. No microcalcifications. No retraction of the surrounding tissue. Nodule right, rich in stroma, poor in cells, radiating. Bleeding foci following thin-needle biopsy. Microcalcifications (only suggested in the mammogram).

157 a, b. *Histology,* magnif 260×.
a) Nodular tumor left. Cellular, solid carcinoma. Little stroma.
b) Radiating nodule right. Relatively acellular, solid, partially scirrhous, growing carcinoma.

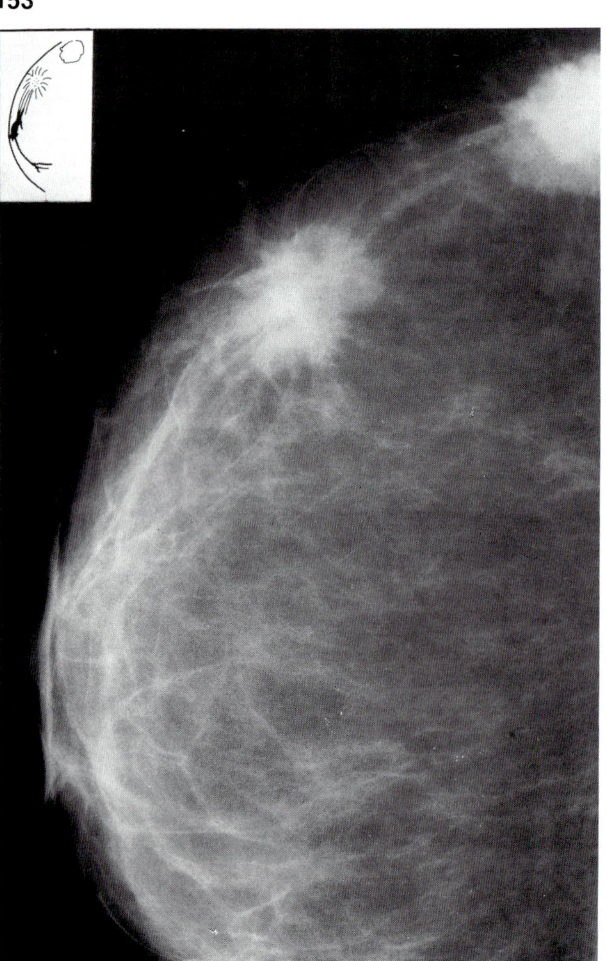

154 a

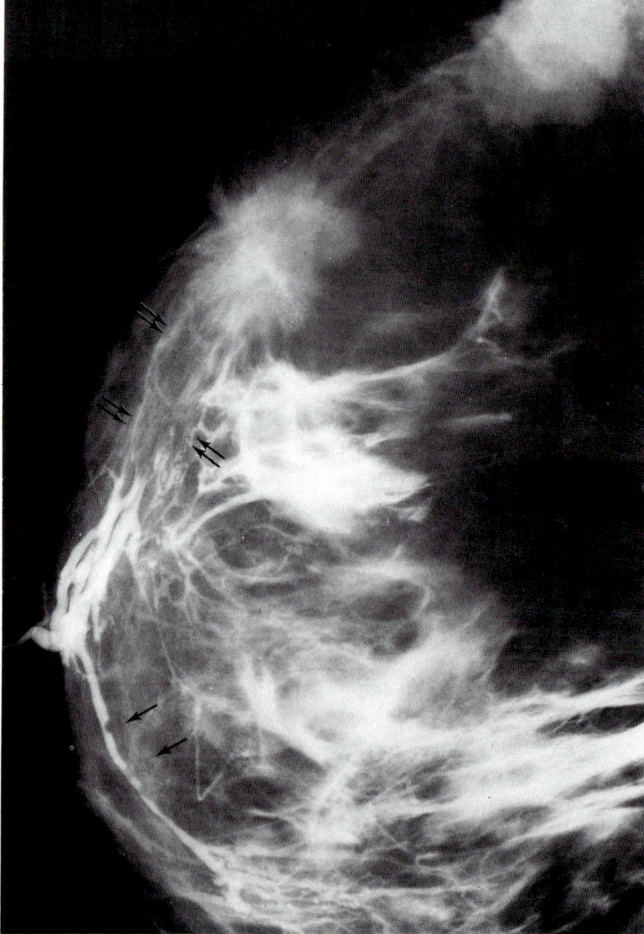

154 b

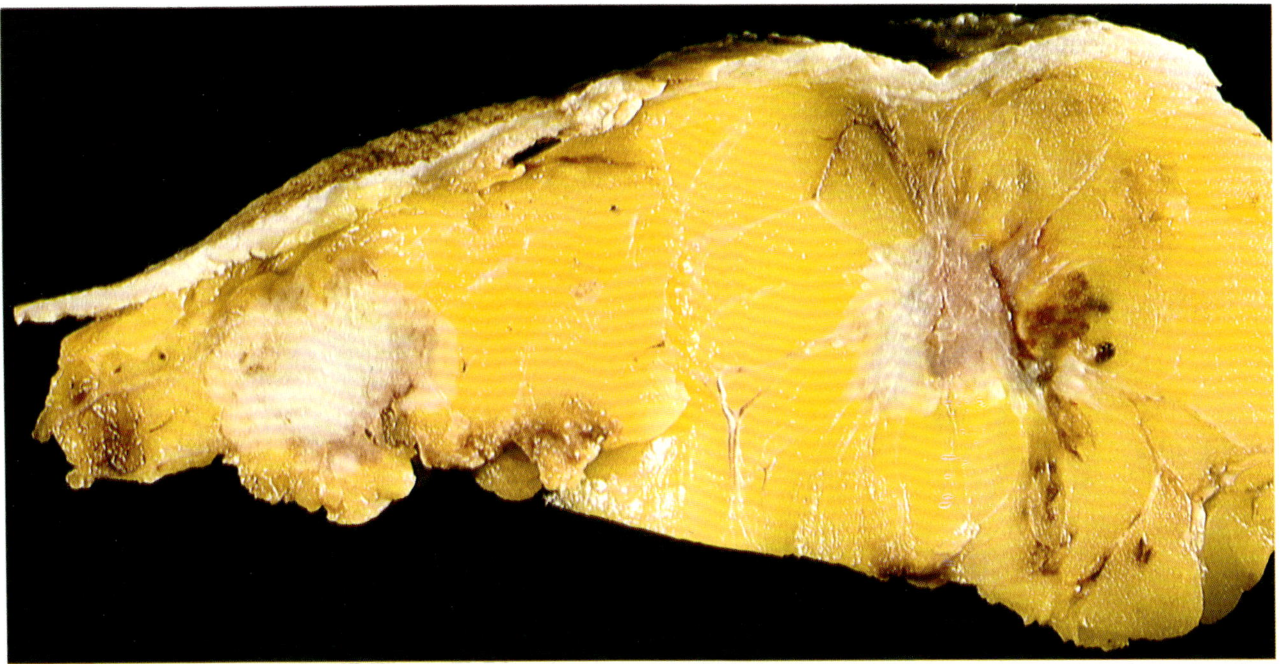

155

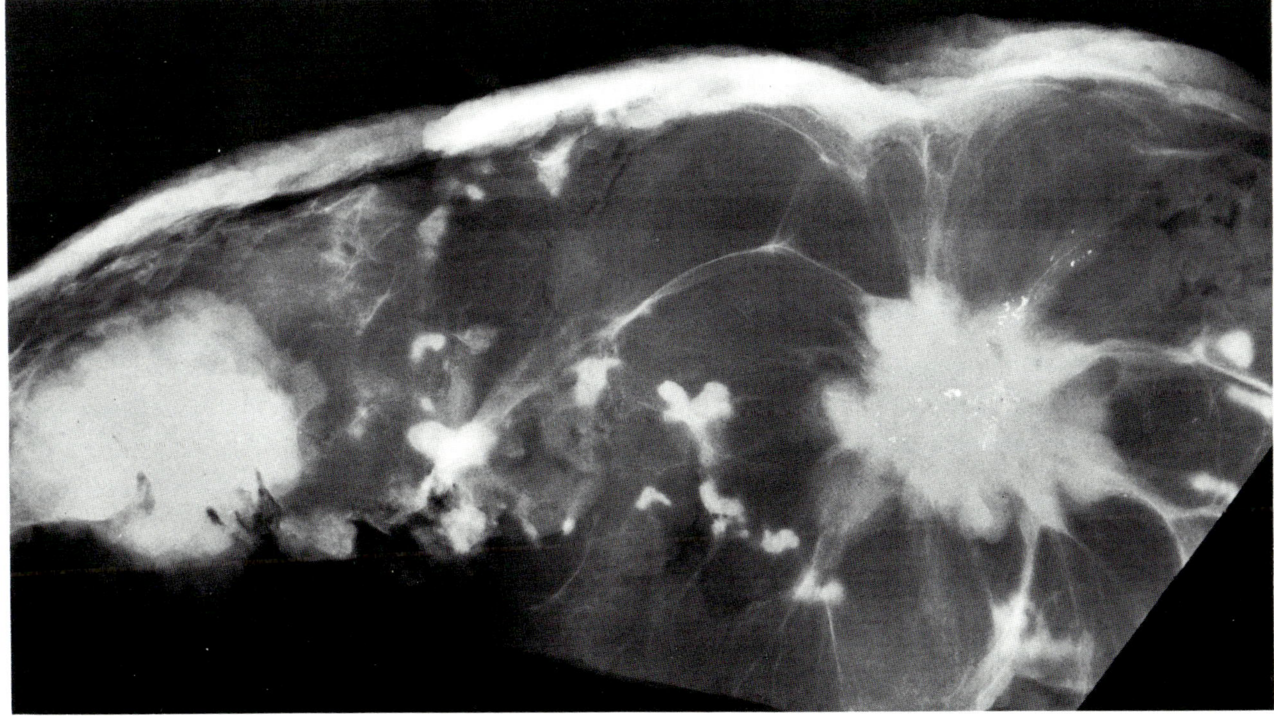

156

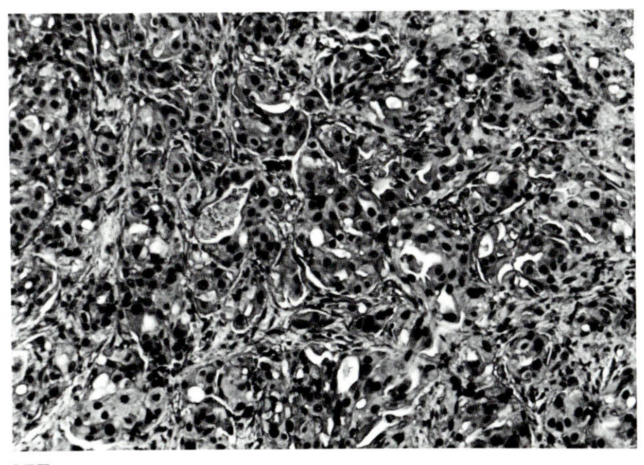

157 a

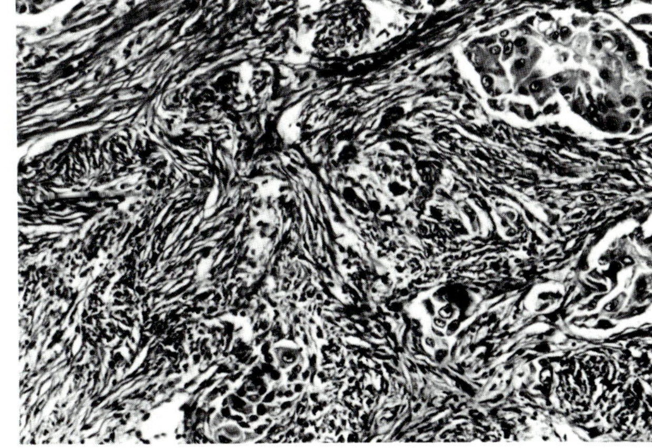

157 b

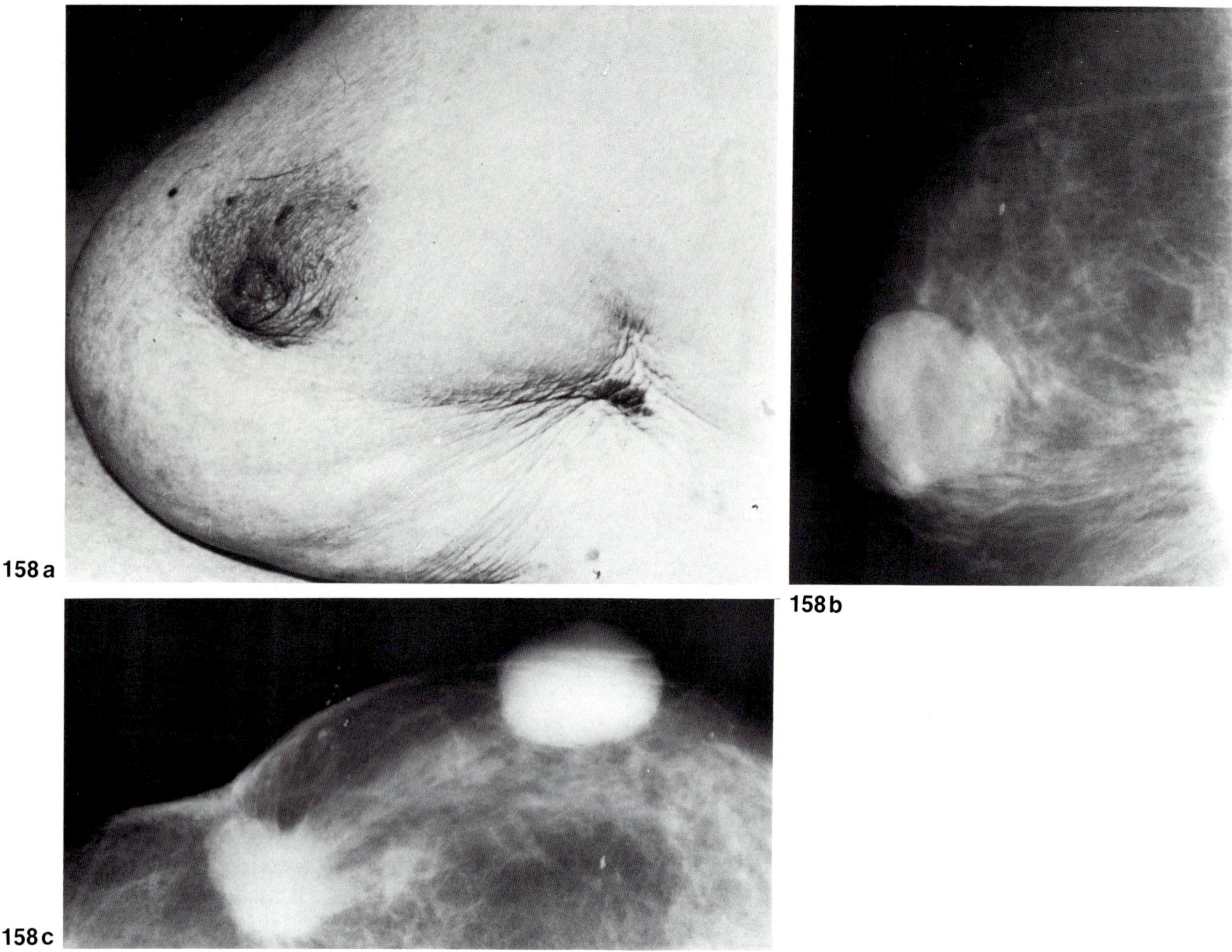

62-year-old female, left breast. For 30 years firm cherry-sized retroareolar nodule. For 2 years nodule in outer upper quadrant with retraction of skin (Figs 158–161).

158 a–c. *Inspection and mammography.*
a) Protrusion and increased pigmentation of skin over nipple with easily movable firm subcutaneous nodule. Lateral retraction of skin. Pigment spots.
b) Mammogram. (Medio-lateral).
c) Cranio-caudal.
Near axilla stellate carcinomatous nodule with retraction of skin. Homogeneous, round, smoothly defined retroareolar opacity (thin-needle biopsy: 6 ml of bloody aspirate).

159 *Macroanatomy.* On left edge of figure stellate carcinoma with retraction of skin and extensions to cyst wall. At the bottom of the cyst is a nodular, papillary tumor with punctate bleeding points. Remaining cyst wall smooth. ▷

160 *Specimen radiograph.* Cyst cavity filled with air. At the bottom is a stellate tumor. Left is an infiltrating carcinoma, vessel below (arrow). ▷

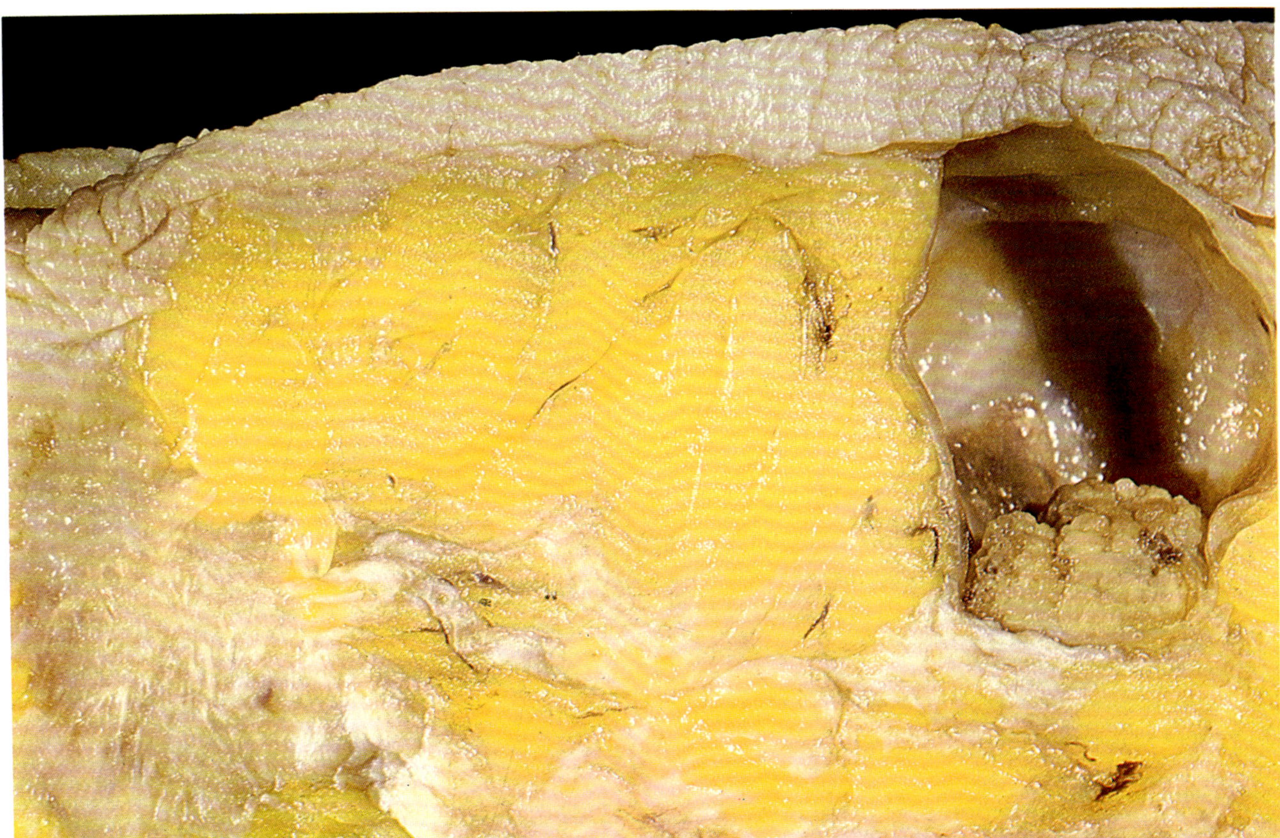

159

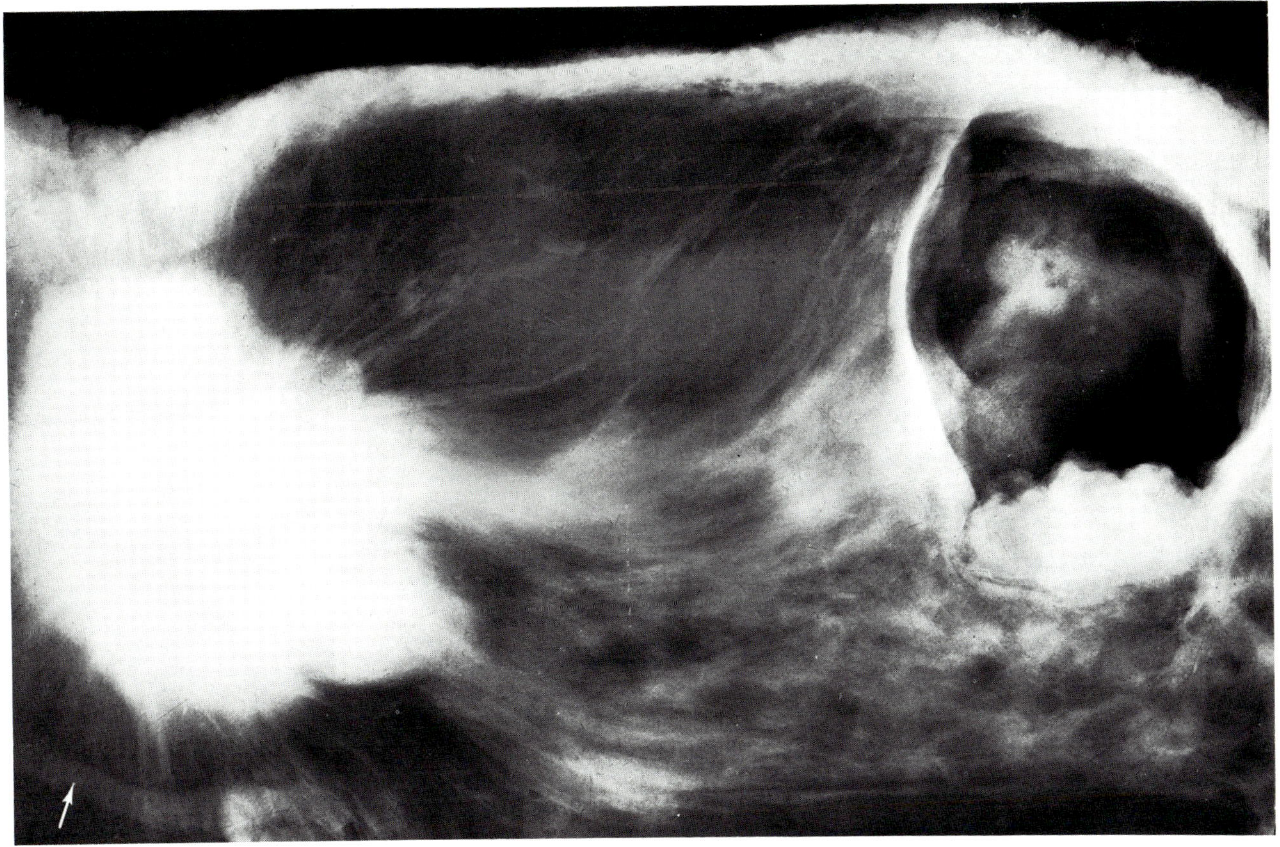

160

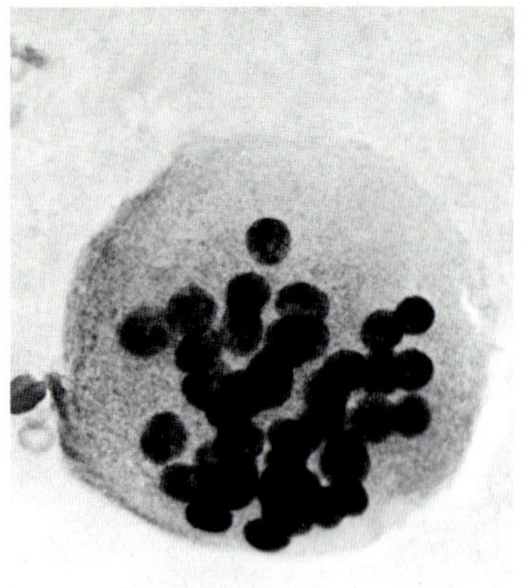

161 a

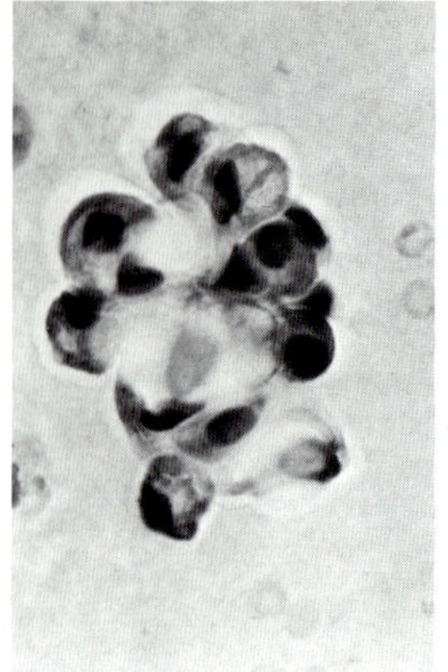

161 b

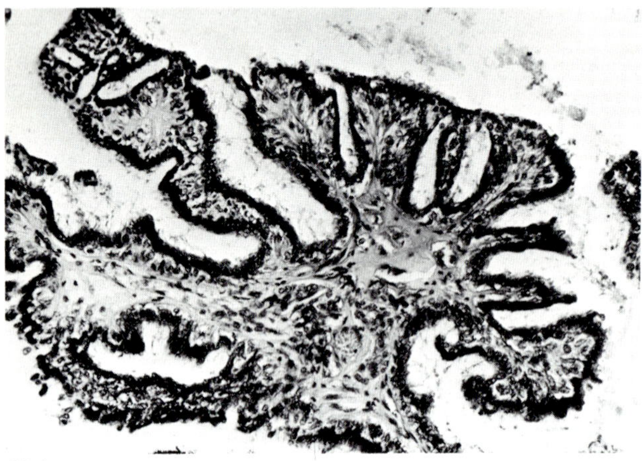

161 c

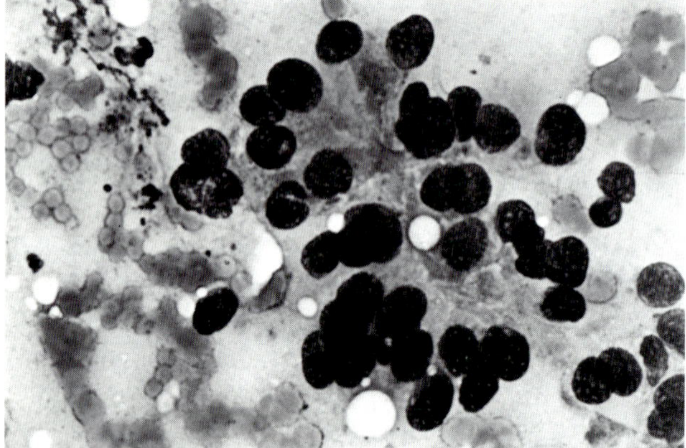

161 d

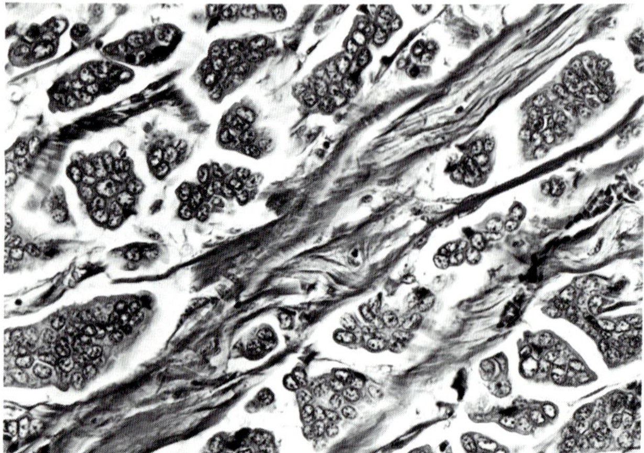

161 e

161 a–e. *Cytology and histology,* magnif 105× each.
a) Cyst aspirate. Multinucleated giant cells (left).
b) Portions of a papilloma with eccentric nuclei and broad bright rim of cytoplasm.
c) Histology. Stroma-rich papilloma with double layer of epithelium. No malignant degeneration.
d) Cytology of carcinoma. Multiple tumor cells with naked nuclei. Only small number of polymorphous nuclei.
e) Histology. Solid strands and nests of tumor cells. Abundant connective tissue (simple solid carcinoma).

38-year-old female. Recent drawing pain in right breast. Palpation: multiple nodules bilaterally similar to mastopathy. Nodule in right outer upper quadrant seems to have become larger (marked with a lead pellet) (Figs 162–163).

162 a, b. *Mammogram.*
a) Medio-lateral.
b) Cranio-caudal.
Fibrous mastopathy with small opacities along ducts. In marked area adenofibrolipoma. No carcinoma. In skin fold a cherry-sized, radiating, nonhomogeneous, palpable (*after* knowledge of its presence in mammogram) tumor nodule.

163 *Cytology,* magnif 105×. Groups of tumor cells. Polymorphous nuclei: nucleus-plasma ratio shifted toward nuclei. Histology: partially solid, partially scirrhous carcinoma. Multiple foci of adenosis in remaining breast.

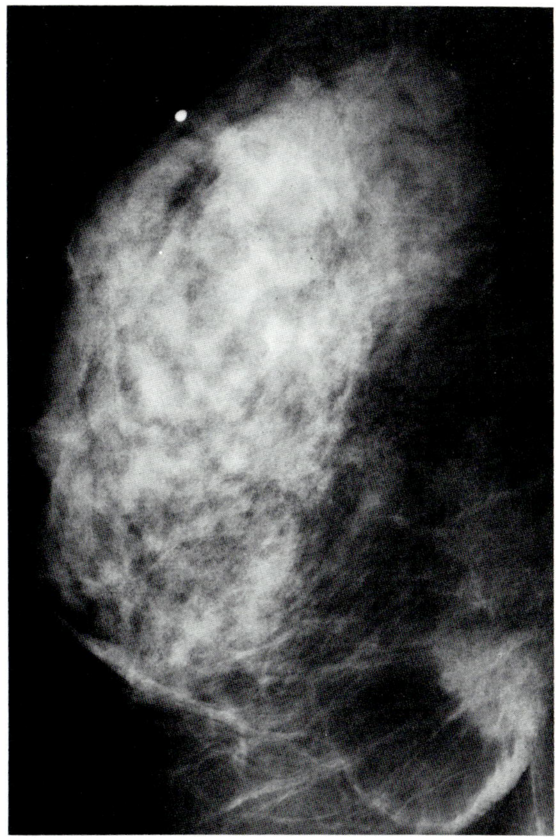

162a

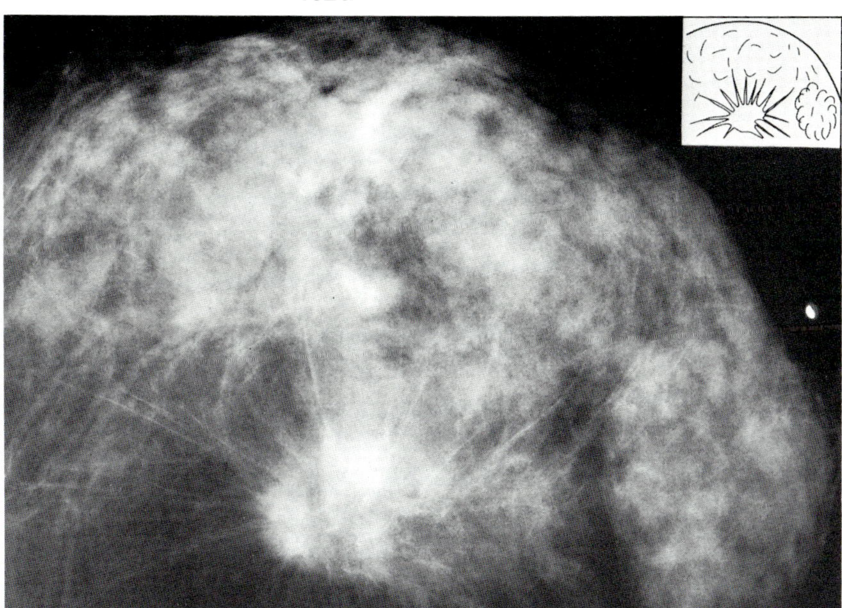

162b

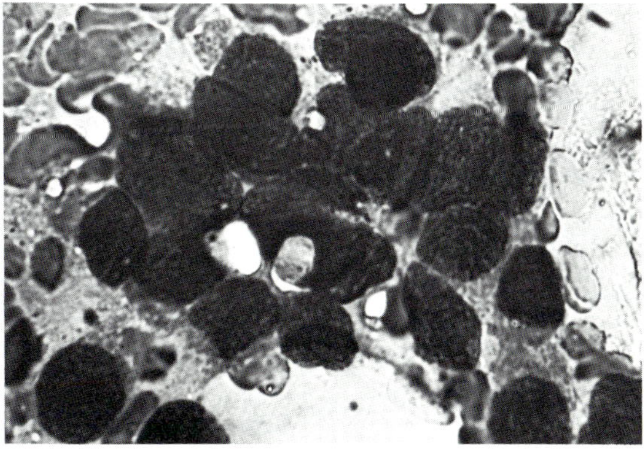

163

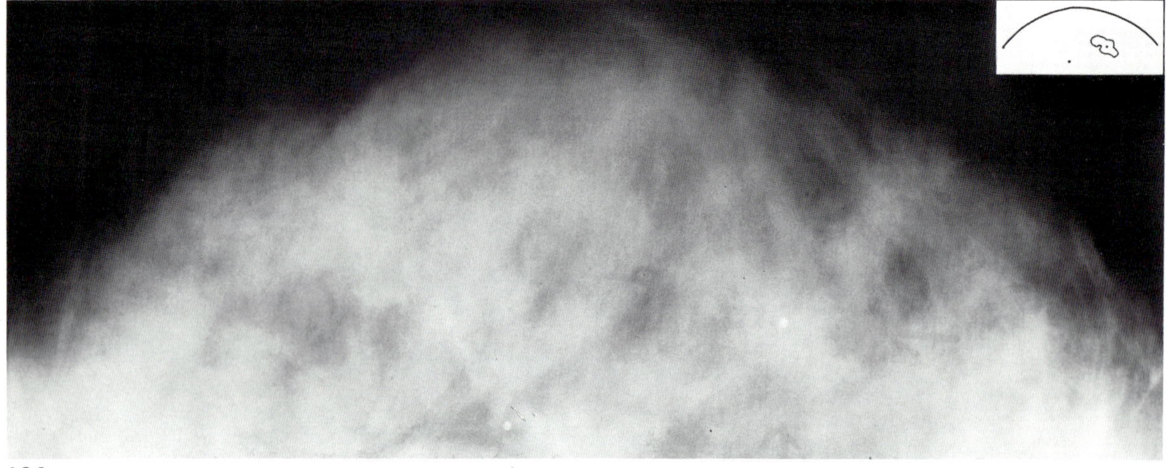
164 a

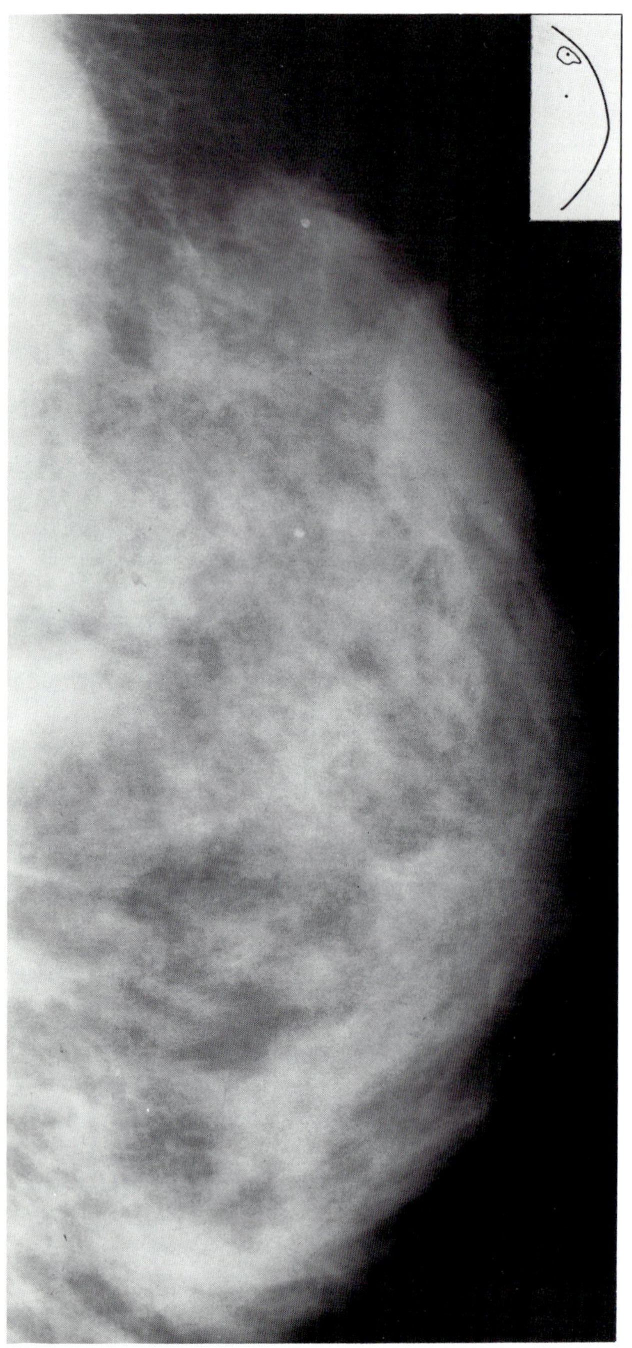
164 b

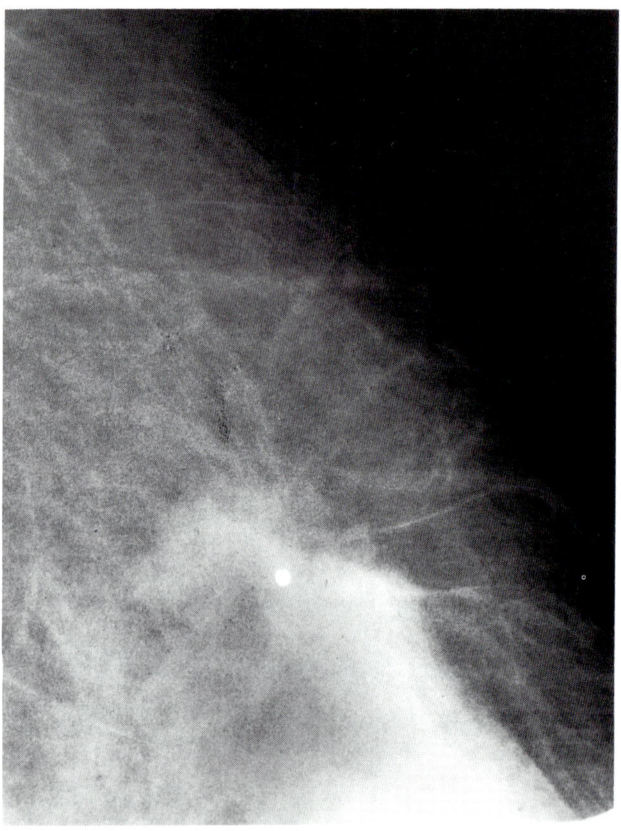
164 c

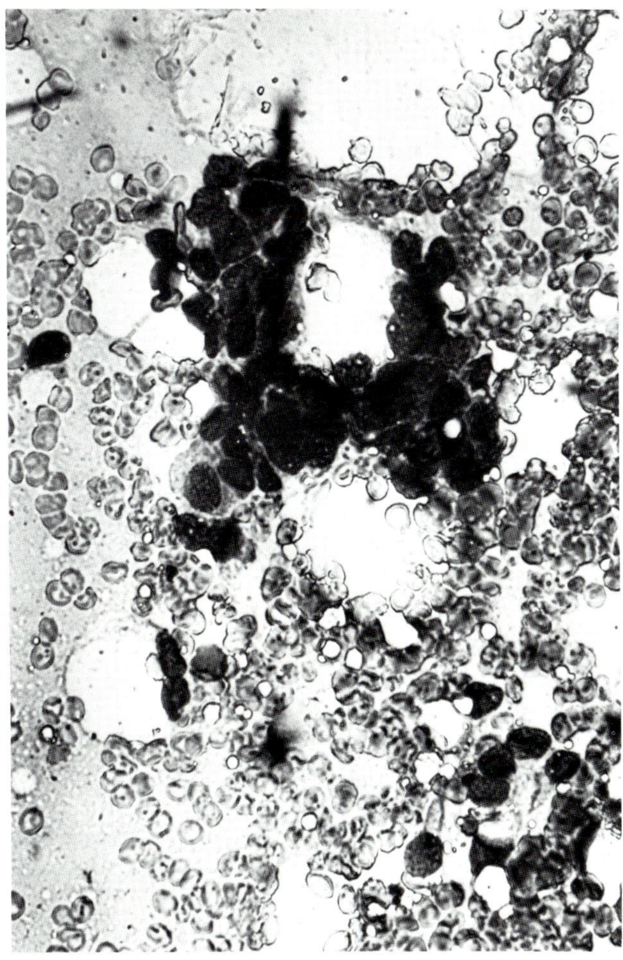

165a

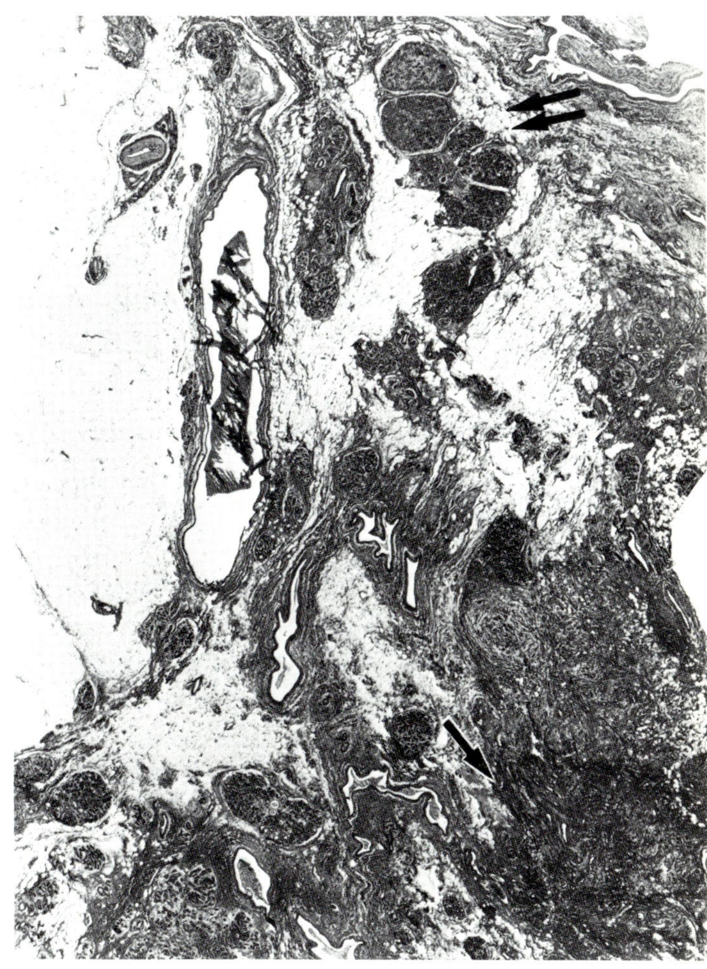

165b

53-year-old female, right breast. For 14 days slightly tender induration of upper outer quadrant. Multiple indurations similar to mastopathy in both breasts (Figs 164–165).

◁ **164** a–c. *Mammogram.*
a) Cranio-caudal.
b) Medio-lateral.
Marked fibrocystic mastopathy with multiple opacities of varying size and extent. Coarse calcium in upper quadrant region (calcified cyst). No microcalcifications.
c) Coned-down view of tender area (latero-medial). Unsharp nonhomogeneous opacity with radiating projections and central, disc-like calcifications.

165 a, b. *Cytology and histology.*
a) Cytology, magnif 60×. Thin-needle biopsy shows multiple plump tumor cells in compact layers. Polymorphous and hyperchromatic nuclei. No mitoses. Erythrocytes.
b) Histology, magnif 10×. Many dilated ducts filled with secretions. Scirrhous breast carcinoma (arrow). Multiple foci of concomitant lobular epithelioses (neoplasia) and adenoses (arrows).

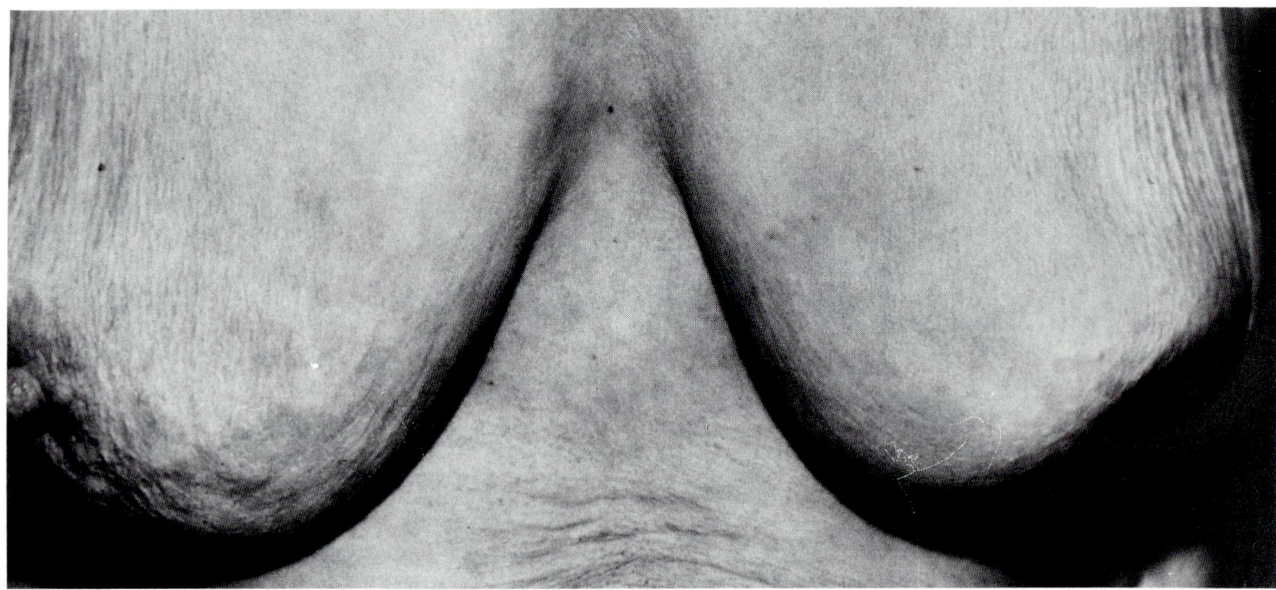

166

83-year-old female. Malignancy in left lower outer quadrant. On right side no abnormal palpation.

166 *Inspection.* Retraction of skin and nipple over carcinoma, left. Wave-like contour of skin over inner lower quadrant of the opposite side. No palpatory findings on right.

167 a, b. *Mammogram.*
a) Left breast (medio-lateral). In the lower-quadrant region nonhomogeneous radiating tumor with thickening and retraction of skin and nipple.
b) Right breast (medio-lateral). In lower-quadrant area nonhomogeneous opacity extending to nipple. Circumscribed thickening of wave-like skin without retraction. Suspicion of malignant tumor.

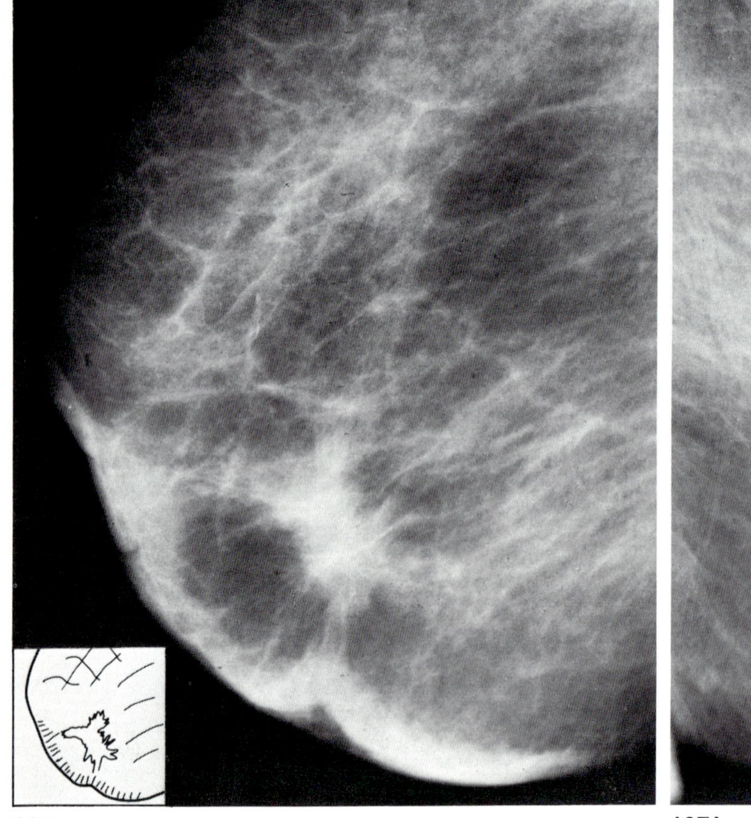

167 a

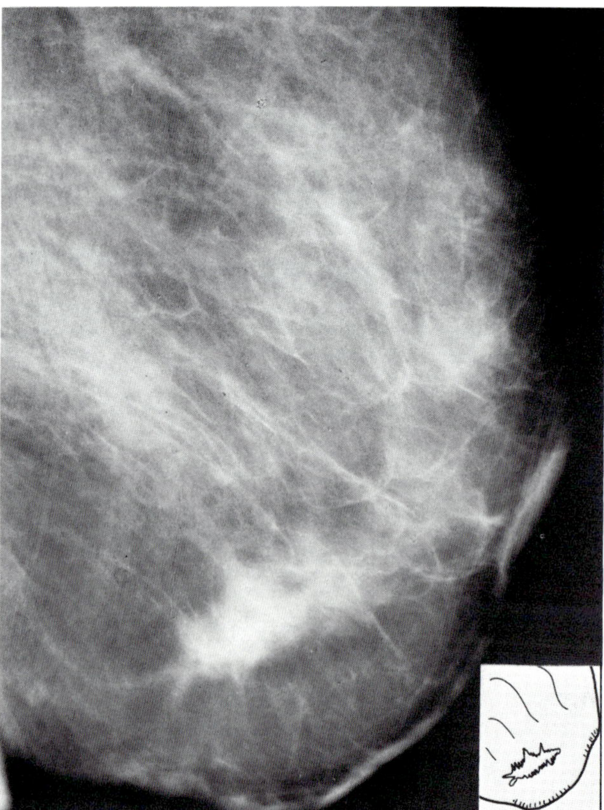

167 b

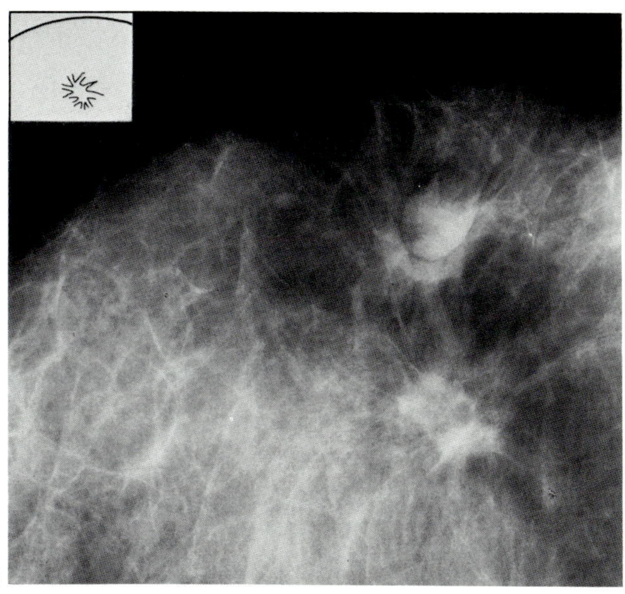
168a

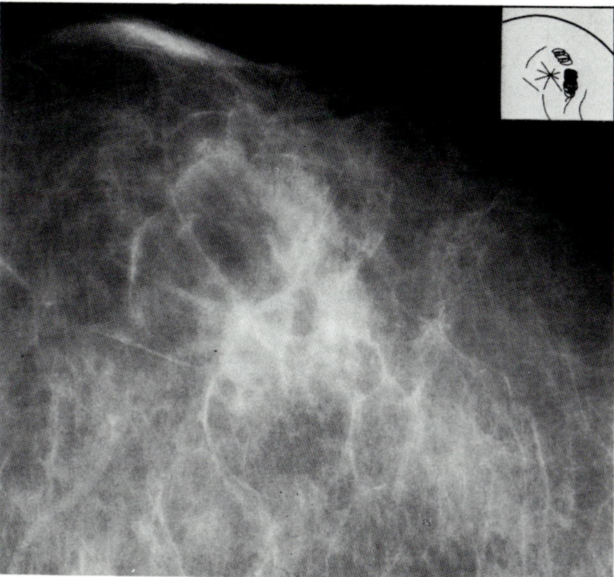
168b

168 a, b. *Mammogram* (cranio-caudal).
a) Left breast. Opacity remains stellate in second position.
b) Right breast. Opacity indicative of cancer in lateral mammogram (Fig 167b) is not identifiable in second position.

169 a, b. *Cytology and histology* of carcinoma shown in Fig 168, left.
a) Cytology, magnif 105×. Dissociated carcinoma cells with moderately polymorphous nuclei and enlarged, plump and confluent nucleoli. Adjacent proliferating normal group of cells.
b) Histology, magnif 80×. Partially solid, partially scirrhous growing carcinoma.

170 a, b. *Cytology and histology* of carcinoma shown in Fig 168, right.
a) Cytology, magnif 105×. Normal epithelial group with uniform nuclei. Between darkly stained bipolar cells (myoepithelial?).
b) Histology. Localized proliferation of acini and of intralobular connective tissue with proliferation of basket cells: sclerosing adenosis. Carcinomas and sclerosing adenoses have similar radiographic appearance in mammogram. Often only biopsy will differentiate the two disease entities.

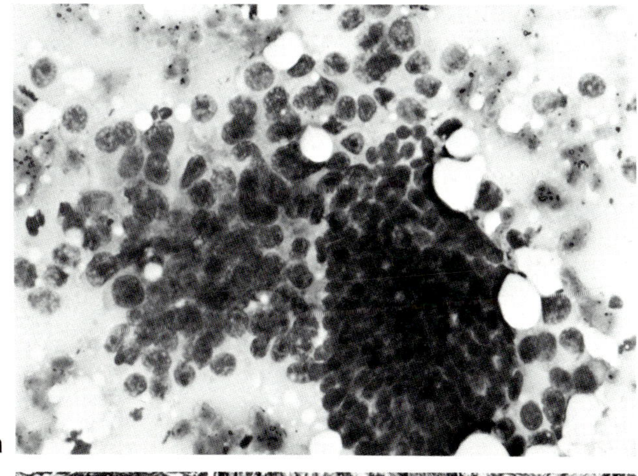
169a

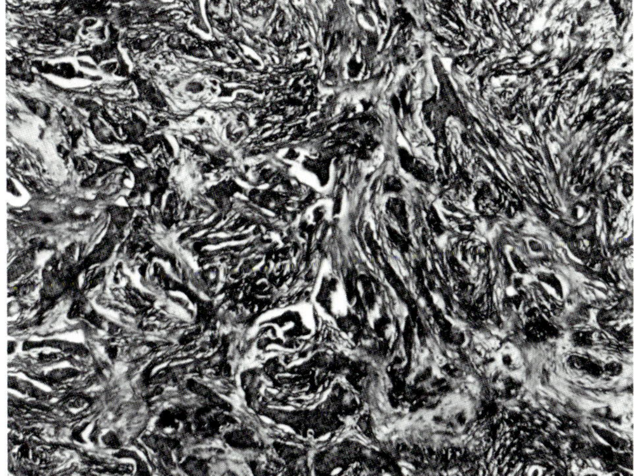
169b

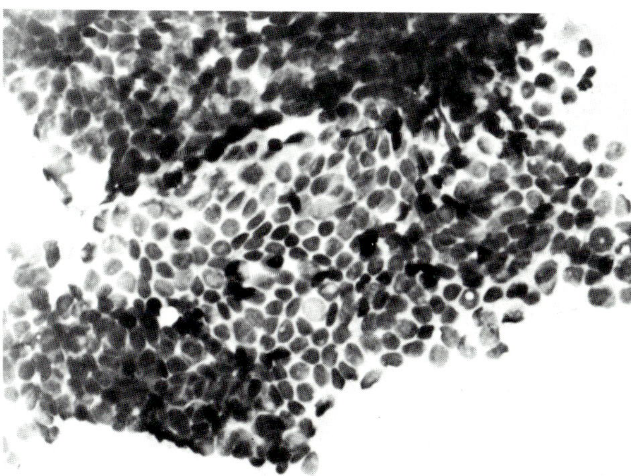
170a

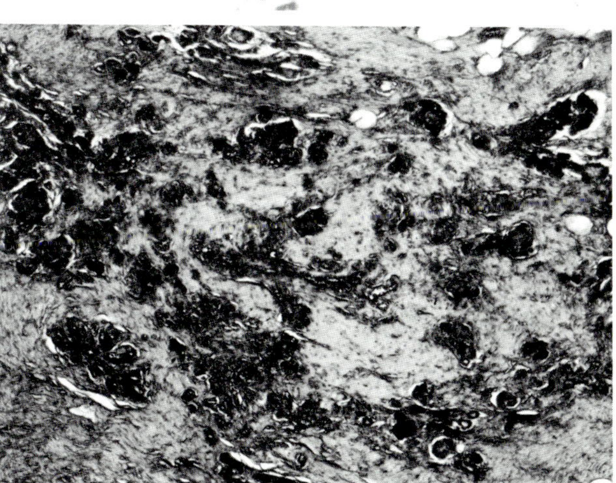
170b

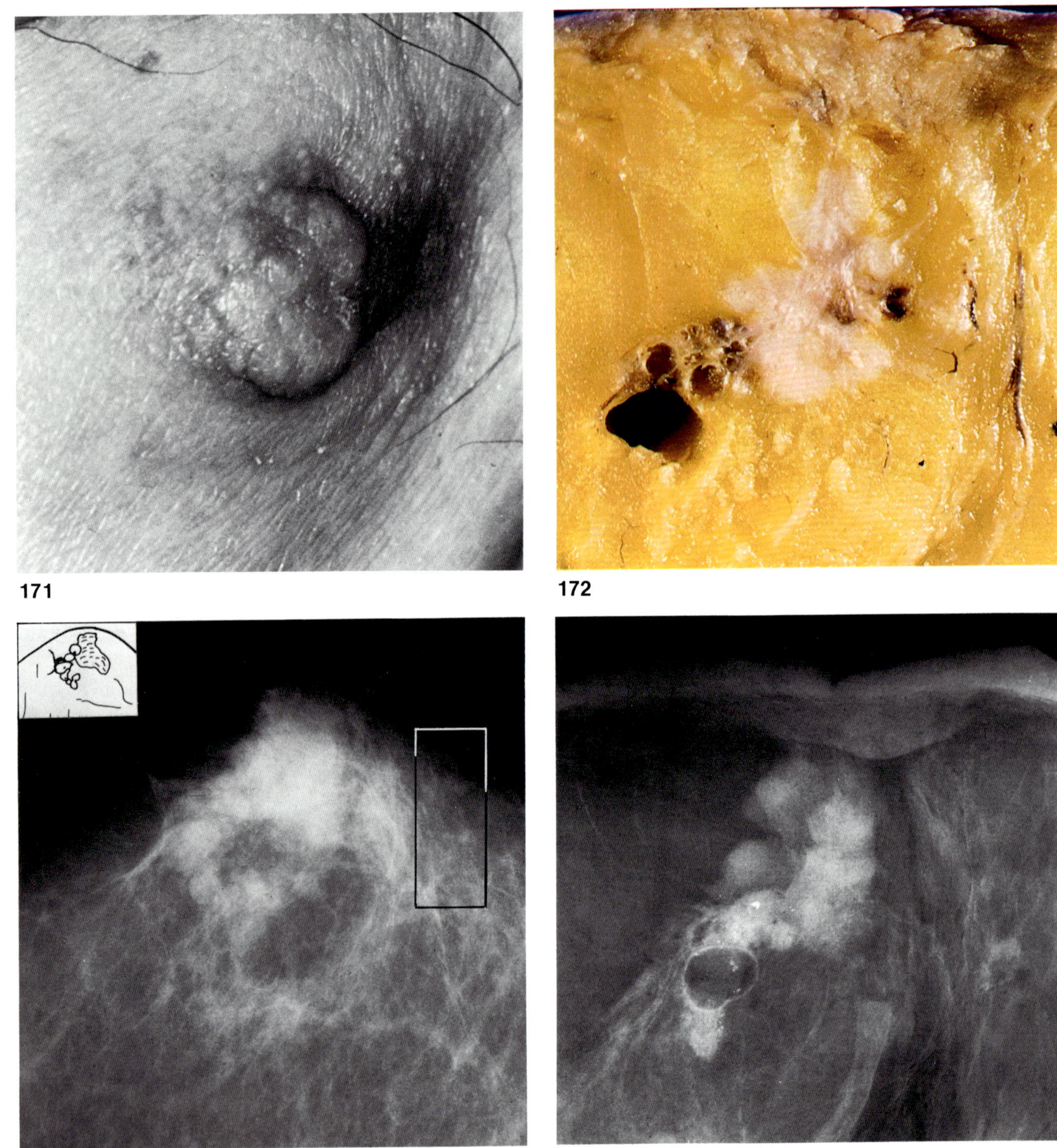

171

172

173 a

173 b

41-year-old female, left breast. Check-up examination. On palpation retroareolar induration (Figs 171–175).

171 *Inspection.* Slight circumscribed retraction of areola.

172 *Macroanatomy.* Cystic dysplasia with conglomerate of multiple smaller cysts. In cysts next to tumor, epithelial proliferations continuing into retroareolar, ill-defined carcinoma nodule.

173 a, b. *Radiographic examinations.*
a) Mammogram (cranio-caudal). Lobulated nonhomogeneous retroareolar opacity with micro- and macrocalcifications.
b) Specimen radiograph. Solitary cyst following emptying. In region of cyst conglomerate, localized micro- and macrocalcifications. Retroareolar lobular carcinoma nodule.

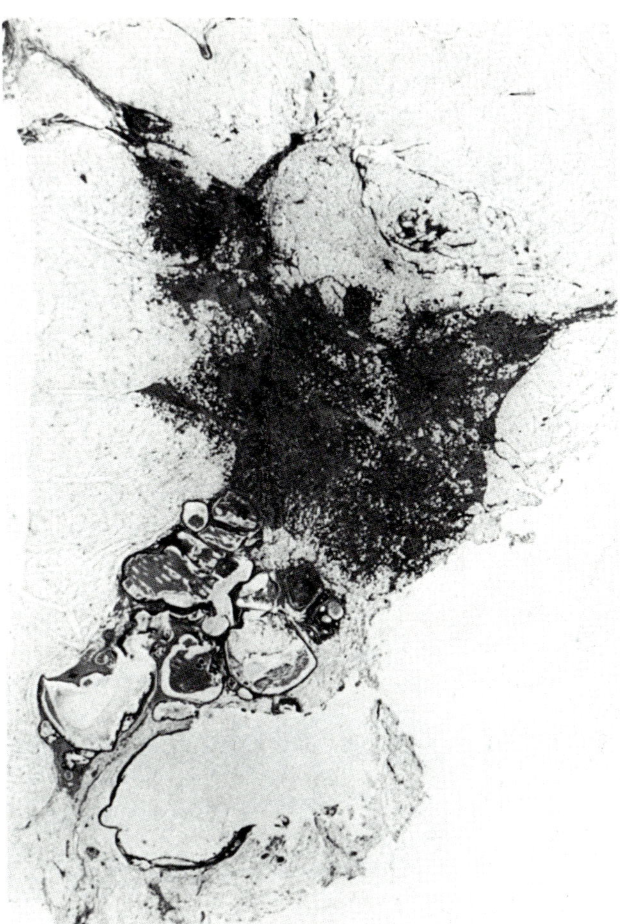

174 *Histological macrosection,* magnif 5×. Partially scirrhous, partially solid carcinoma. Several cysts partially filled with secretions below. In smaller cysts epithelial proliferations next to tumor.

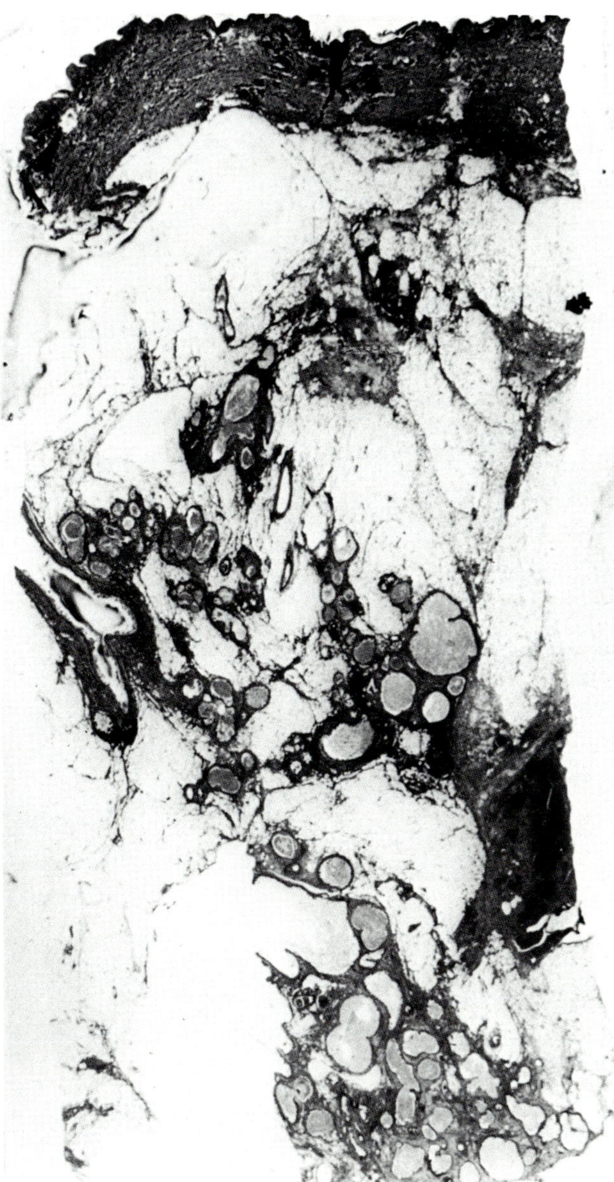

175 *Histological macrosection* from normal parenchyma (region marked in Fig 173a). Small cystic dysplasia with multiple ectatic ducts and cystically degenerated acini.

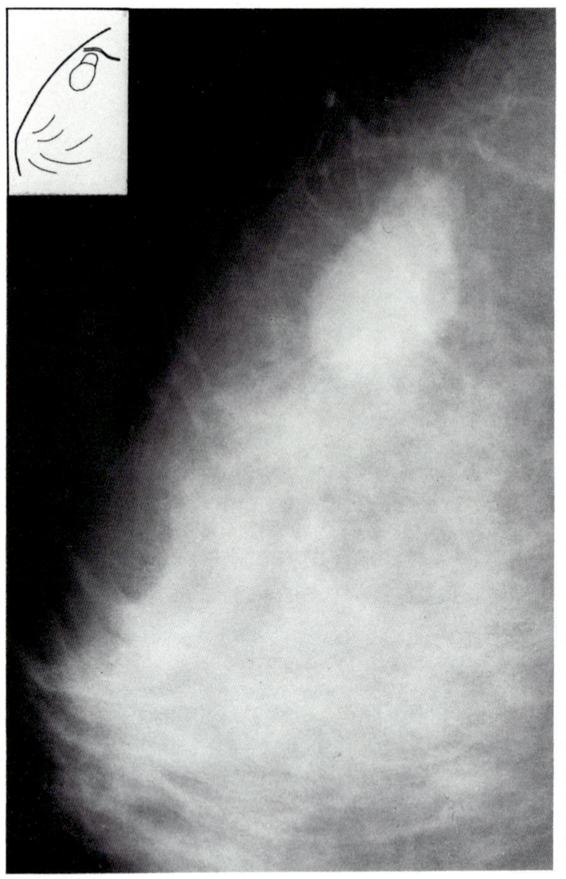

176a

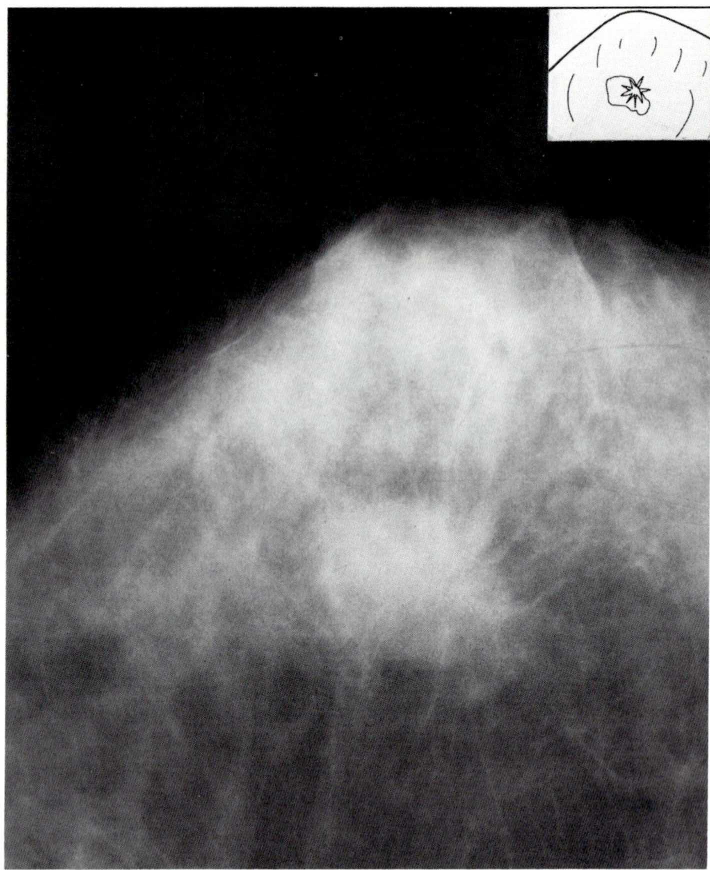

176b

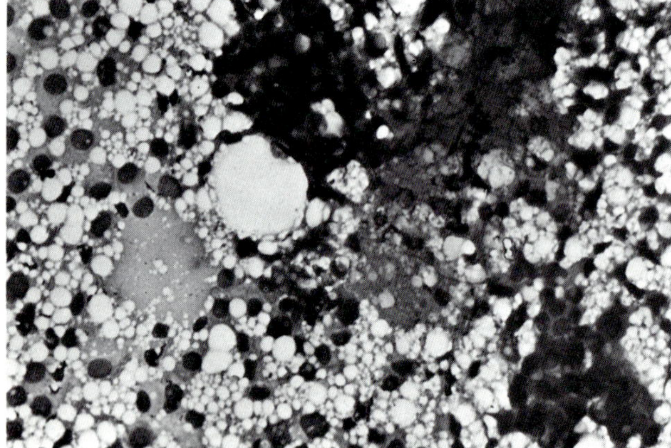

177

29-year-old female, right breast. For 3 weeks cherry-sized, palpable, easily movable nodule in upper outer quadrant. Slight skin retraction (Figs 176–179).

176 a, b. *Mammogram.*
a) Medio-lateral. Smooth, double shadows of homogeneous density.
b) Cranio-caudal. Smooth, round tumor density with superimposed radiating opacity. Suspicion of malignant degeneration of a cyst.

177 *Cytology.* On aspiration 3 ml of hemorrhagic fluid. Cytology shows polymorphous and hyperchromatic layers of tumor cells. Dissociated cells, some with naked nuclei. Secretion, debris and erythrocytes.

178 a, b. *Anatomic-radiographic comparison.* ▷
a) Macroanatomy. Partially nodular, partially radiating carcinoma nodule with central necrotic cavity appearing in mammogram as a cyst. Irregular cavity wall. Next to tumor some hemorrhage following thin-needle biopsy.
b) Specimen radiograph. Partially nodular, partially radiating tumor. Air-filled tumor cavity with irregular contour.

179 *Histology.* Cranial portion of the tumor. Nodular portion of the carcinoma (right edge of figure). Cellular solid carcinoma right of stroma-rich scirrhus. Ectatic blood vessels and ducts. Necrosis in tumor center (light). (Cavity not shown.) ▷

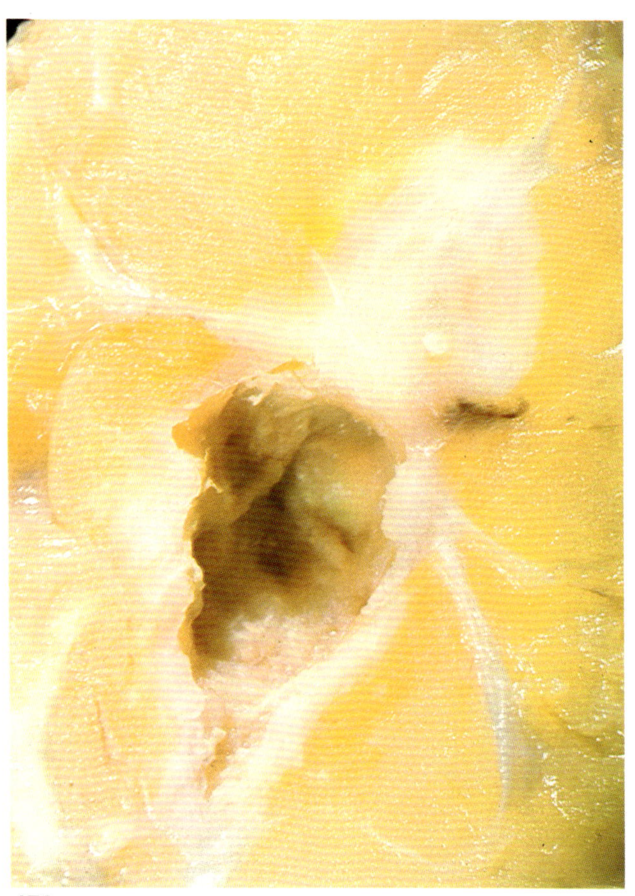

178 a

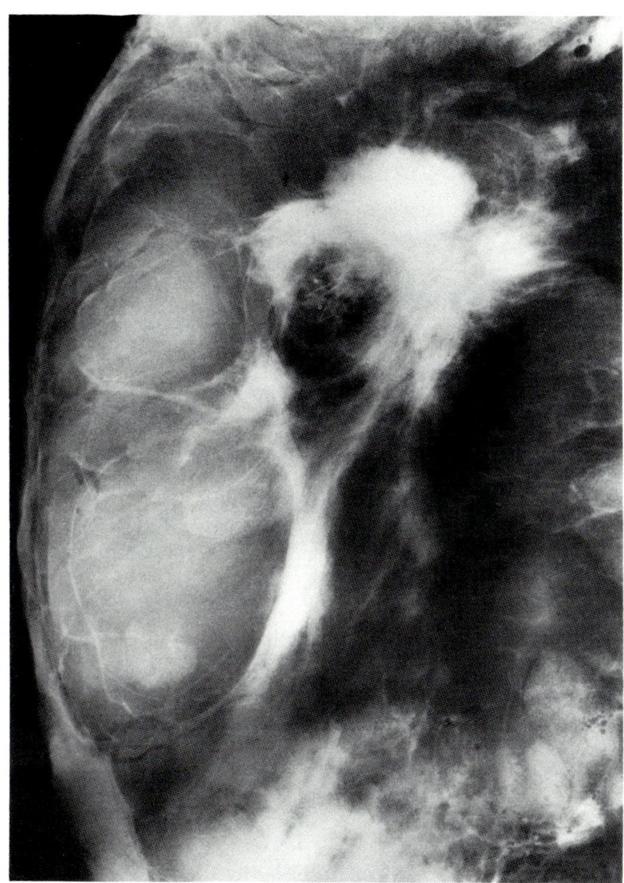

178 b

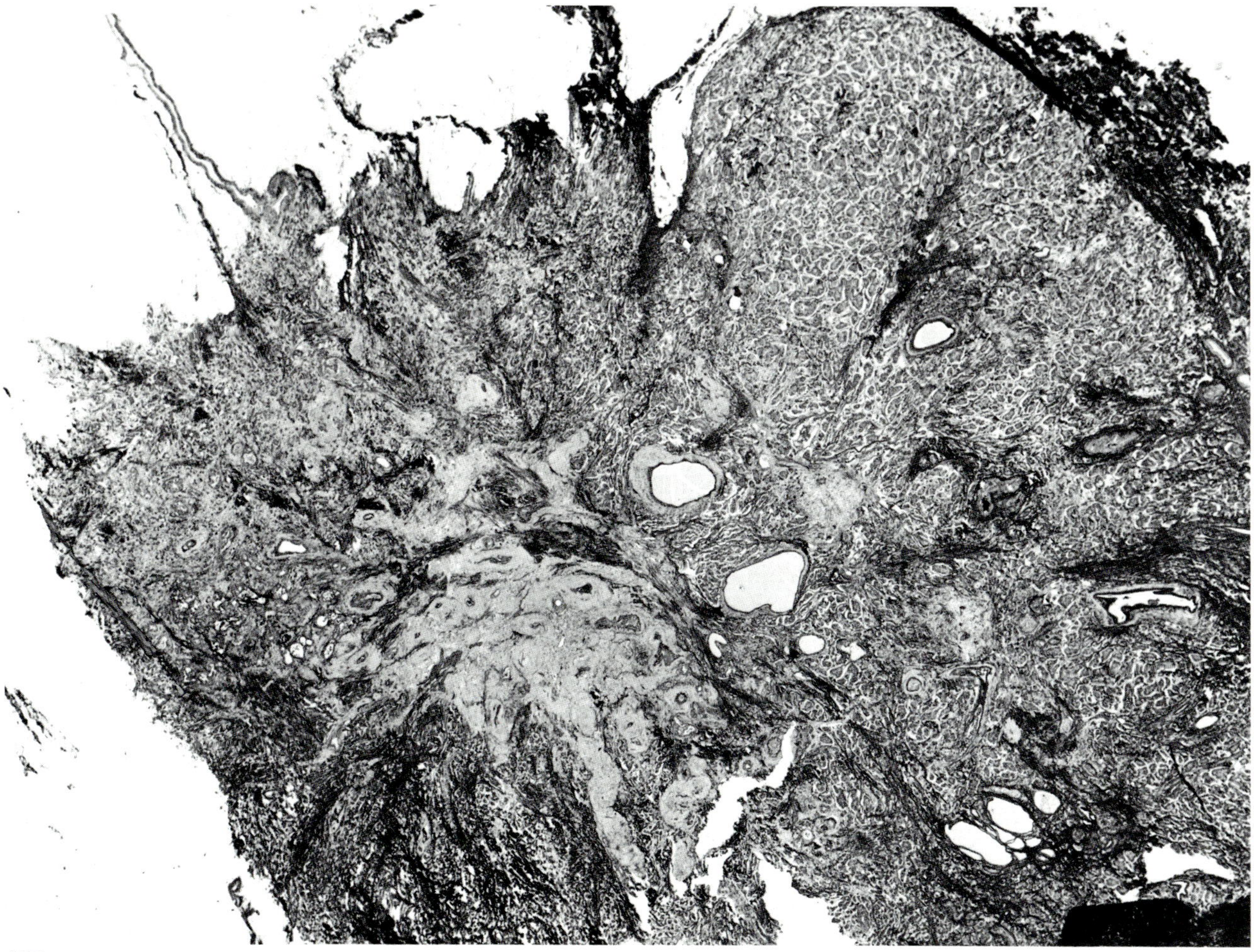

179

Nodular, smoothly-defined malignancies

Medullary and mucinous carcinomas (Figs **180–202**) are typical of this group. In addition, malignant, degenerated papillomas (Fig **202**), cellular sarcomas (Fig **206**) and cellular metastases from tumors of other organs (Figs **203**, **271**) belong to this group of tumors with typical nodular appearance in the mammogram.

There is no retraction of surrounding tissue, so surrounding architecture is not distorted. There is no peritumoral lucency. The tumors are well vascularized and show circumscribed hyperthermia with temperatures of 1 to 3 °C above the normal parenchyma in the thermogram (Figs **185**, **272**, **284**). Microcalcifications are rare. Coarse calcifications secondary to regressive changes may occur following therapy (Fig **203**).

The tumors are easily movable and may be confused with cysts and fibroadenomas (Figs **184**, **202**).

The radiographic findings of nodular, growing carcinomas are as follows:

a) round or oval, smooth or lobulated, homogeneous opacities without microcalcifications;
b) no retraction of surrounding breast structures, no retraction of skin or nipple;
c) no tumor projections, palpable findings corresponding to radiographic findings;
d) less radio-opacity than connective tissue and water, possibly overlooked in stroma-rich breasts;
e) rapid enlargement by multiplication of cells, by bleeding into the tumor (medullary carcinoma) or by production of mucus (mucinous carcinoma);
f) increased vascular pattern in surrounding breast parenchyma (hyperthermia in the thermogram).

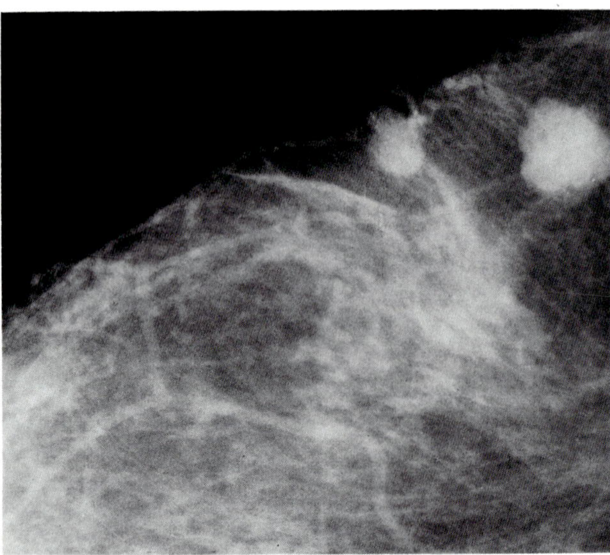

180 *Mammogram.* Two homogeneous, smooth but lobulated nodules in region of outer upper quadrant. No retraction of surrounding morphological structures, increased peritumoral vascular pattern. (Histology: medullary carcinoma with cellular satellite tumor).

Nodular, growing *primary* carcinoma has a relatively favorable prognosis as compared to other primary carcinomas. On the other hand, sarcoma and metastases which are also nodular, growing tumors have a very poor prognosis.

Sarcoma of the breast (mesenchymal tumors) are rare. Their incidence among malignant tumors is less than 1%. Peak incidence is between 45 and 55 years of age. Rapid growth is characteristic.

According to VON ALBERTINI (1974) the most common form of sarcoma in the breast is *spindle cell sarcoma*, probably originating from stroma of a fibroadenoma. In addition, there are *polymorphocellular sarcomas* and *round cell sarcomas*. Liposarcomas and myxomatous sarcomas are rare.

Because of their cellularity many sarcomas grow in nodular fashion and are smoothly defined from surrounding tissue (Fig **206**). There are also, however, *diffusely* growing types.

At *palpation* the sarcoma is a movable tumor and, in spite of its size, is contiguous with neither skin nor musculature. Skin and nipple retractions are rare. In contradistinction to remaining nodular tumors (mucoid carcinoma, medullary carcinoma), these tumors have a very poor prognosis. They metastasize early.

In one case a polymorphous giant cell sarcoma in a 53-year-old woman metastasized to the right heart. The metastasis grew as a nodular, lobulated tumor from the right atrium through the tricuspid valve into the right ventricle and pulmonary outflow tract. Clinically the predominant feature was a superior vena cava syndrome. The patient died with acute right heart failure. The tumor in the breast was diagnosed as sarcoma during life; the *metastasis* in the heart was found at autopsy (Figs **204–208**).

Metastases from malignancies of other organs to the breast are rare. Occasionally, metastases from a malignant melanoma are found both in males and in females. In one case the metastasis grew nodularly in the right breast and diffusely in the left. They showed cytologically an identical picture similar to a small cell breast carcinoma.

Lymphatic systemic diseases may manifest themselves in the breast. These types of tumors usually are very cellular, resulting in nodular, sharply-defined and ill-defined opacities in the mammogram. Necrotic areas of the tumor may calcify (Fig **203**).

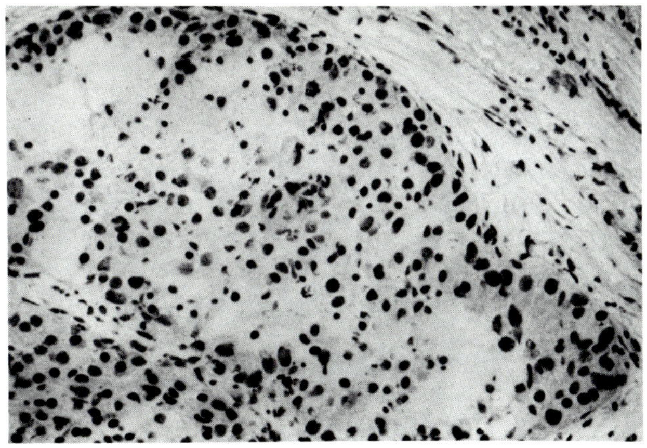

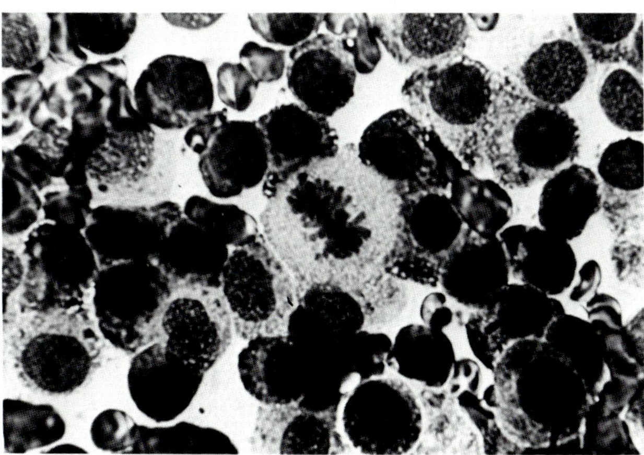

181 a, b. Medullary carcinoma.
a) *Histology,* magnif 105×. Very cellular tumor. No stromal septa. Polymorphous and polychromatic nuclei. Sharp delineation from normal surrounding tissue.

b) *Cytology,* magnif 260×. Numerous moderately polymorphous tumor epithelioses. Mitoses. No cellular coherence.

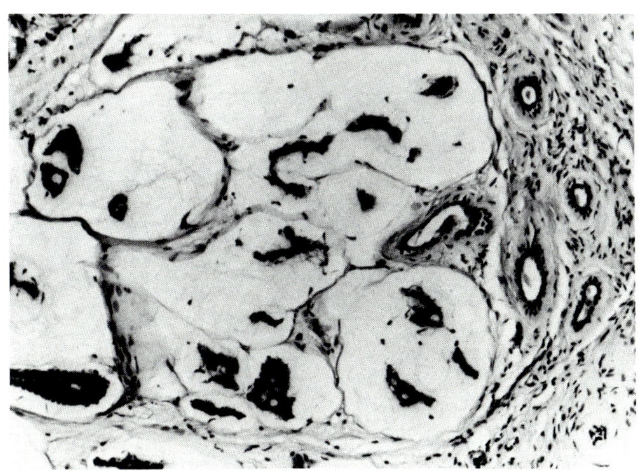

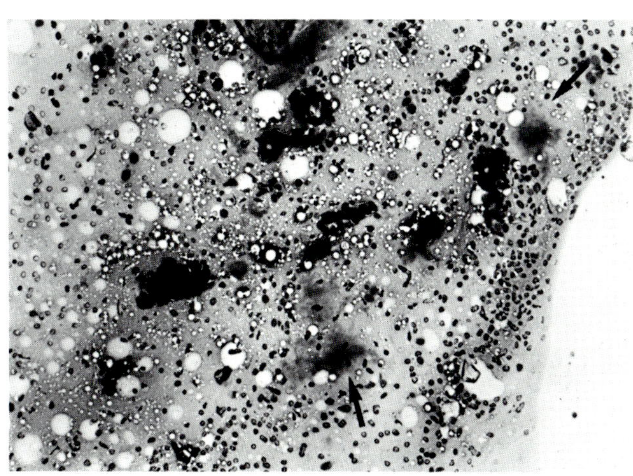

182 a, b. Mucoid carcinoma.
a) *Histology,* magnif 40×. Mucus-filled chamber-like areas (clear) with clusters of tumor cells within.

b) *Cytology,* magnif 80×. Multiple compact epithelial layers. Mucus (arrow). May be confused with degenerating fibroadenoma.

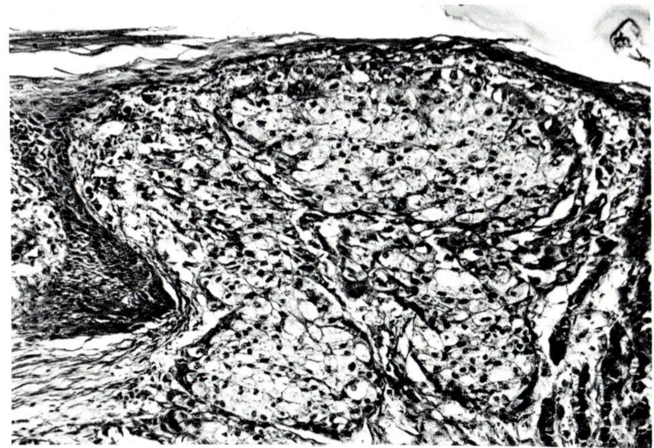

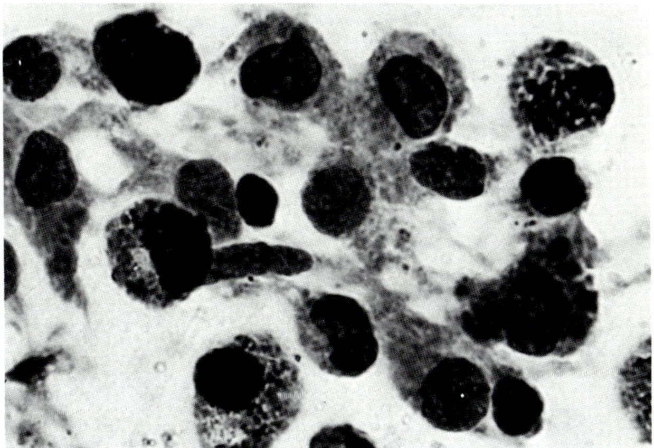

183 a, b. Subcutaneous metastasis of a cellular hypernephroma.
a) *Histology,* magnif 40×. Large confluent layers of plant-like cells with eccentric polymorphous nuclei. Sharp delineation from breast parenchyma and skin (left in figure).

b) *Cytology,* magnif 260×. Many tumor cells with broad rim of cytoplasm. Polymorphous nuclei. Differentiation from primary breast carcinoma not possible.

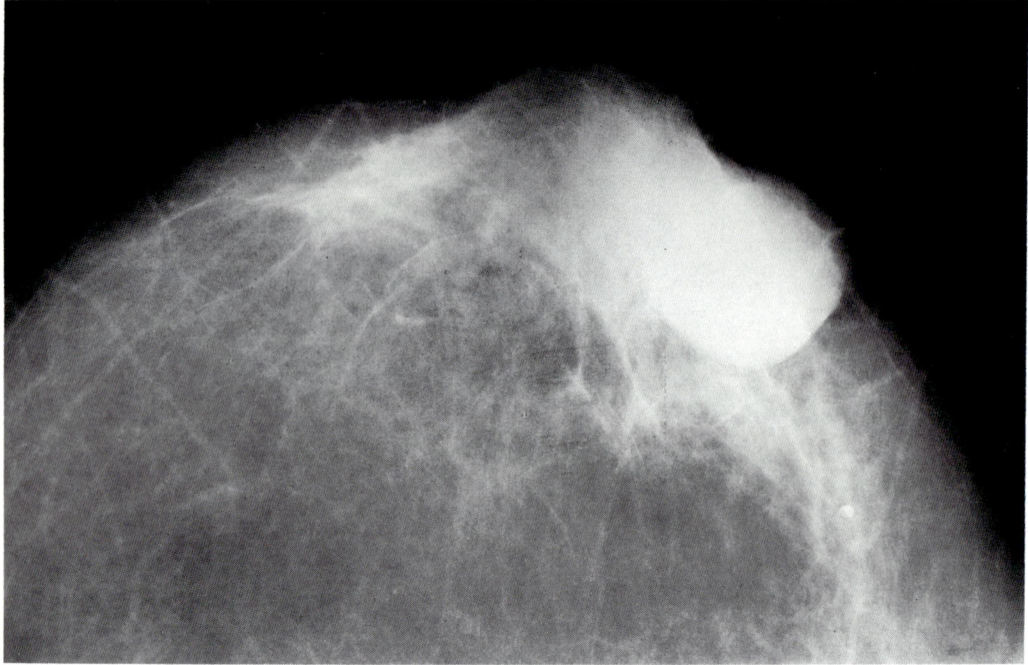

184 a

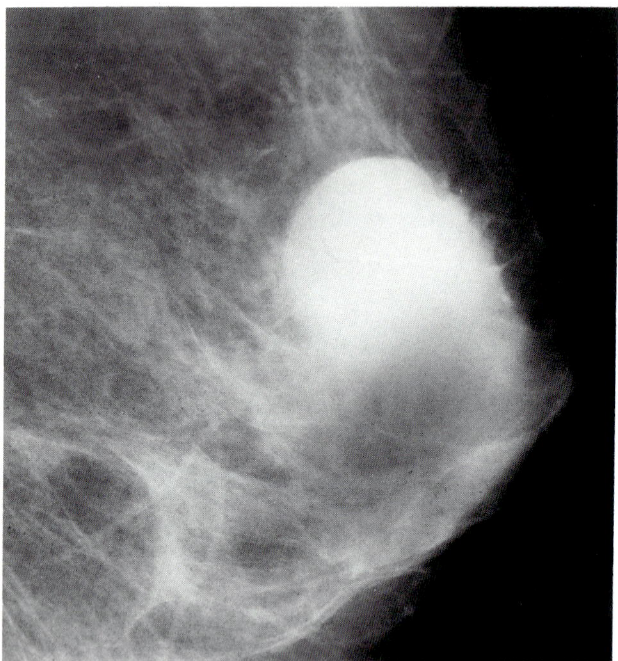

184 b

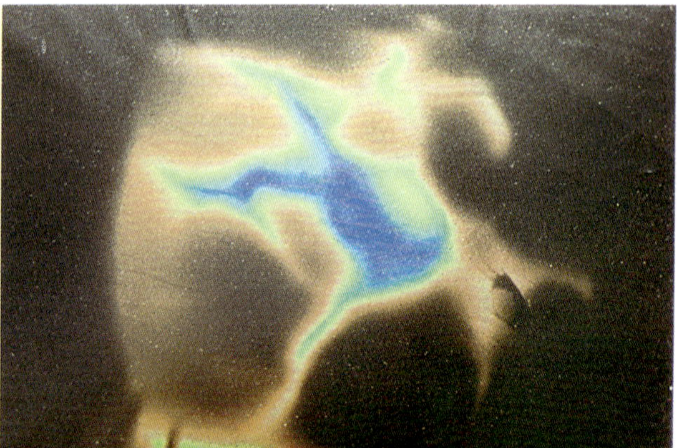

185

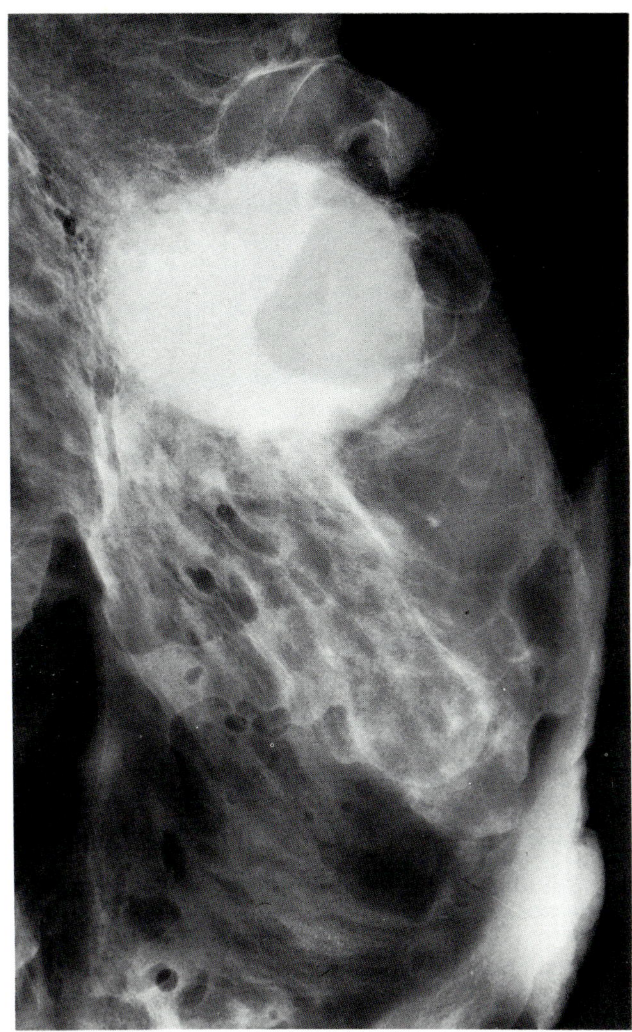

186

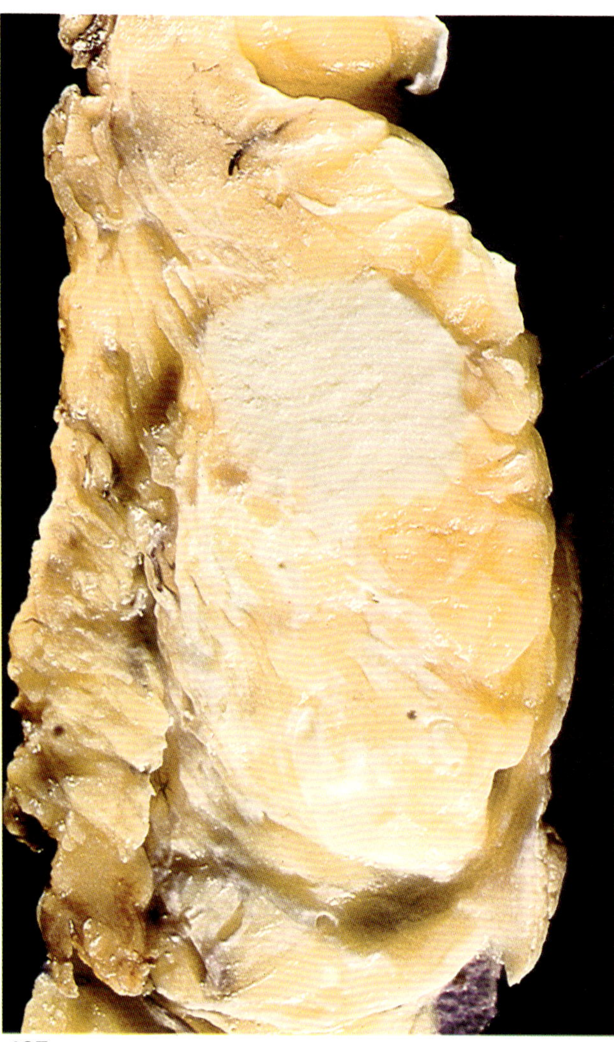

187

49-year-old female, right breast. For 14 days palpablc nodule in upper outer quadrant. Tumor is easily movable. No skin retraction. Presumed fibroadenoma or cyst (Figs 184–187).

◁ **184** a, b. *Mammogram.*
a) Cranio-caudal.
b) Medio-lateral.
Homogeneous, predominantly smoothly defined opacity, poorly-defined delineation from retroareolar area. No retraction of surrounding tissue. Presumed benign tumor.

◁ **185** *Plate thermography* right. Stellate, atypical neovascularization over nodule (left breast thermographically "cold").

186 *Specimen radiograph.* Right tumor edge smooth, above-left somewhat irregular. No radiolucent rim around tumor. Below tumor are dilated, visibly empty lactiferous ducts.

187 *Macroanatomy.* Smoothly-defined carcinomatous nodule; only cranial border has somewhat sawtooth-like contour. Breast rich in fatty tissue with band-like fibrosis. Nipple below to right. Histology and cytology (see Fig 181).

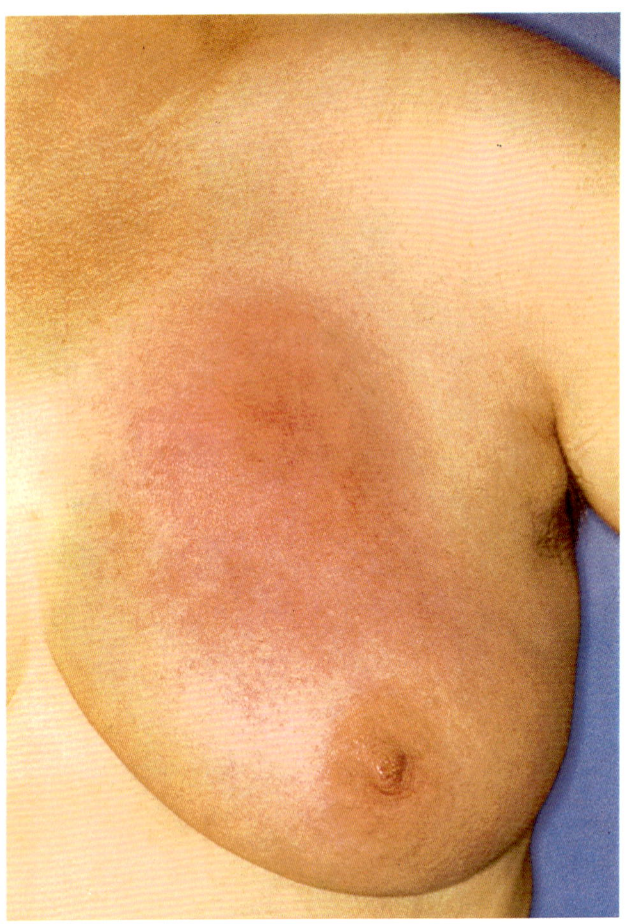

188

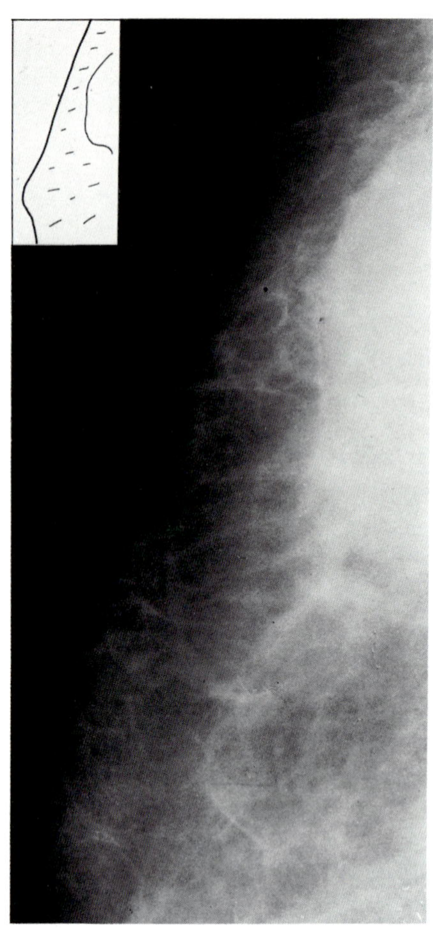

189

47-year-old female. For 14 days slowly enlarging reddish-blue changes in left breast (Figs 188–190).

188 *Inspection.* Large hematoma with bulging skin. Palpation negative for tumor. Swelling axilla. Thermography: diffuse hyperthermia (4 °C) of discolored skin.

189 *Mammogram* (medio-lateral). Smoothly-defined, somewhat pointed homogeneous opacity adjoining chest wall. Net-like appearance in mammogram produced by hematoma in tissue surrounding tumor. Thin-needle biopsy: aspiration of blood.

190 a, b. *Anatomic-radiological comparison.* ▷

a) Macroanatomy. Round, yellowish tumor with hemorrhagic necrosis. Connective tissue capsule. Localized bleeding in parenchyma surrounding nodule. Histology: medullary carcinoma with hemorrhagic necrosis.

b) Specimen radiograph. Nonhomogeneous, round, sharply-defined tumor opacity. Increased translucency of recent hemorrhage. No microcalcifications.

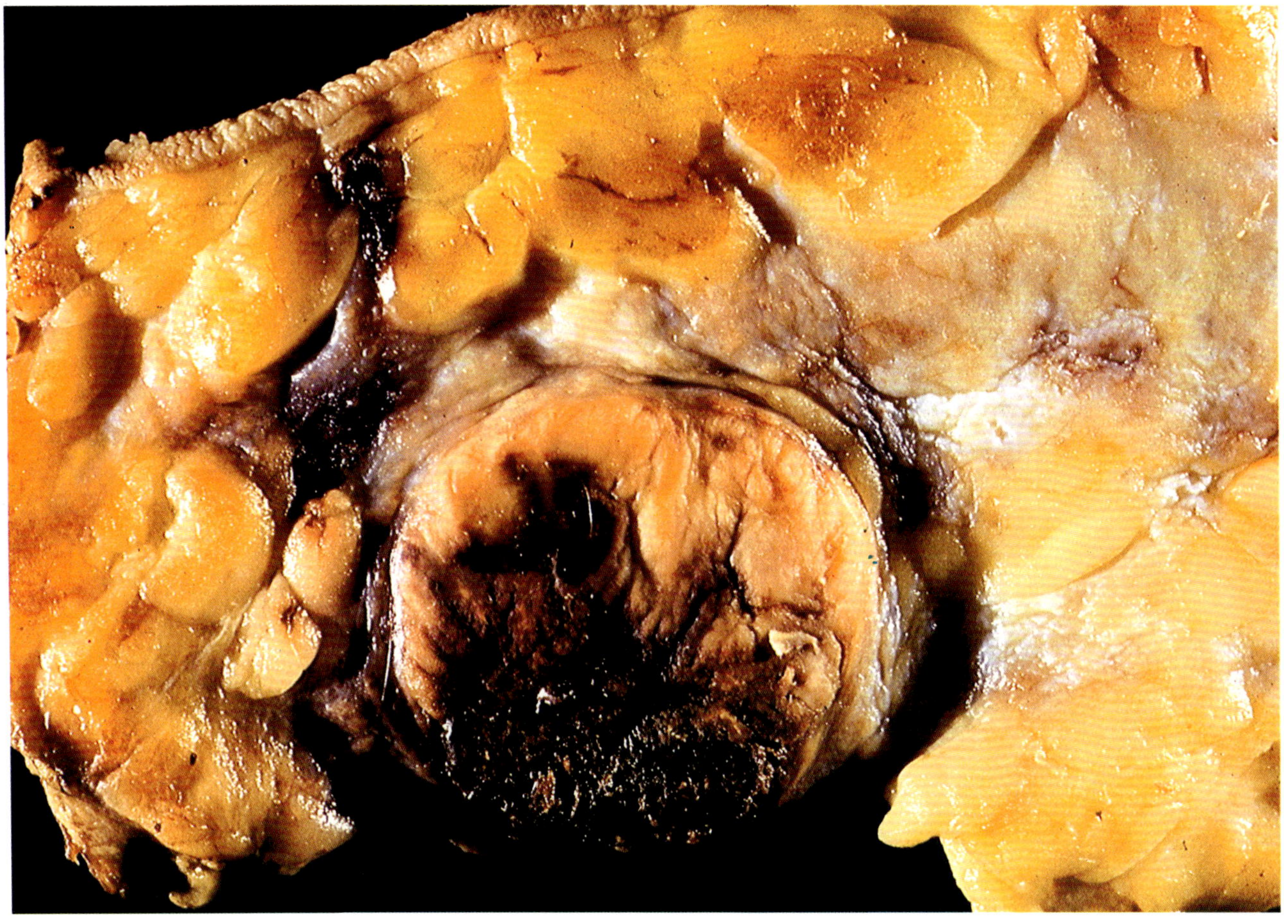

190 a

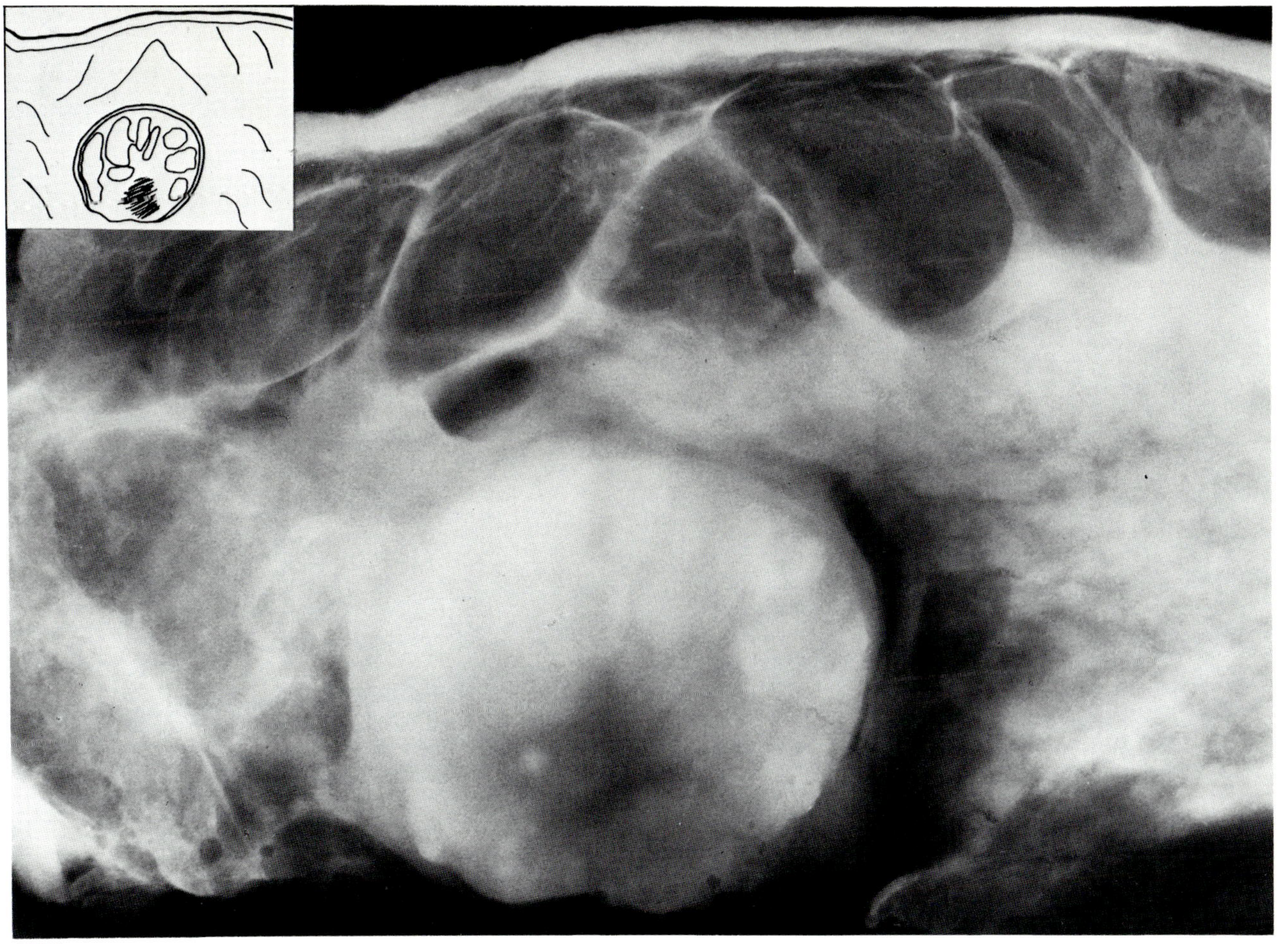

190 b

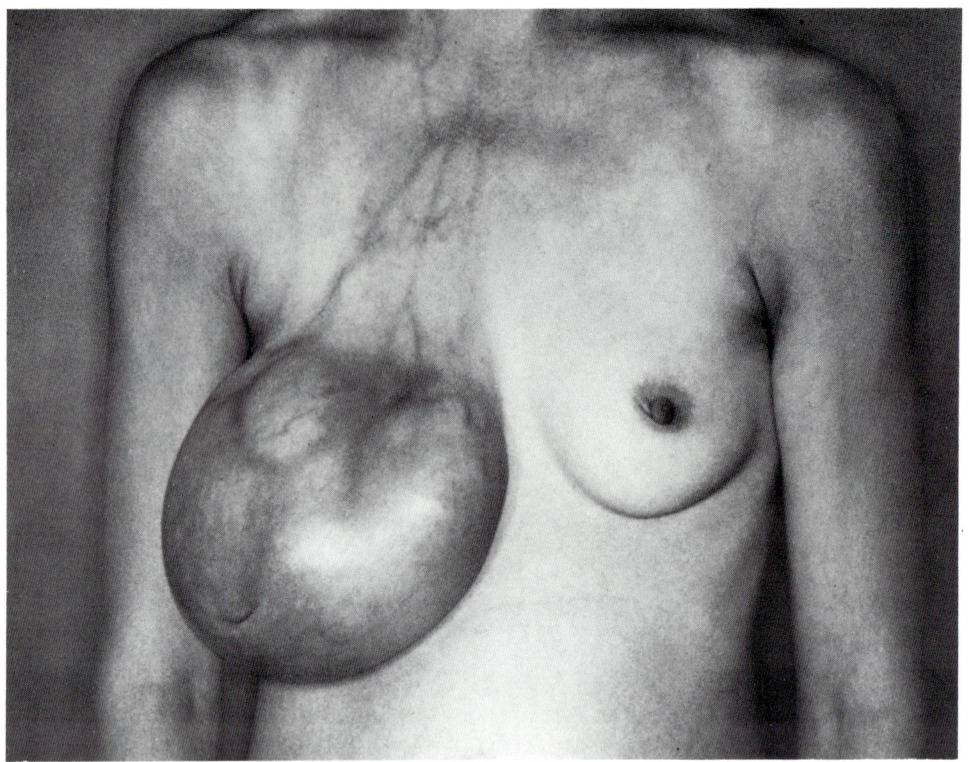

191

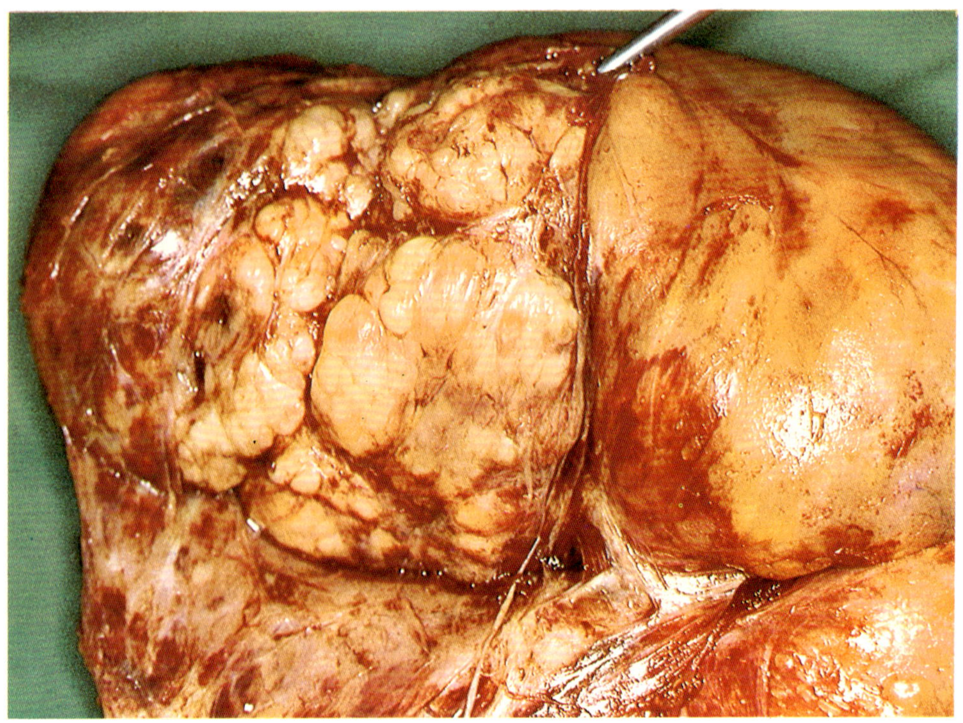

192

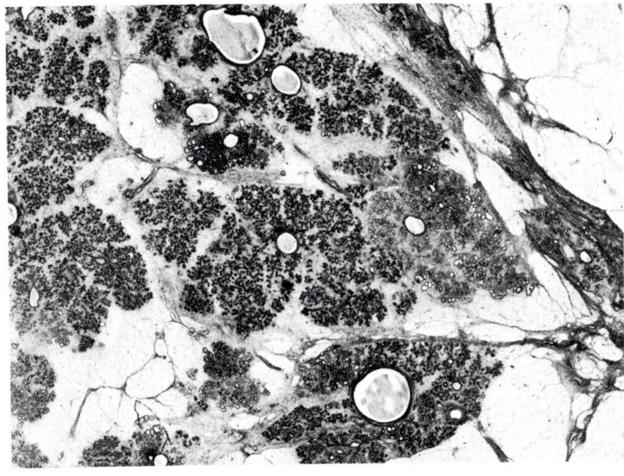

193 a

193 b

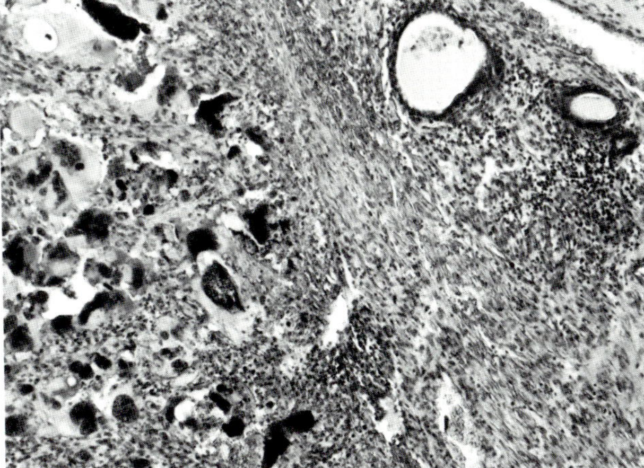

193 c

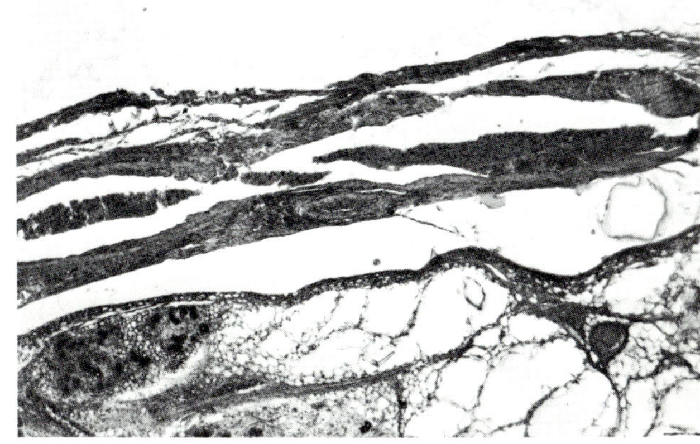

193 d

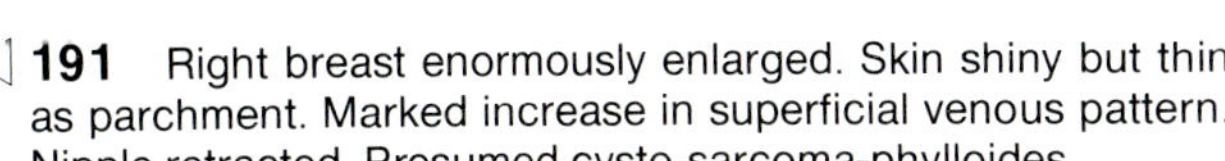

32-year-old female. Right breast allegedly has always been somewhat larger than left. For 3 months (!) marked increase in size (Fig 191–197).

◁ **191** Right breast enormously enlarged. Skin shiny but thin as parchment. Marked increase in superficial venous pattern. Nipple retracted. Presumed cysto-sarcoma-phylloides.

◁ **192** *Macroanatomy.* Surgical removal of a 1400-gr tumor. After opening of tumor capsule, protrusion of soft lobulated nodular tumors.

193 a–d. *Histology.* (Sections of Fig 197, magnif 105×.)
a) Adenosis. Marked proliferation and neoformation of acini in one lobule. In center of lobule ectatic lactiferous ducts filled with secretions.
b) Smoothly defined satellite nodule in breast. Tumorous thrombosis of peripheral veins (Fig 197).
c) Border of apple-sized, giant-cell, anaplastic, cellular, medullary primary carcinoma. Remaining parenchyma (right) with ectasia and round cell infiltration of ducts.
d) Tumor embolus in capsular vein of tumor (Fig 197).

194 *Mammogram* (mastectomy specimen). Very dense breast with large opacity and multiple coarse densities (adenoses and satellite tumors). Primary tumor (above left in figure).

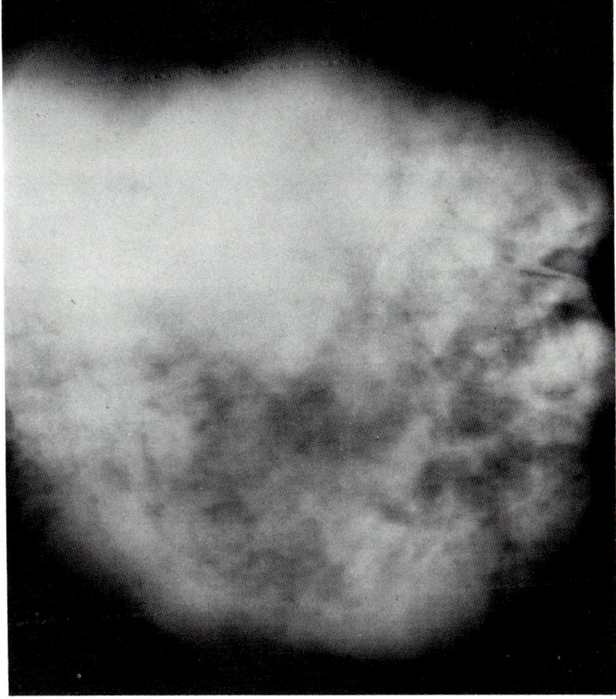

194

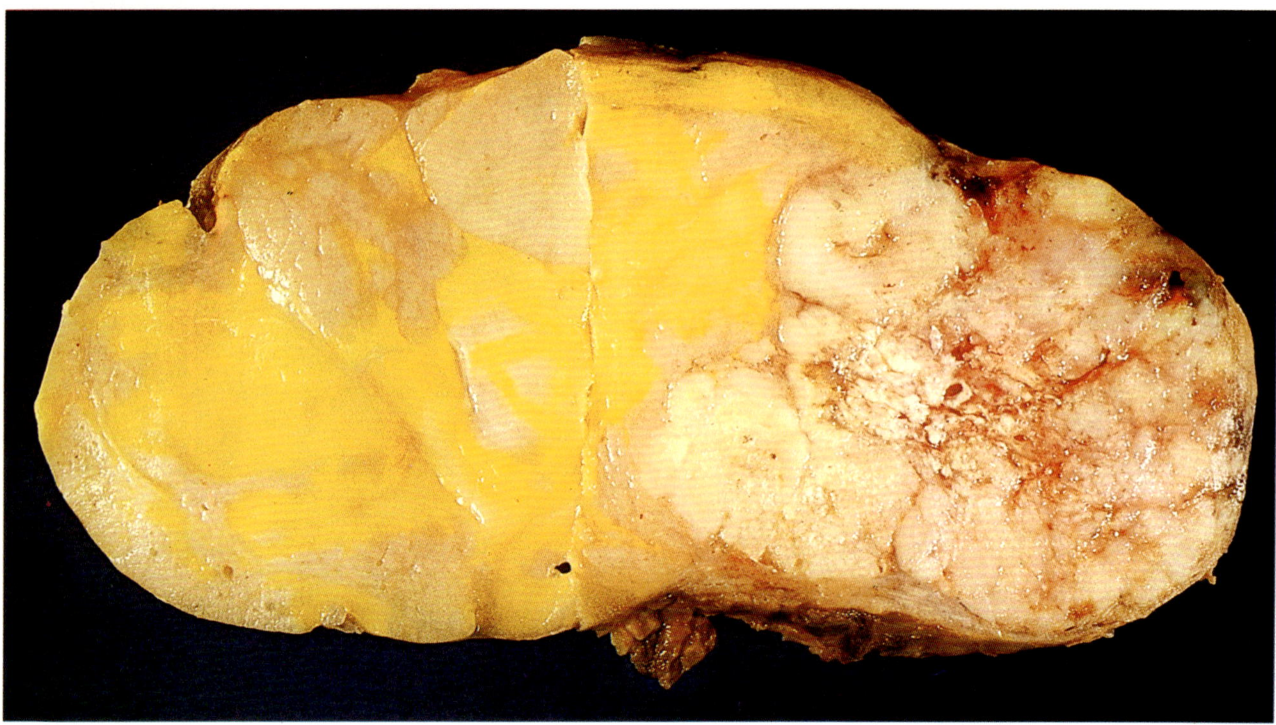

△
195 *Macroscopic cross-section* of breasts. Right: lobulated, multilobular carcinoma with multiple small hemorrhagic necroses. Left: breast parenchyma with fatty tissue (yellow) and gray-brown vitreous areas particularly at edge of breast (foci of adenosis).

196 *Specimen radiograph.* Tumor with central necrosis. ▷ Nonhomogeneous radio-opacity. Nodular contour. Confluent and markedly enlarged lobules in the breast, causing smooth oval opacities in less radiopaque fatty tissue. They are confluent at edge of specimen to form nonhomogeneous, large opacity.

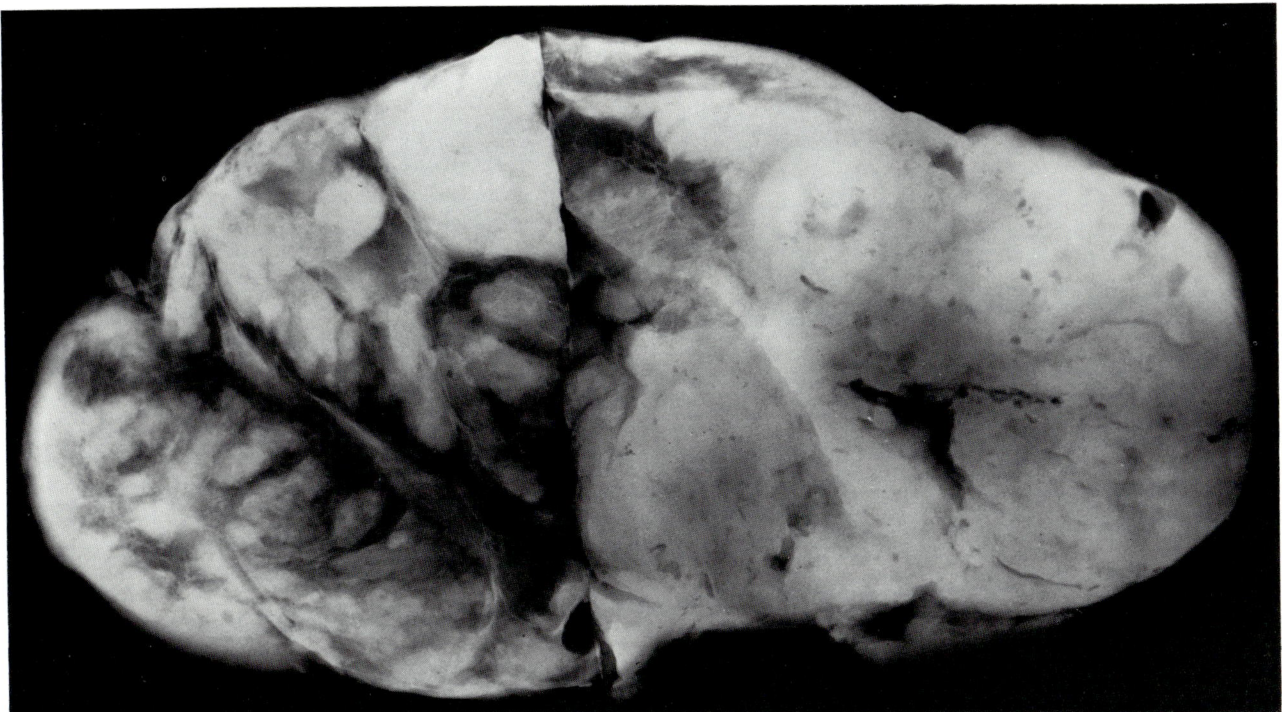

196

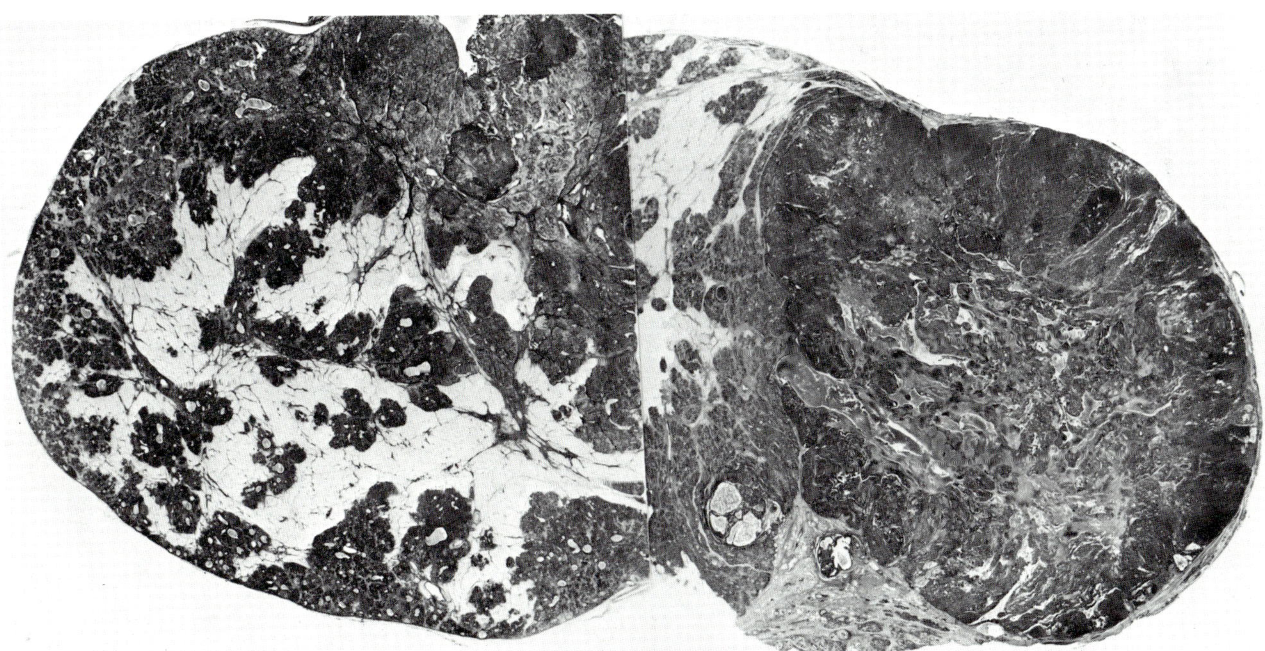

197

197 *Histological macrosection.* Carcinomatous nodule with band-like, central necrosis (cross hatched in drawing). Smooth delineation from breast parenchyma (compare Fig 193c). Markedly enlarged lobules with centrally located dilated ducts (dotted in drawing) (adenoses, compare Fig 193a). At upper edge (left of midline) and at left-lower edge of main tumor (arrow), five metastatic satellite tumors, partially necrotic (compare Fig 193b). Marked proliferation of entire breast with multiple carcinomatous nodules and adenoses of lobules caused marked enlargement of breast within a period of 3 months. At upper edge on right, tumorous thrombosis in a capsular vein (two arrows) (Fig 193d).

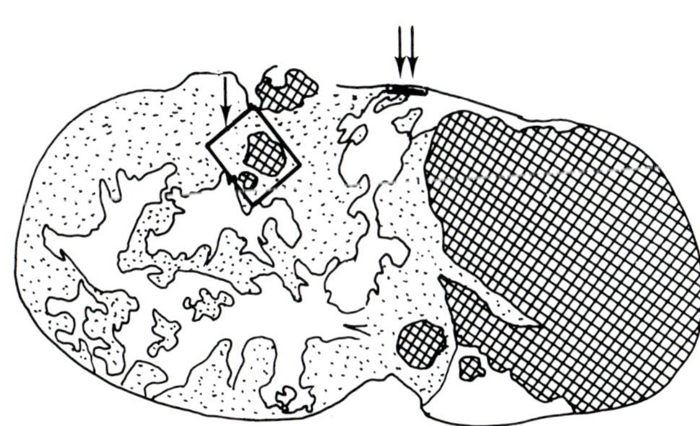

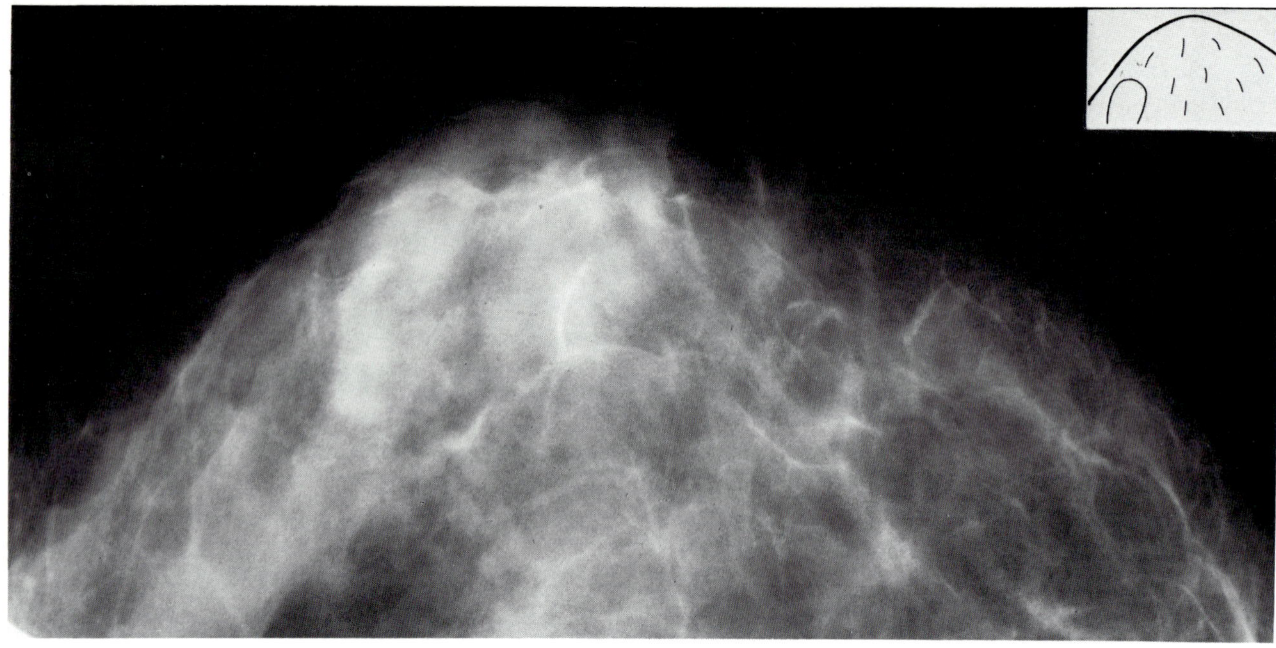

198

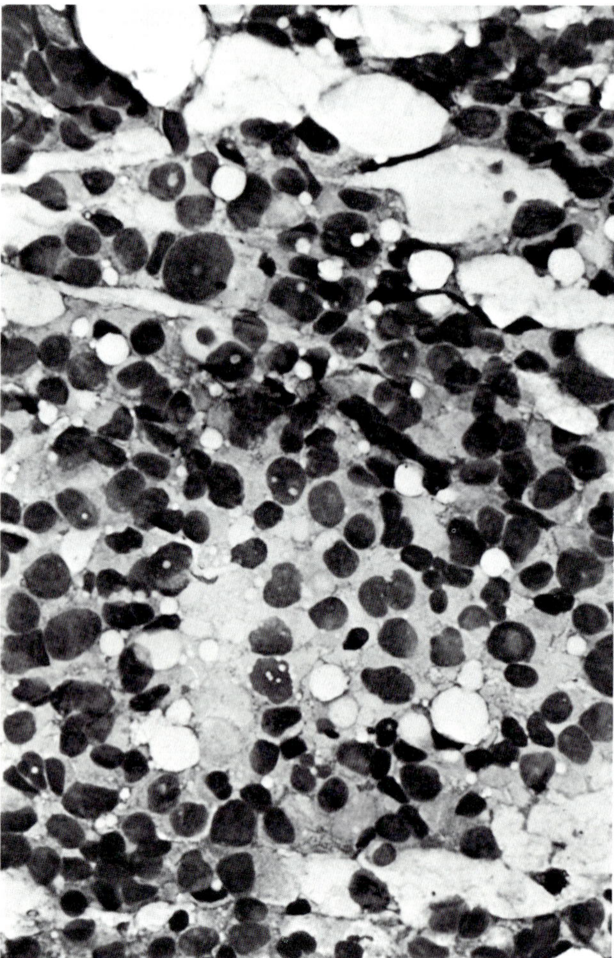

199

30-year-old female, left breast. Easily movable, walnut-sized, soft tumor in outer-upper quadrant (Figs 198–199).

198 *Mammogram* (cranio-caudal). Breast structure normal for age. Faintly radiopaque, walnut-sized, sharply defined opacity laterally, apparent only after learning of its presence by palpation. Presumed cyst. Thin-needle biopsy: no cyst but solid tumor. Large number of cells.

199 *Cytology.* Numerous tumor cells, partially without cytoplasm. Polymorphous nuclei with regressive changes (vacuoles in nucleus and plasma). Histology: medullary carcinoma without metastasis to axillary lymph nodes.

52-year-old female, right breast. Small, easily movable nodule in lower outer quadrant (Figs 200–201). ▷

200 *Mammogram* (cranio-caudal). Partially smooth-, partially ill-defined opacity. No microcalcifications. Suspicious for carcinoma. Histology: mucoid carcinoma.

201 a, b. *Histological-microradiographic comparison.*
a) Histology, magnif 20×. Mucoid carcinoma nodule with abundant mucus (light) and lobulated smooth contour. To its left, solid carcinoma with abundant stroma (dark).
b) Microradiograph, magnif 20×. Mucoid carcinoma is less radiopaque than stroma-rich solid carcinoma. The tumor has multiple stromal septa and is chamber-like. These septa have the same radio-opacity as those of solid carcinoma. It would appear that they have an identical matrix. Circumscribed mucoid nodule within solid carcinoma, secondary to production of mucus with increased radiographic lucency.

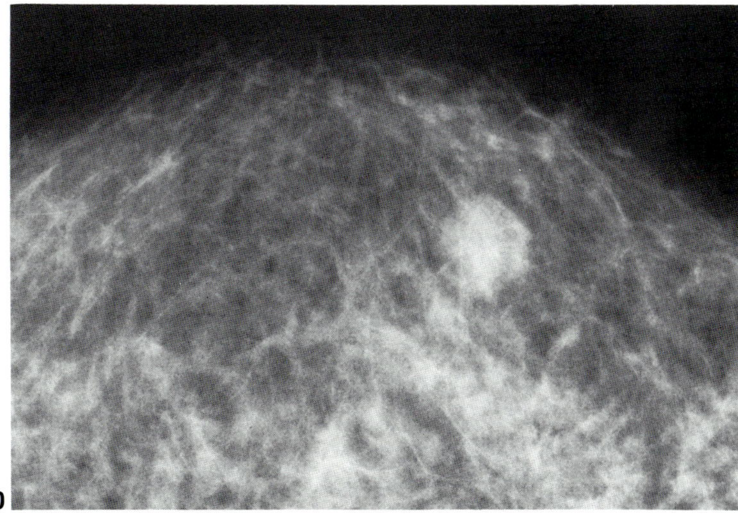

200

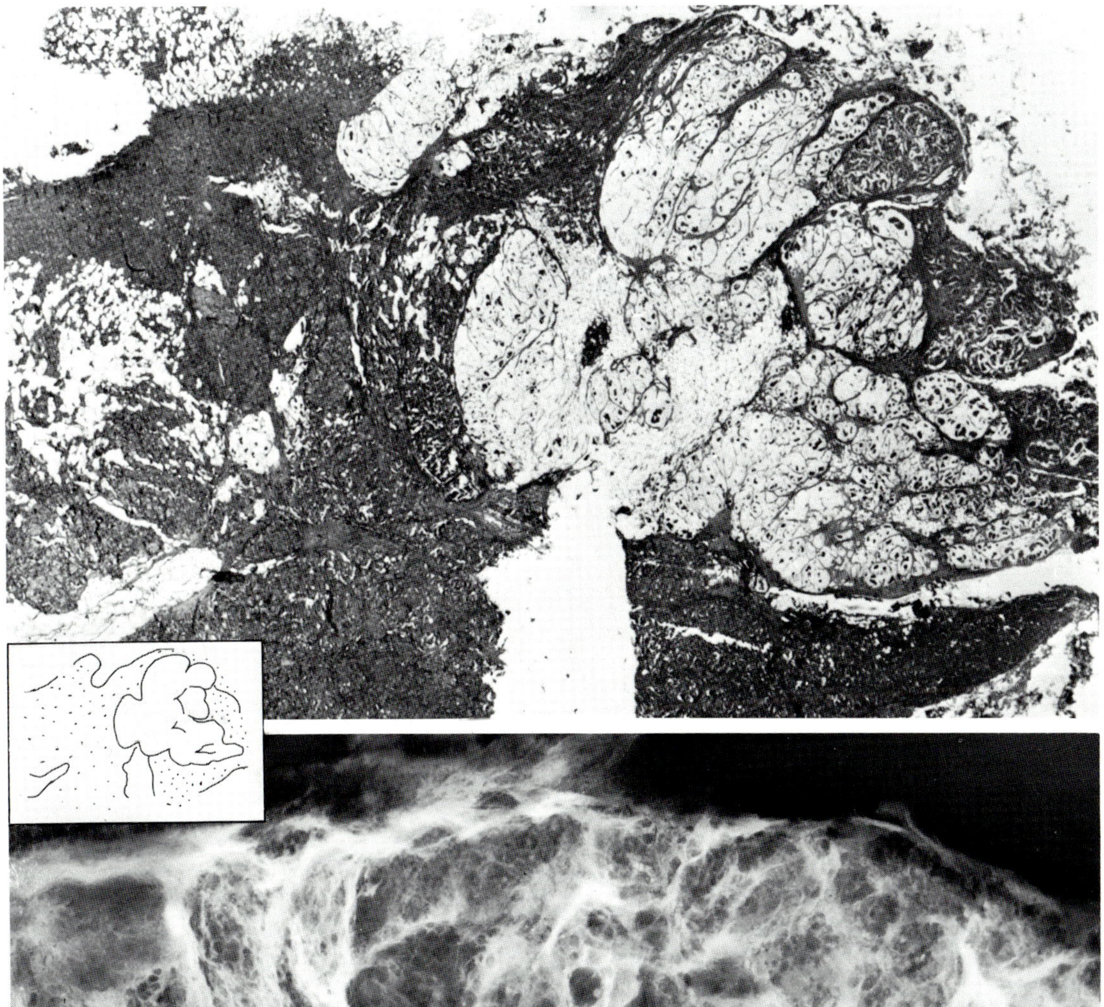

201 a

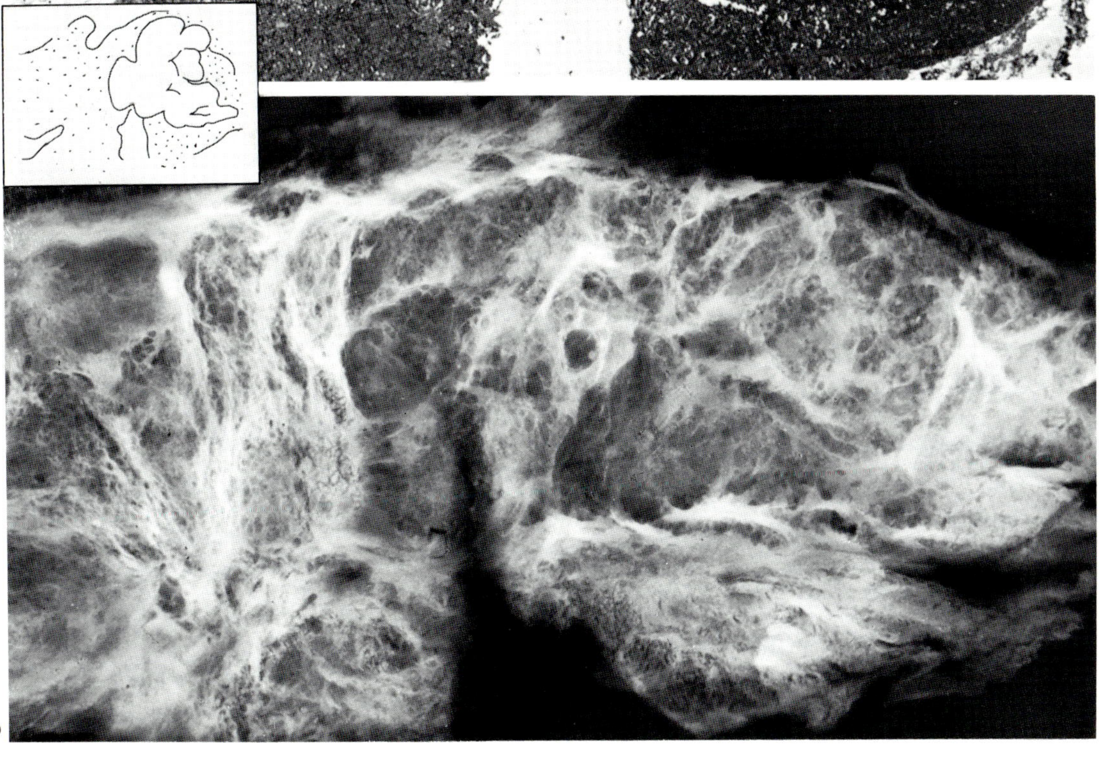

201 b

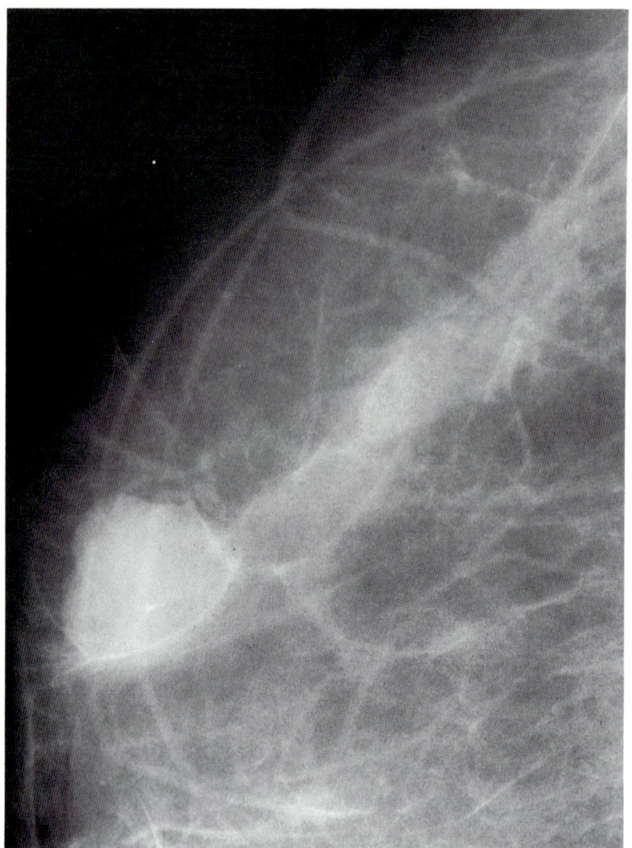

202 a

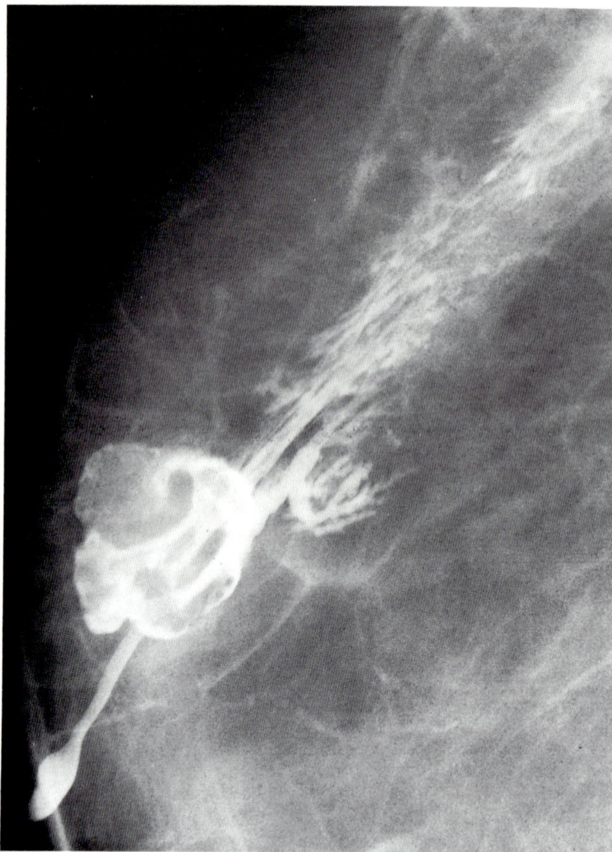

202 b

38-year-old female, right breast. For 4 weeks cherry-sized nodule in upper outer quadrant. Easily movable on palpation. Presumed fibroadenoma or cyst. For many years serous secretions from duct (Fig 202).

202

a) *Mammogram* (medio-lateral). Lobulated homogeneous opacity resting on broad base, a band-like opacity. Some comedocalcifications.

b) *Galactography* (medio-lateral). An intraductal tumor is outlined by contrast medium. In region of band-like opacity an increased number of peripheral ducts with peripheral defects in column of contrast medium. Diagnosis: papilloma of duct. Peripheral intraductal proliferations. Thin-needle biopsy.

202

c) *Cytology.* Ductal macrophages and large, benign-appearing uniform sheets of epithelium. Hyperchromatic nuclei.

d) In addition to normal epithelial layers, small groups of cells with markedly polymorphous, hyperchromatic nuclei. Broad rim of cytoplasm. Multiple nuclei. Suspicion of malignant degeneration.

e) *Histology.* Base of intraductal papilloma with dilated duct. In lumen of one duct are desquamated tumor cells. Diagnosis: papilloma with transformation into papillary ductal carcinoma.

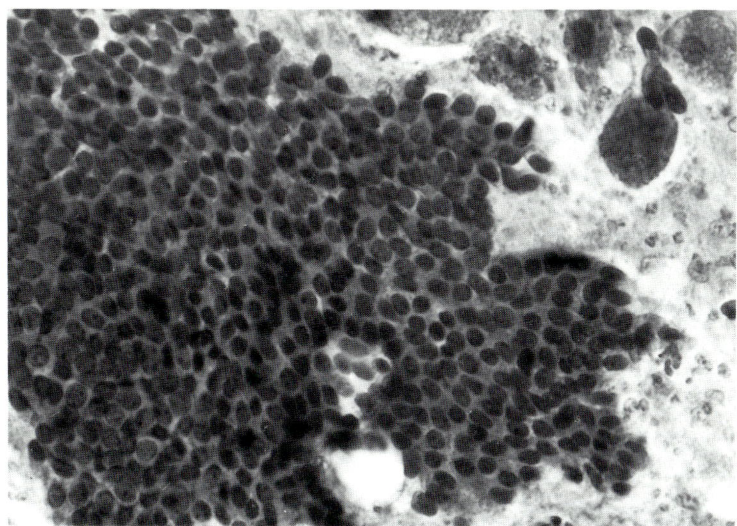

202c

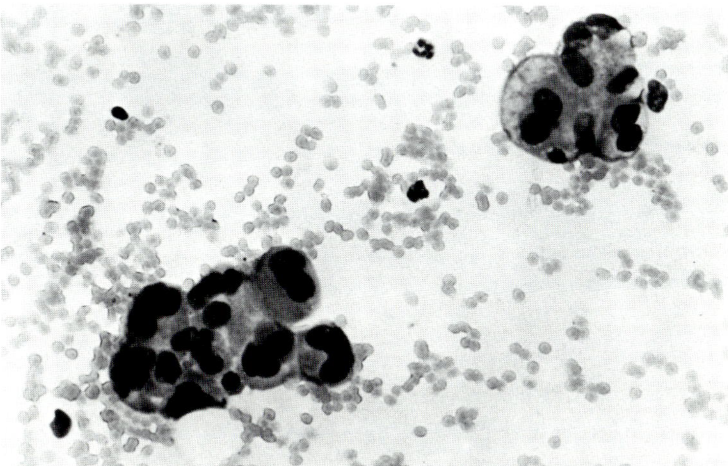

202d

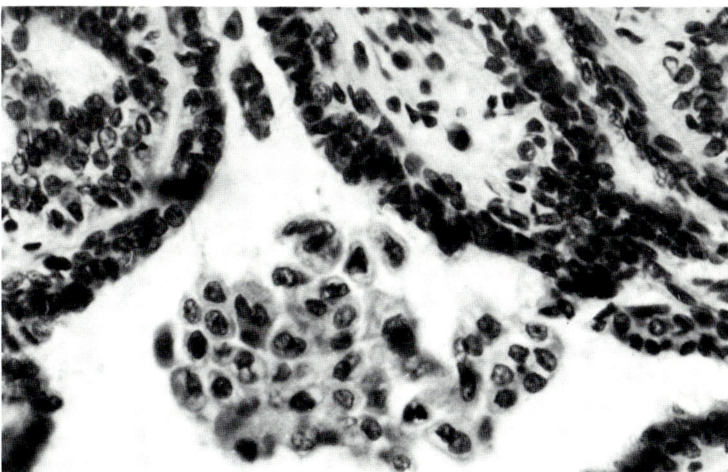

202e

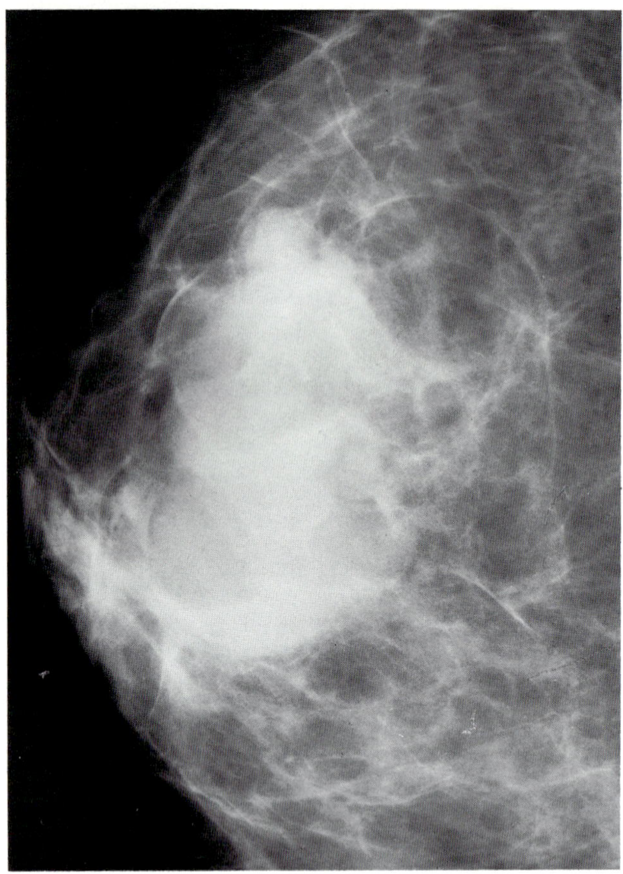
203a

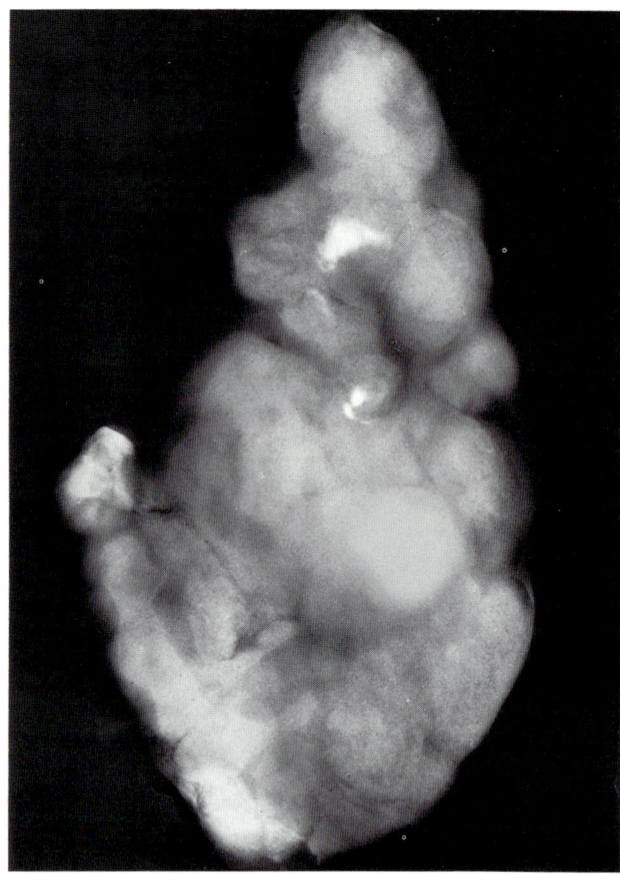
203b

55-year-old female, left breast. Treatment for malignant lymphoma for 5 years. Involvement of left supraclavicular and axillary lymph nodes. Cherry-sized tumor in left breast for past 4 years. Regression of this nodule after repeated chemotherapy treatments. In past 6 months renewed increase in size. Current palpation shows walnut-sized, retroareolar, easily movable nodule. No tenderness (Fig 203).

203
a) *Mammogram.* Nodular, homogeneous, dense tumor, predominantly smooth. In dorsal portion, however, ill-defined delineation from breast parenchyma. In upper part of nodule are coarse calcifications.
b) *Specimen radiograph.* Conglomerate of multiple small nodular opacities. Coarse calcium deposits.

c) *Histological macrosection.* Lymphomatous tumor. At lower edge new tumor parenchyma. At upper edge marked necrosis with necrotizing and calcified cell remnants (after chemotherapy).
d) Enlarged section (from c), magnif 260×. Malignant lymphatic cells with polymorphous and polychromatic nuclei. Little stroma. At upper edge of figure necrotic epithelium clearly separated from active tumor (less pigmented).
e) *Surgical specimen.* Nodular tumor dissected from fat and cut open. Active parenchyma reddish-brown. Necrotic tumor grayish-white, well defined from the active cellular portion of the tumor. ▷

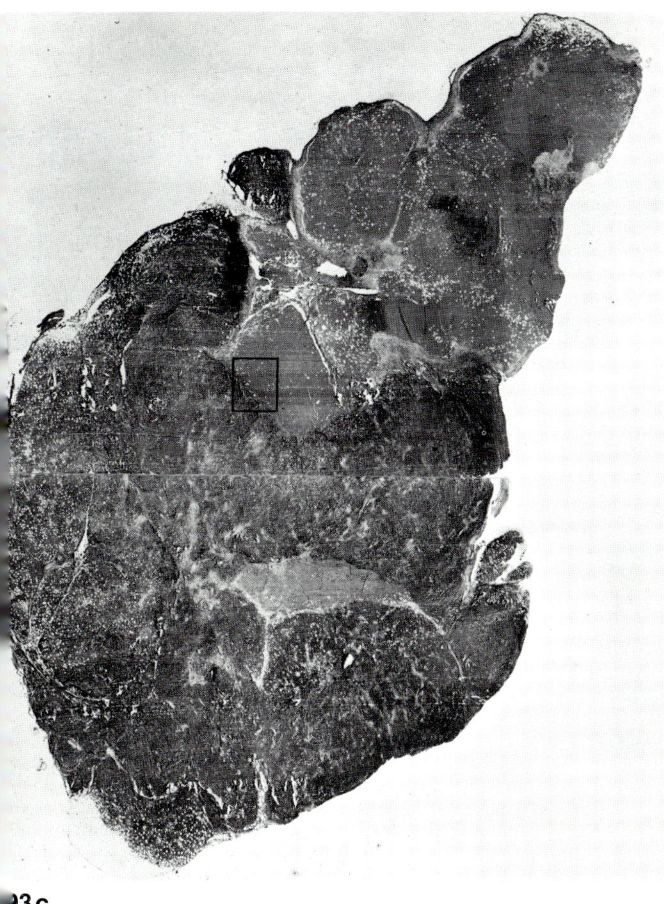

03c

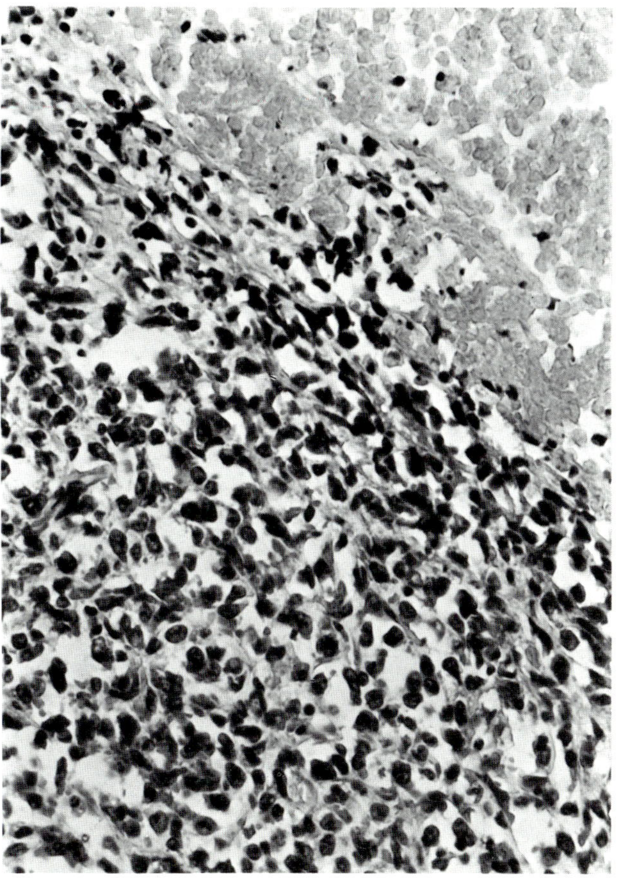

203d

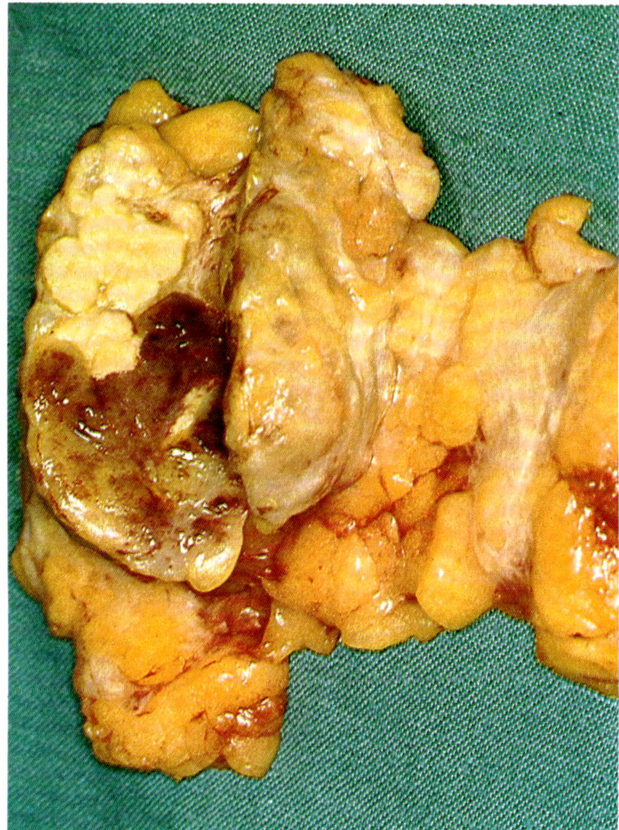

203e

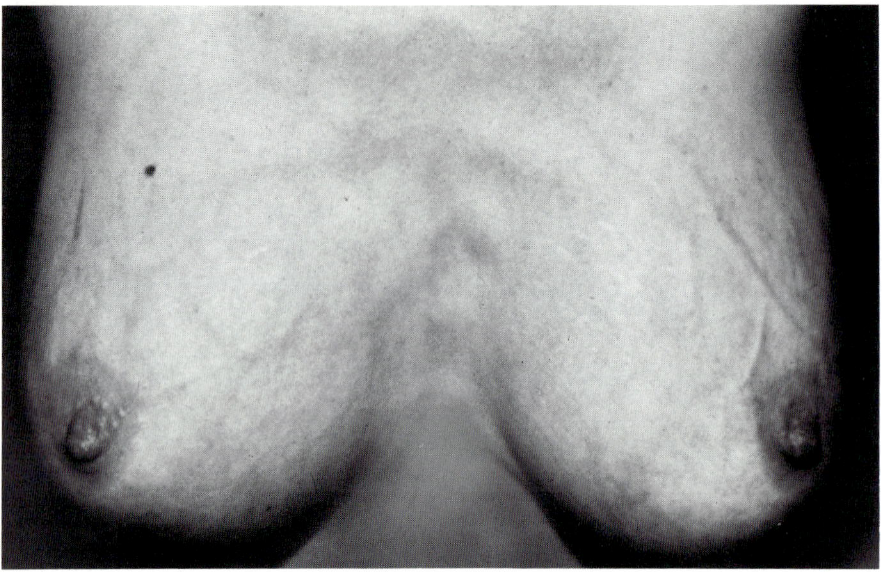
204

53-year-old female, left breast. Hospitalized for 4 weeks because of right heart failure. Superior vena cava syndrome. Moderate enlargement of left breast. Enlarged superficial veins. Firm, poorly movable tumor in upper outer quadrant. Death secondary to right heart failure (Figs 204–208).

204 Appearance of both breasts. Moderate enlargement of left breast. Increased superficial venous pattern.

205 a, b. *Mammogram* (medio-lateral).

a) Left breast 2 years earlier. Fibrocystic mastopathy. No evidence of malignancy.

b) Mammogram, follow-up examination. Homogeneous opacity of entire right breast. Tumor density in upper quadrant area with smooth and ill-defined contours. No microcalcifications.

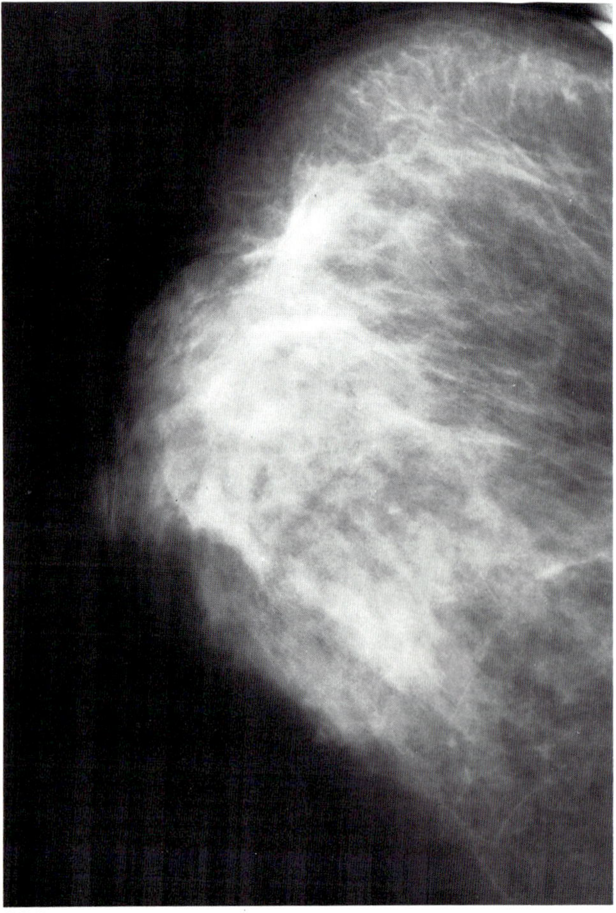
205 a

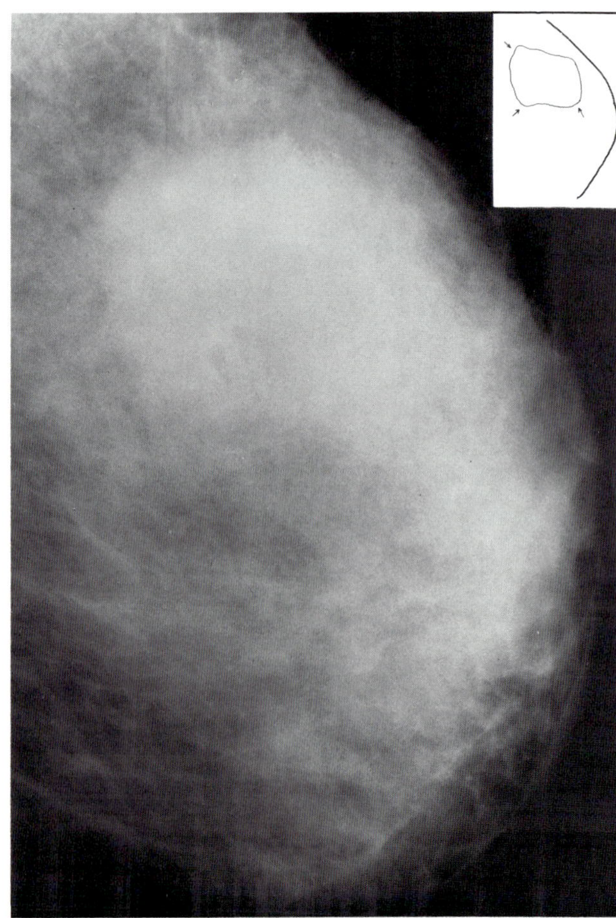
205 b

206 *Surgical specimen.* Nodular, lobulated tumor with hemorrhagic foci. Sharp delineation from breast parenchyma.

207 a, b. *Cytology and histology.*
a) Cytology. With thin-needle biopsy numerous, partially spindle-shaped tumor cells. Marked lymphocytic infiltration. In right corner multinucleated giant cells.
b) Histology. Mesenchymal tumor with spindle-shaped, mesenchymal cells having ill-defined borders. Abundant delicate fiber formation. Many lymphocytes. Multinucleated giant cells. Diagnosis: cellular, spindle-cell sarcoma with many giant cells.

208 Tumor metastasis in right ventricle. Ventricle and atrium opened, posterior cusp of tricuspid valve recognizable between atrium and ventricle. Apex of heart below. Cylindrical, nodular tumor grown from right atrium through posterior cusp of tricuspid valve into right ventricle. The tumor extends to apex of heart and projects into pulmonary outflow tract (not visible). Superior vena cava syndrome and cause of death explained by these findings.

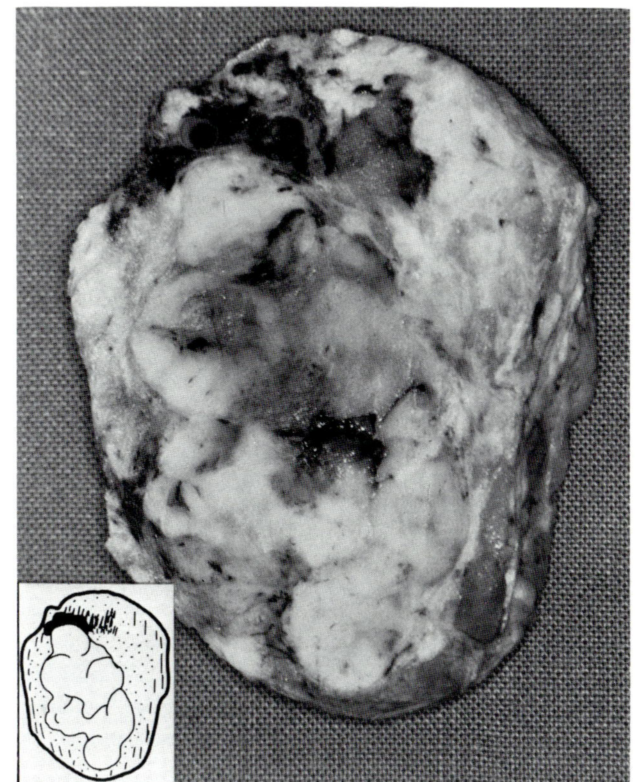

206

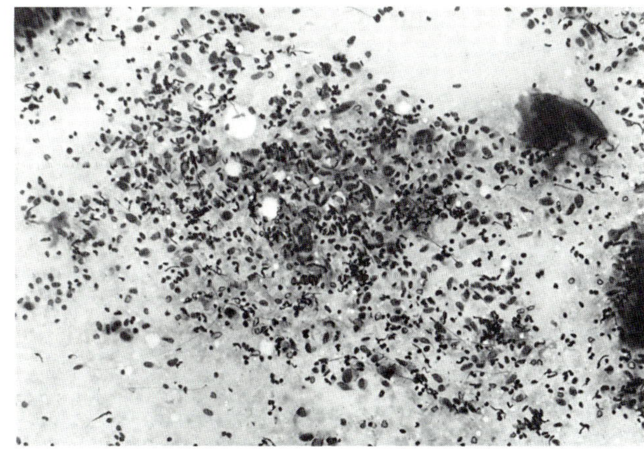

207 a

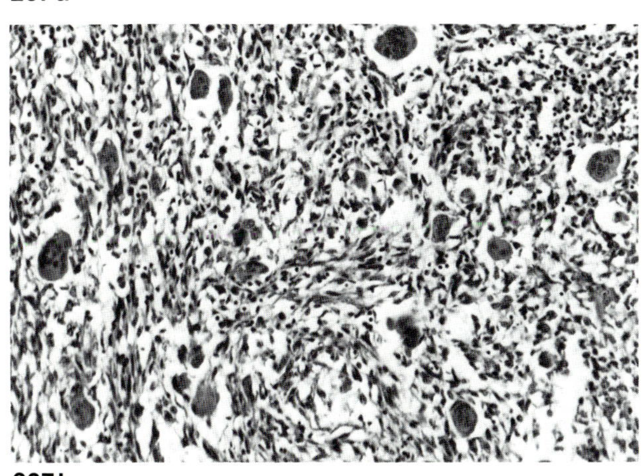

207 b

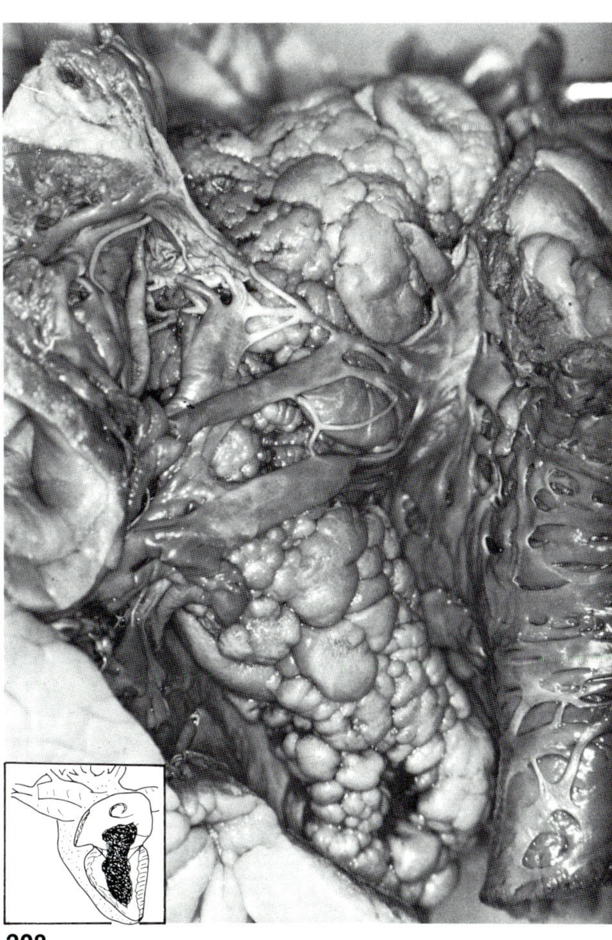

208

Predominantly ductal spread of tumor

There are tumors *with* (Fig **209**) and *without* calcifications (Fig **216**) because not all ductal carcinomas tend to become necrotic with deposition of calcium.
This type of tumor causes characteristic radiographic-anatomic changes in the breast. If associated with calcifications, it allows diagnosis; if not, the diagnosis is delayed.
In the absence of calcifications there are radiographically curvilinear, band-like, partially net-like opacities without solid tumor density. Ectatic and double-contoured ducts are also noted (Fig **110**). Diagnosis in early stages is difficult since similar densities also may occur with atypical or benign changes of ducts from periductal fibrosis. In the stroma-rich breast, particularly with central location of the tumor, retraction of the nipple may be the first and only sign of malignancy (Fig **216**).
Calcified tumors, however, are recognizable radiographically very early, prior to clinical changes in the breast. The calcium deposits often are needle-like and in groups. At times they are arranged as fine, stipple-like calcifications following the course of the ducts (Fig **209**). Tumor density is always absent at first. In early stages no nodule or induration is palpable. In very late and already infiltrating stages, there are circumscribed nodular indurations in the breast; a single circumscribed nodule is not palpable.
Only a few duct carcinomas cause abnormal secretion. When it occurs, usually it is serous, occasionally milky and rarely bloody (Fig **210**). Bloody secretion is found more frequently with duct *papilloma*.
Intraductal, neoplastic, epithelial proliferations may cause increased nipple temperature—thermographically 0.5 to 1 °C higher than normal (hot nipple). Normally the nipple is cold in comparison to the areola and remaining breast. A unilateral, even minimally increased temperature (0.5 °C) is indicative of intraductal epithelial proliferation (Figs **114** d, **248**).

Mammographic prognosis of a carcinoma

Radiological classification of carcinomas as "stellate," "nodular" and "intraductal" has prognostic significance. According to von Albertini (1974) all undifferentiated carcinomas with the exception of medullary carcinoma have similarly poor prognosis (scirrhus, solid carcinoma, adeno-scirrhus). Mammographically these are the stellate neoplasias. Only medullary carcinoma has a more favorable prognosis among undifferentiated tumors. Radiographically this tumor shows nodular growth without calcifications. The pure mucoid carcinoma has a similar appearance. The latter and pure comedocarcinoma have the best prognosis among all cancers. The comedocarcinoma can be recognized early radiographically if associated with calcifications which, according to Hassler (1969), can be expected to occur in two thirds of all cases.
There is continuous radiographic transition between stellate, nodular and intraductal growth with relatively little significance regarding prognosis. The stellate-growing carcinomas have the poorest prognosis. Prognosis is more favorable with nodular, smoothly-defined tumors and is best with pure comedocarcinoma which in two thirds of all cases can be recognized radiographically by typical calcifications.

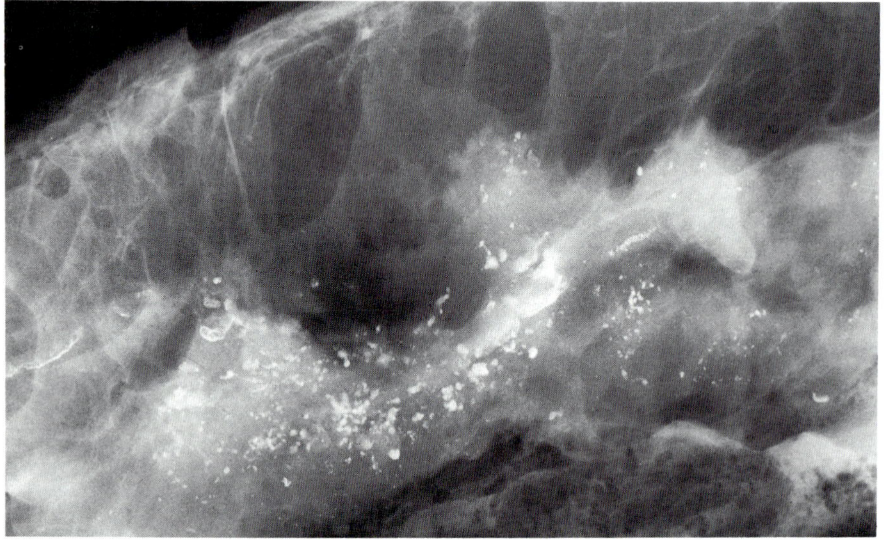

209 Comedocarcinoma with various-sized calcifications in ground-glass, nonhomogeneous, indistinct opacity of breast. No circumscribed tumor density. At left edge of figure are calcified vessels.

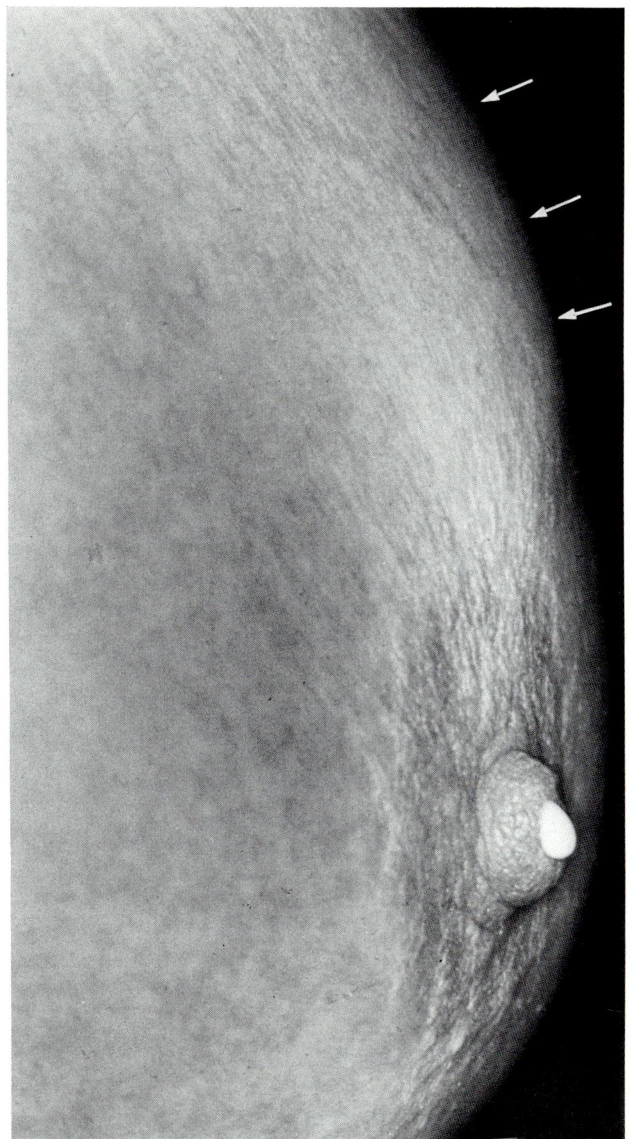

210

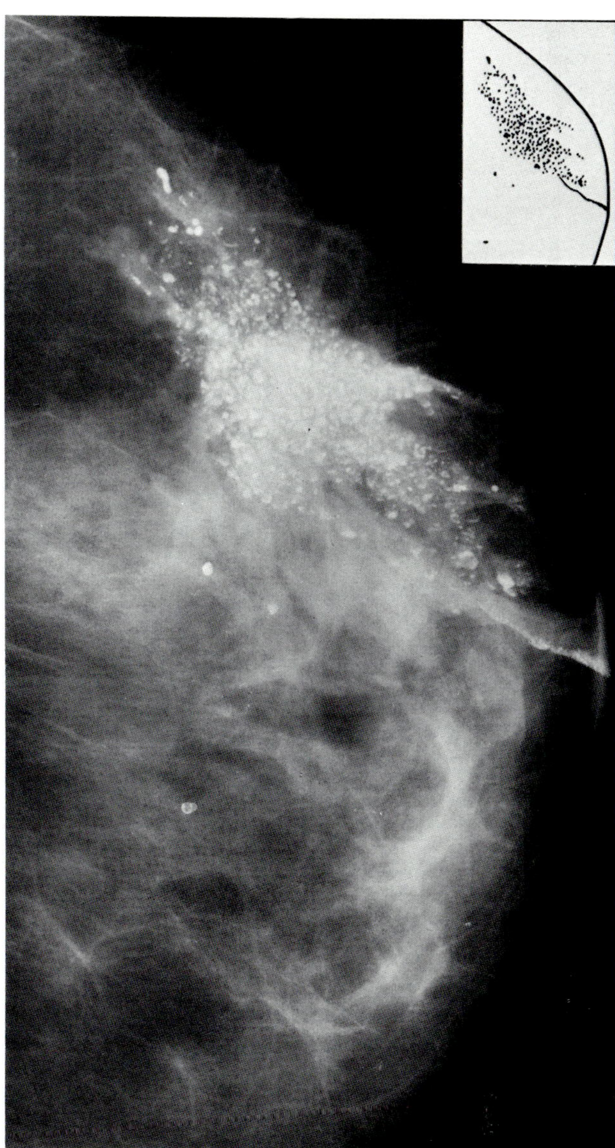

211

64-year-old female. For 2 years secretion of milk from the left breast. Firm, easily movable nodule above nipple with protrusion of skin (Figs 210–213).

210 *Inspection.* Tumor protrusion of skin. A drop of milky secretion at nipple.

211 *Mammogram* (medio-lateral). Extensive coarse group calcifications. Extension along ducts and Cooper's ligaments. Calcifications can be traced into nipple.

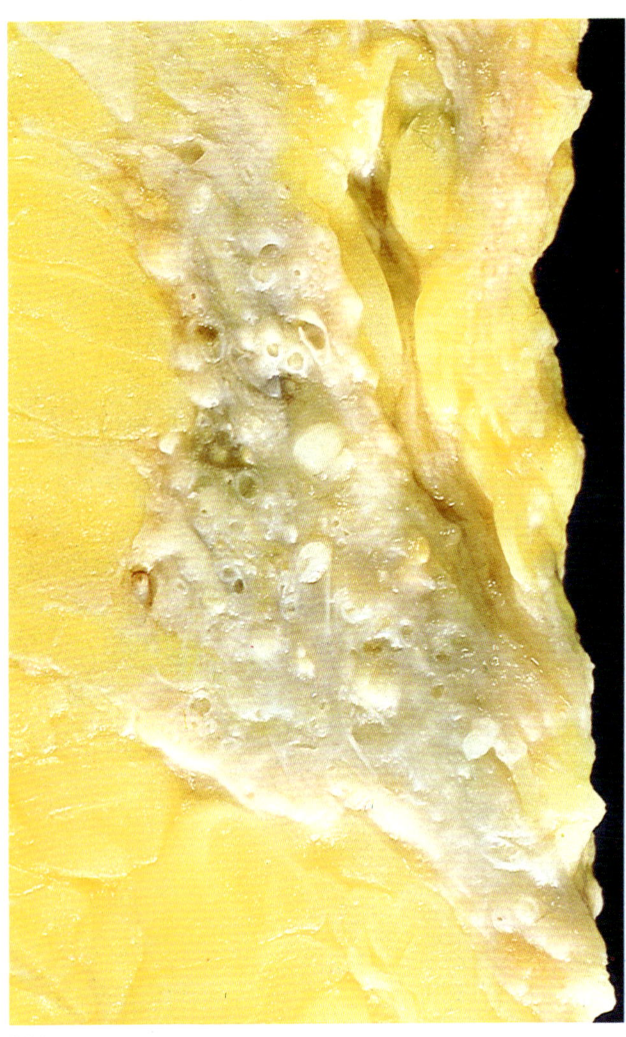

212

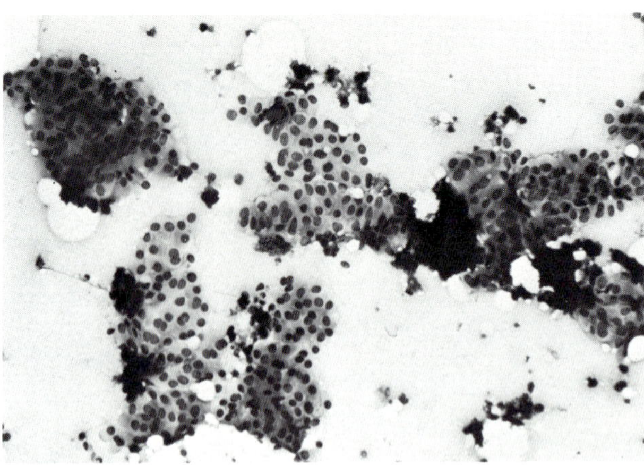

213 a

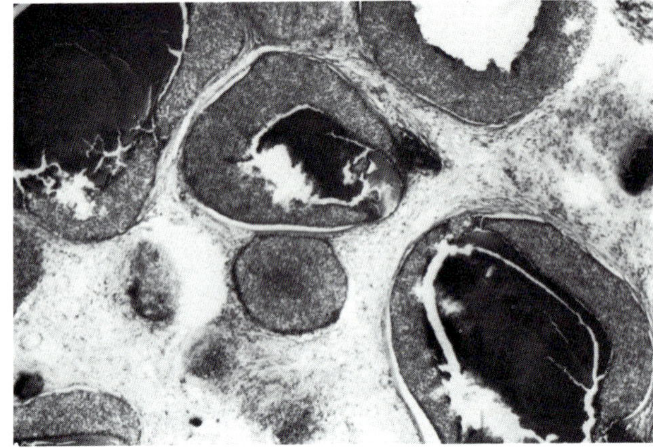

213 b

212 *Cut section of tumor.* Ectatic and partially ruptured gray-white ducts with yellowish calcium plugs.

213 a, b. *Cytology and histology.*

a) Cytology. With thin-needle aspiration, multiple layers of tumor cells of ductal origin with broad cytoplasm. Only slightly polymorphous nuclei. Multiple bizarre calcium particles (black).

b) Histology. So-called comedocarcinoma with markedly dilated ducts; in contiguous tumor parenchyma coarse calcifications. Magnif 25×.

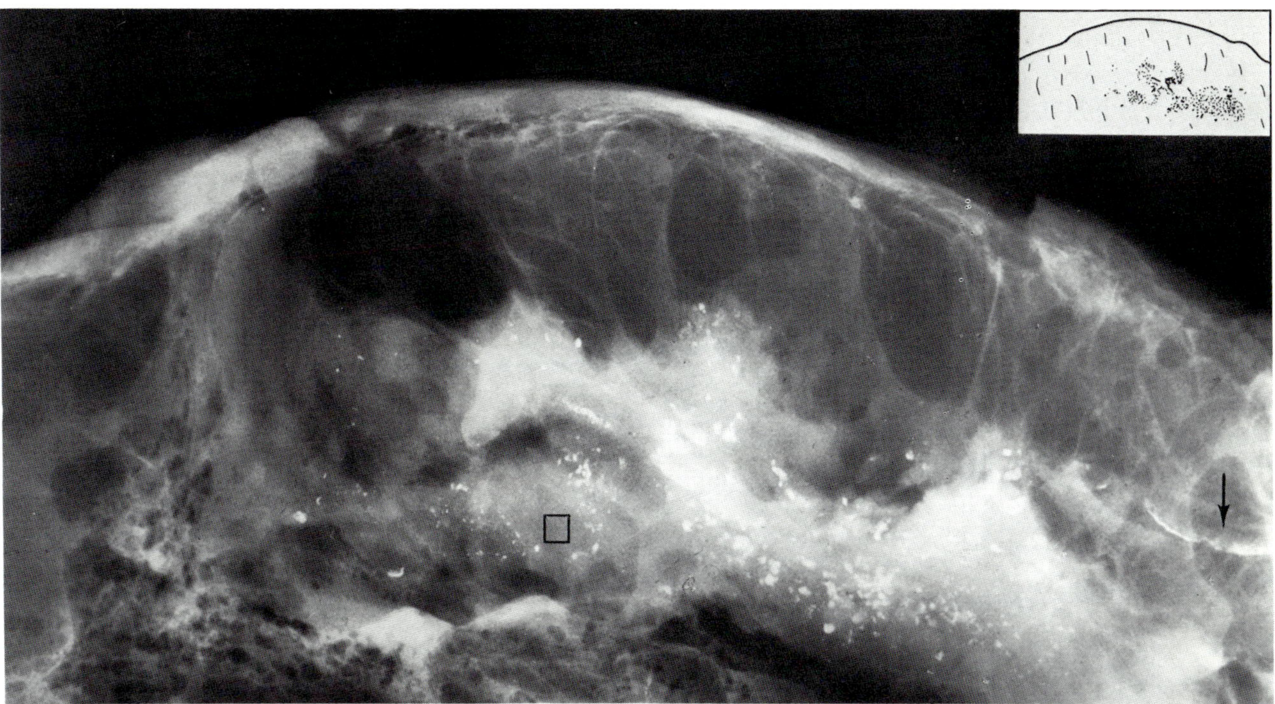

△
214 *Specimen radiograph* of comedocarcinoma. Coarse and tiny calcium deposits in entire breast. Faintly radio-opaque, small, low contrast tumor density with nonhomogeneous cloudy opacities next to ducts. At right side of figure vascular calcifications (arrow). Histologically: infiltrating duct carcinoma with marked calcium deposits in ducts.

215 *Microradiograph,* magnif 105× (from Fig 214). Multiple, slightly dilated ducts (dark spotty areas) containing partially round, partially bizarre appearing calcium particles (white opacities). Among microscopic calcium particles only those larger than 0.2 mm are recognizable in mammogram. ▷

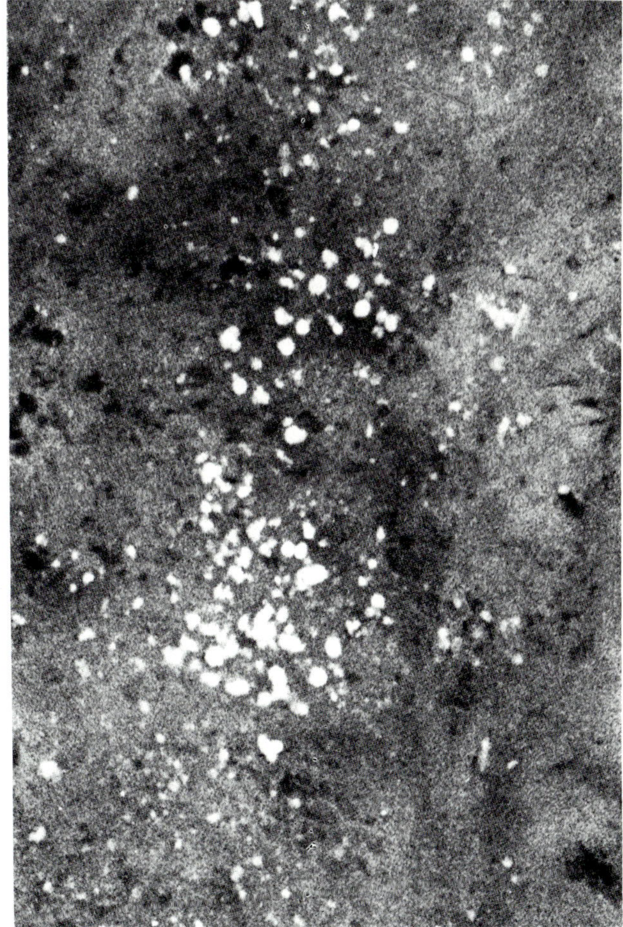

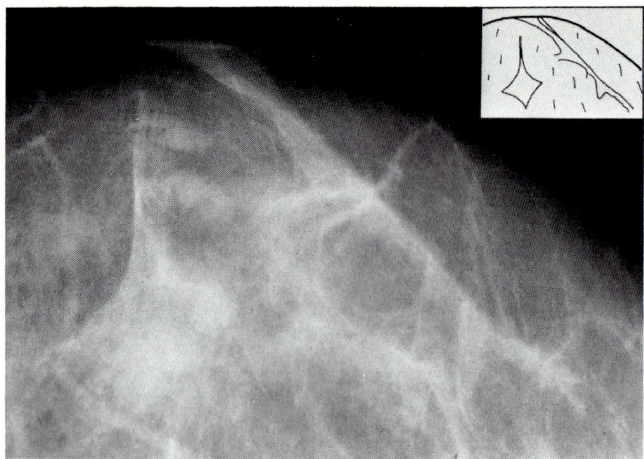

216

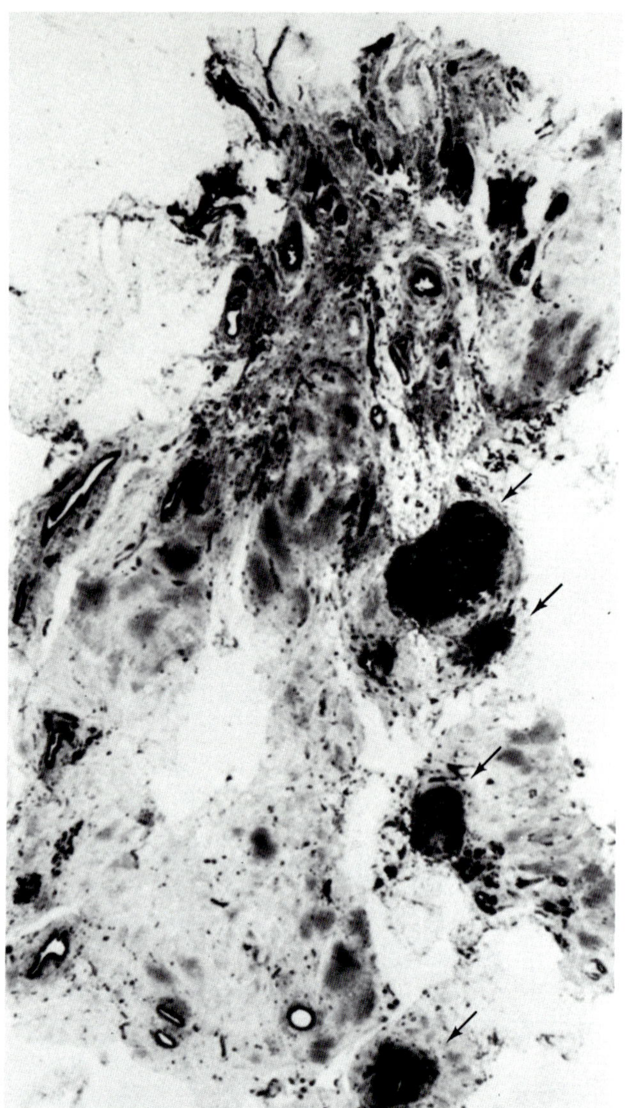

217

65-year-old female, right breast. Nipple retraction for several weeks. Negative palpation (Figs 216–221).

216 *Mammogram* (cranio-caudal). Band-like opacity originating from the nipple. Wrong diagnosis: fibrosis of breast.

217 *Histological macrosection* of retroareolar space (nipple above). Multiple dilated ducts filled with tumor (arrows). Because of intraductal spread, no homogeneous tumor density seen in mammogram (may be confused with fibrosis).

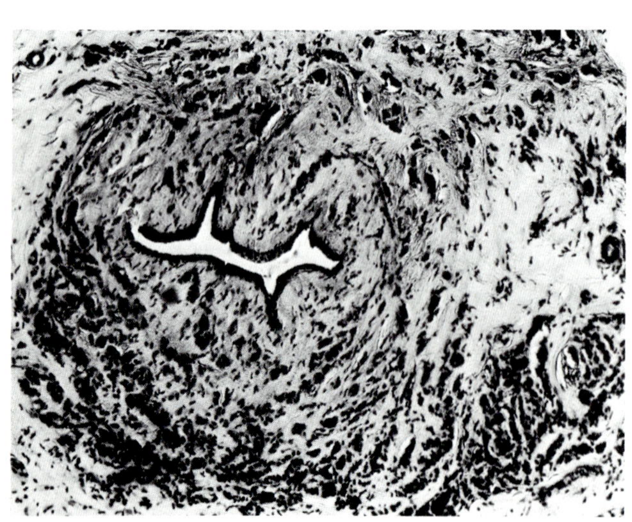

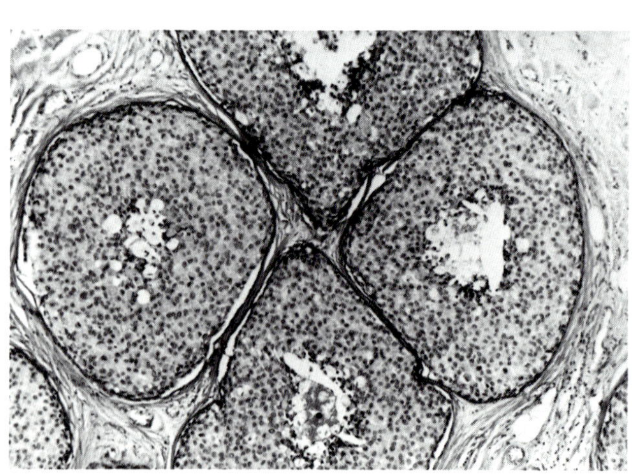

218 a, b. *Histology.*
a) Survey, magnif 40×. Main duct. Tumor cells (dark) in periductal stroma, lymph channels and small ducts. Diffuse infiltration of surrounding parenchyma (radiographically: ductal dilatation without circumscribed nodule).

b) Histology of an area distant from the nipple, magnif 105×. Small-cell, intraductal carcinoma. Ducts dilated and filled with tumor tissue. Basal membrane intact.

219 *Macroanatomy.* Partially lobulated, partially unsharp gray-white area with demonstration of ducts dilated by tumor plugs shown in cross-section.

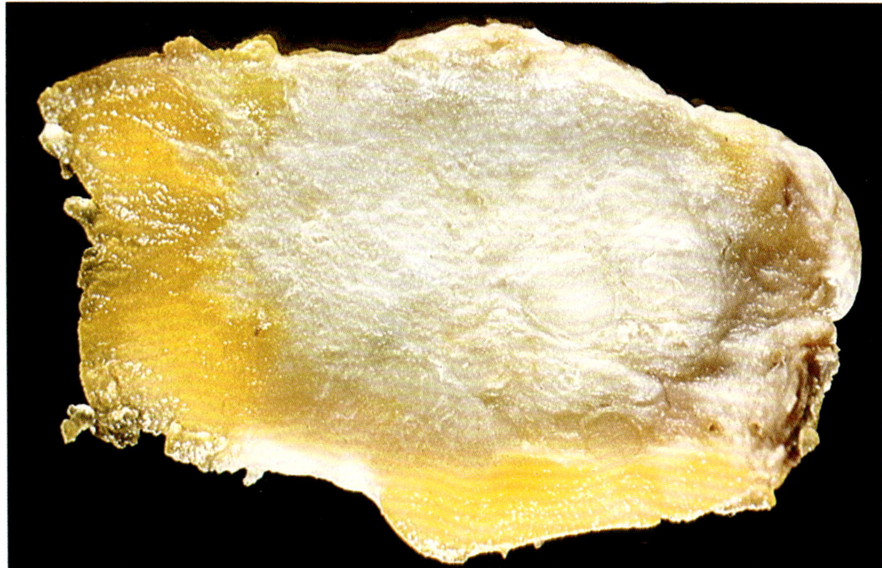

220 *Histology,* magnif 40×, van Gieson stain. Connective tissue reddish-brown. Ducts dilated by dark tumor masses (lower portion of figure). Fibrosed wall of ducts. At upper edge of figure many small ducts and lobules infiltrated by tumor (secondary lobular carcinoma).

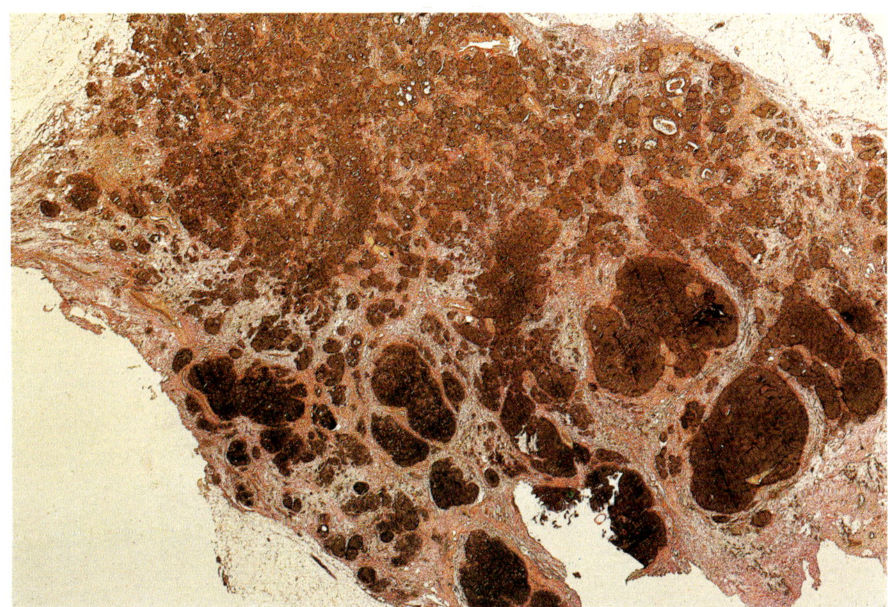

221 *Microradiograph,* magnif 40×. Tumor cells in dilated ducts are less radiopaque than fibrotic walls of ducts. In lobular carcinoma close by, likewise, less radio-opacity of infiltrated terminal ducts and lobules.

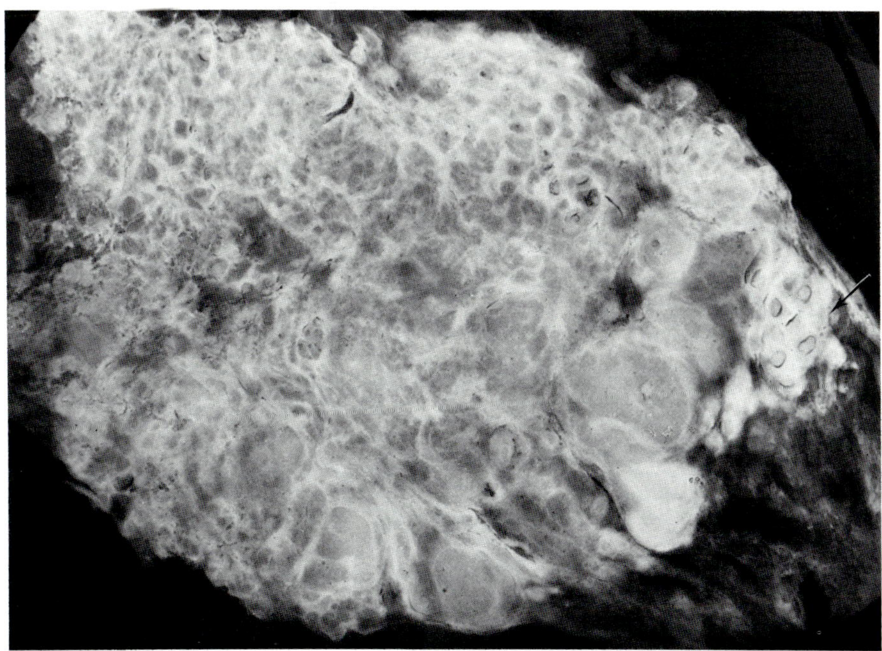

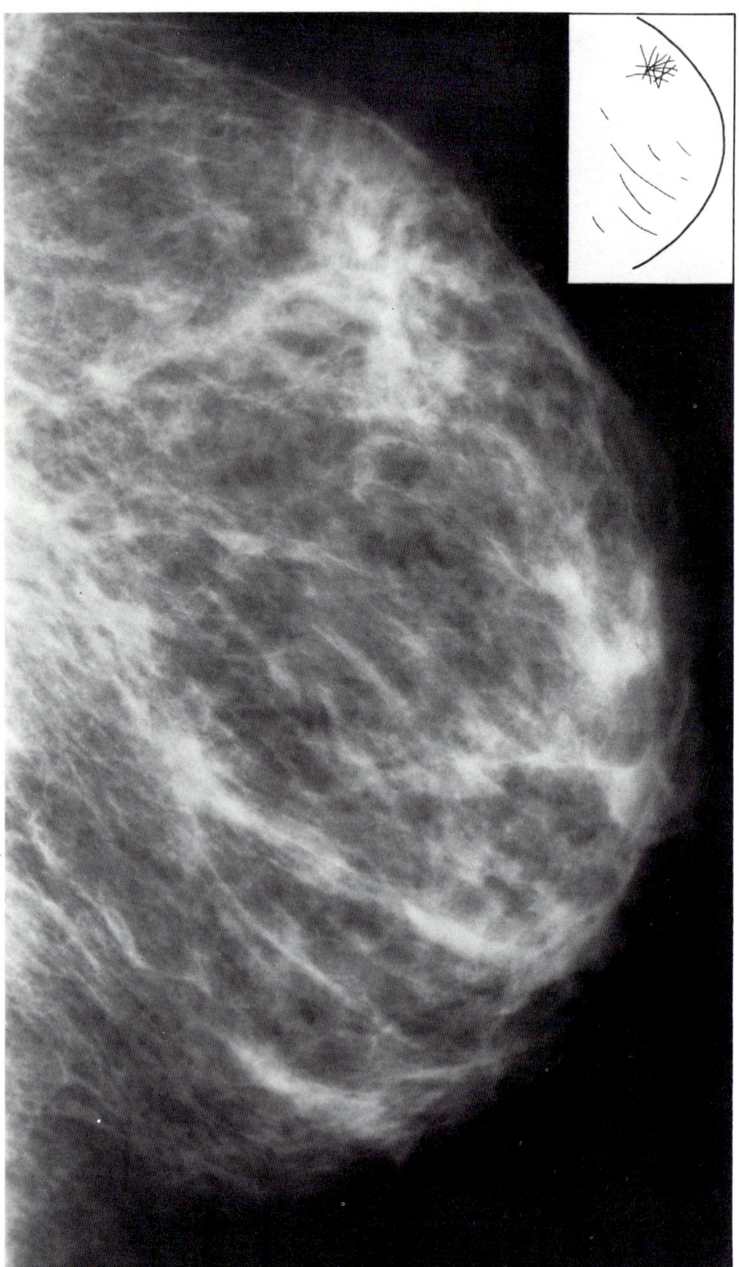

59-year-old female, left breast. On palpation circumscribed soft swelling in inner upper quadrant (Fig 222).

222 *Mammogram* (medio-lateral). Thickening of ducts of entire breast. In upper portion of breast nonhomogeneous, net-like thickening of breast structure. Histology: infiltrating duct carcinoma. No microcalcifications.

Special growth patterns of malignant breast tumors

Paget's disease, all other tumors of the nipple (Fig **223**) and cornifying, squamous-cell carcinoma arising from the epidermis belong to this group.
Paget's disease occurs after age 50. Clinically there is an eczematous change of the nipple. Cytological examination of secretions will differentiate it from inflammatory eczema.

A 63-year-old patient with generalized psoriasis was found to have scaling skin lesions over the entire body and both breasts. There had been eczematous changes of the left nipple for 2 years believed to be secondary to psoriasis and left untreated. After 3 years a large, coarse, painful tumor was found in the left breast with metastases in the axilla (Figs **229–231**).

The nipple radiographically is thickened in Paget's disease. Slight changes may be overlooked in mammograms of this area because it is commonly overexposed. In more advanced stages the retroareolar space becomes thickened. On occasion there may be comedo-calcifications (Fig **228**). Commonly a clinically occult duct carcinoma is found in mammograms in the retroareolar area or deeper. Nevertheless, when there is eczema of the nipple, absence of a tumor in the radiograph does not exclude Paget's disease.
Lymphosarcoma. The primary manifestation of a lymphosarcoma in the nipple region is shown in Fig **257**.
According to HAAGENSEN (1971) only 75 cases of primary breast lymphosarcoma have been reported in the world literature.
Histologically *reticulum-cell, lymphocytic, mixed* and *follicular* types can be distinguished.
The tumor can not be differentiated from carcinoma by palpation (Fig **203**). Skin retraction is rare.
Lymphosarcoma can be confused in frozen section with an undifferentiated, small-cell carcinoma resulting often in radical mastectomy (HAAGENSEN, 1971). The therapy of choice is rather *radiation* as lymphosarcomas are very radiosensitive.

A cylinder-like, painless swelling in the areola region occurred in a patient over a period of six months. The lesion was hyperthermic. Originally an inflammatory lesion was believed to be present and treated as such (oxyphenbutazon, antibiotics). There was no improvement within three weeks. Mammographically the nipple was thickened. The remaining breast was normal. Examination of cells from *thin-needle biopsy* suggested presence of a leukemic infiltrate. The *histological* examination of the nipple showed a lymphosarcoma of the lymphocytic type.

Lymphosarcoma of the areola and skin must be differentiated from benign skin lymphadenosis *(lymphadenosis benigna cutis)*. According to VON ALBERTINI (1974) in benign skin lymphadenosis there are extensive lymphatic infiltrates with localized nodules which may extend into subcutaneous tissue. These infiltrates are lymphatic tissue and not lymph nodes. The etiology is unclear. The tumor regresses after treatment with antibiotics.

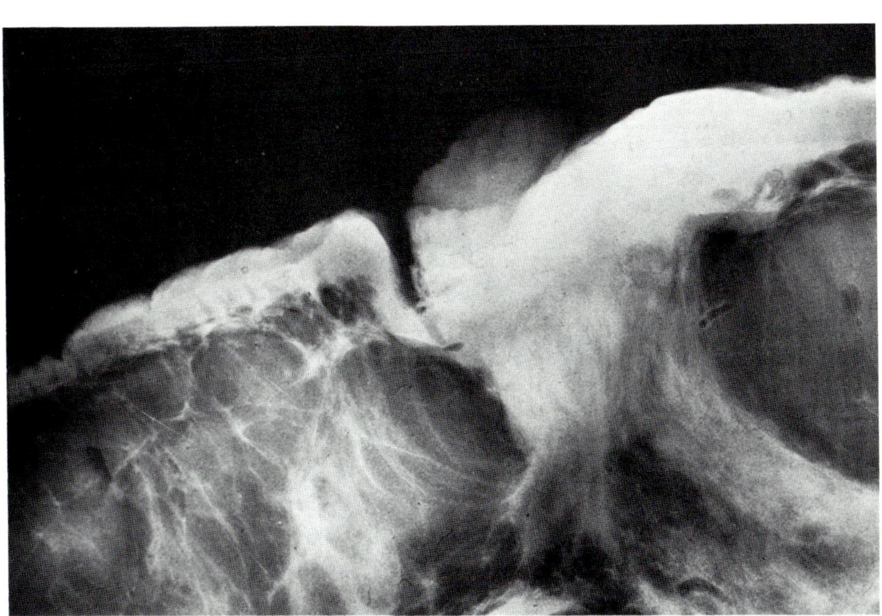

223 Scirrhous carcinoma in areola with nipple retraction.

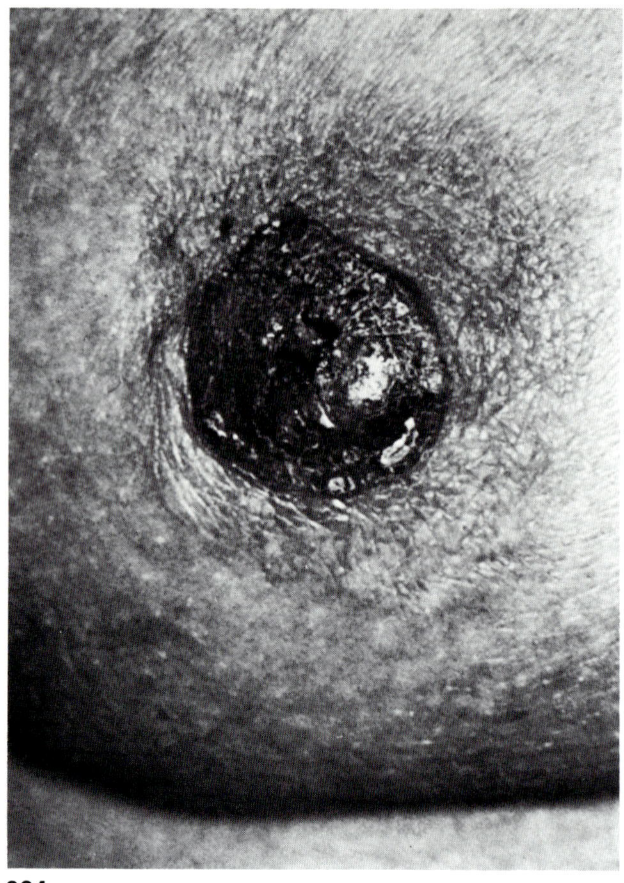

224

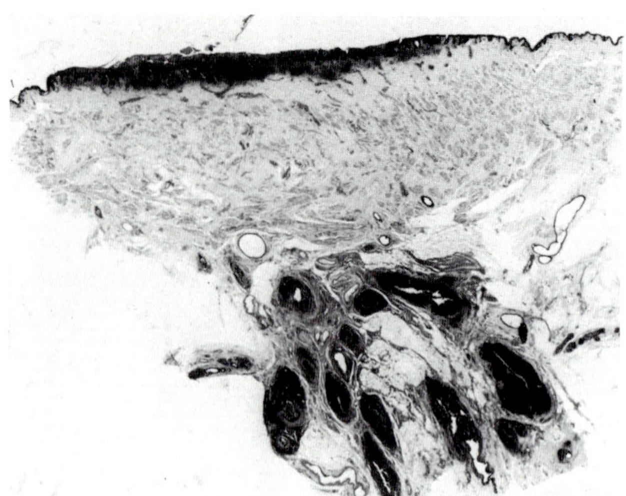

225

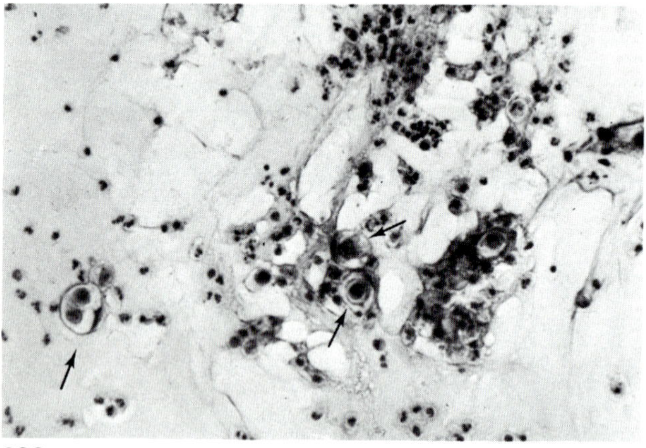

226a

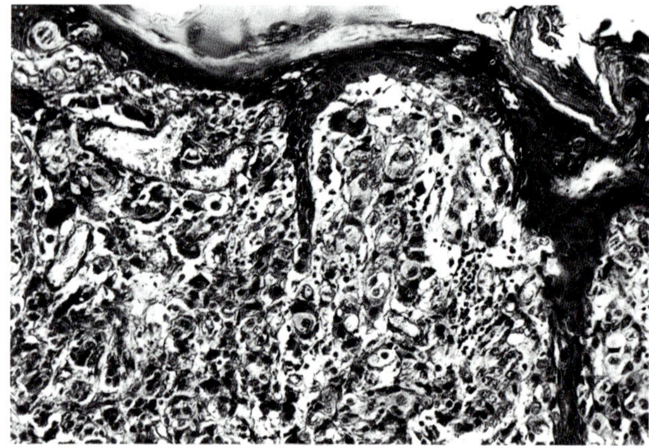

226b

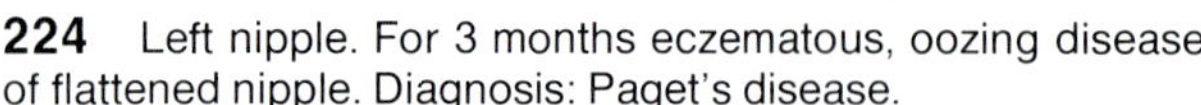

53-year-old female, left breast (Figs 224–226).

224 Left nipple. For 3 months eczematous, oozing disease of flattened nipple. Diagnosis: Paget's disease.

225 *Histological survey picture,* magnif 20×. Circumscribed thickening of epidermis by tumor epithelium. No infiltration of subcutaneous tissue. Tumor growth in retroareolar ducts (noninvasive duct carcinoma).

226 a, b. *Cytology and histology.*

a) Smear from nipple, magnif 105×. Uninucleated and multinucleated Paget's cells. Polymorphous and polychromatic nuclei. Water-clear broad cytoplasm (arrow). Granulocytes and lymphocytes.

b) Histology, magnif 105×. Paget's disease with tumor cells in basal epithelial layer and diffuse infiltration of corium (dermis) by nests of tumor cells of vesicular clear epithelium. Polymorphous and hyperchromatic nuclei.

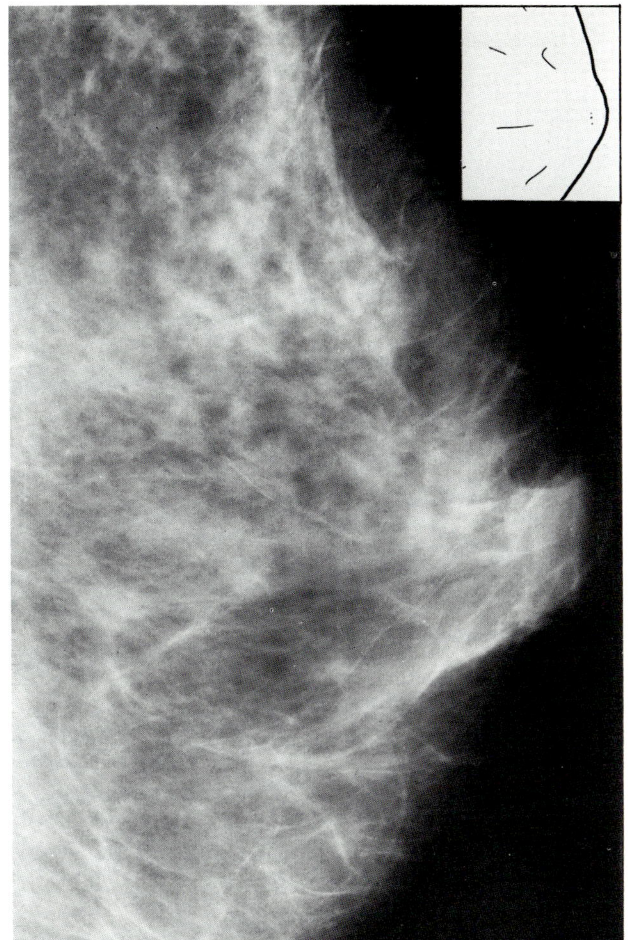

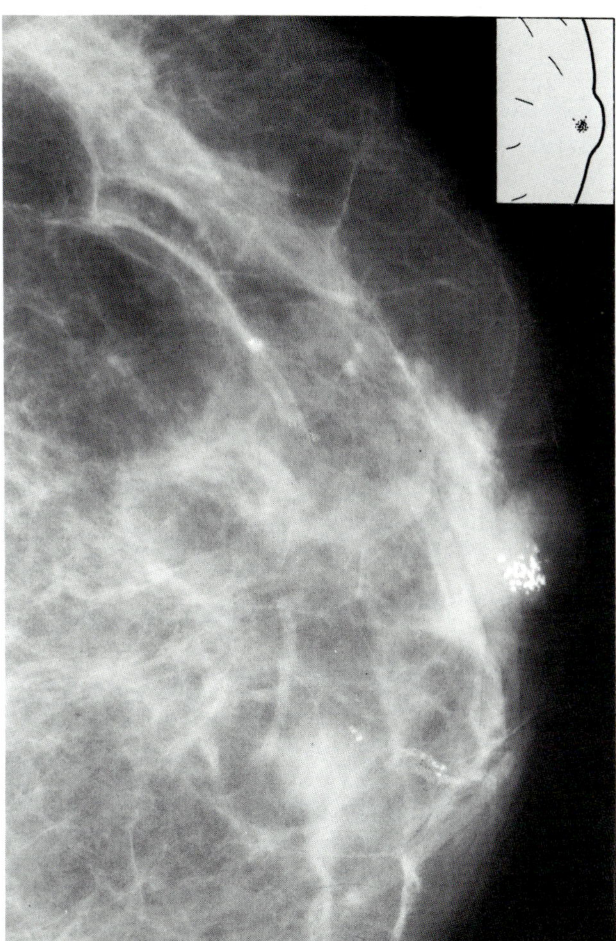

227 *Mammogram* (medio-lateral) of 50-year-old female with Paget's disease of nipple. Stipple-like, barely recognizable calcifications in region of nipple which is not thickened. No evidence of retroareolar tumor or tumor in remaining breast. Normal mammographic findings (diagnosis by inspection, cytology and histology).

228 *Mammogram* (medio-lateral) of 63-year-old female with Paget's disease of nipple. Retroareolar microcalcifications suspicious for an intraductal carcinoma. Minimal nipple retraction. Groups of microcalcifications also in remaining parenchyma.

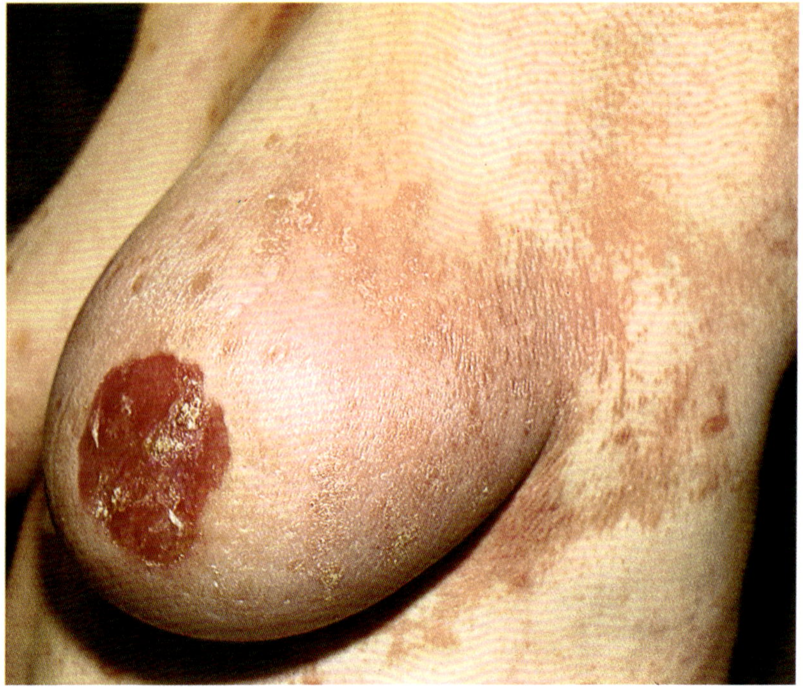
229

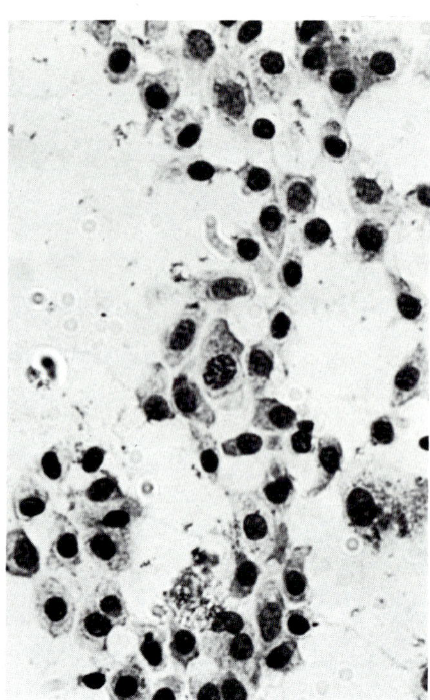
230

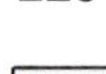

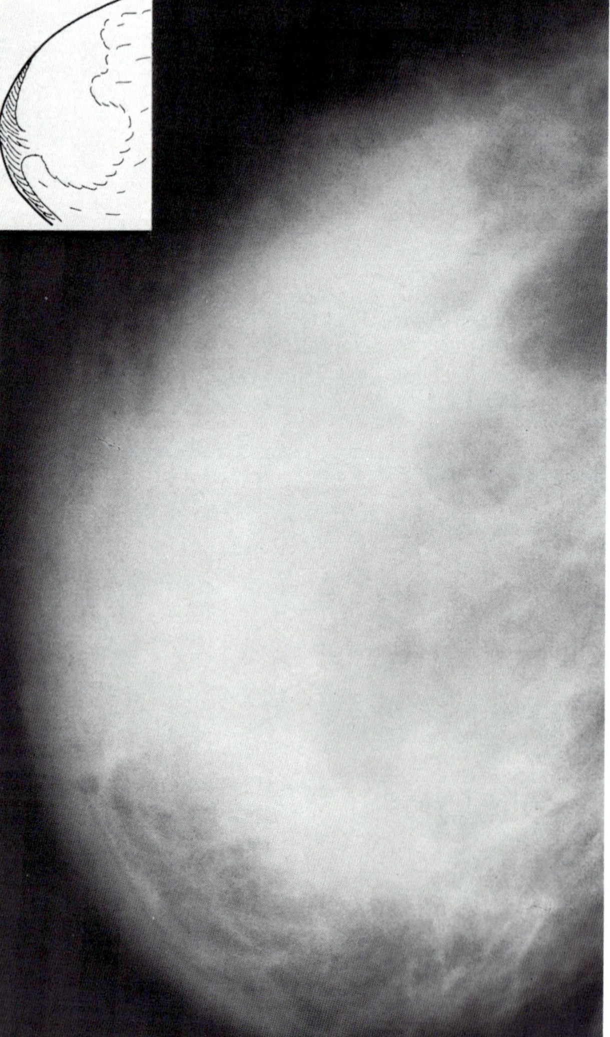
231

63-year-old female, left breast. For 30 years generalized psoriasis of entire body. For 2 years eczema of left nipple misdiagnosed as psoriasis. Enlargement of breast. Enlarged lymph nodes in left axilla (Figs 229–231).

229 Left breast. Small, palm-sized, weeping eczema of areola. Nipple no longer identifiable. Fist-sized tumor with enlargement of left breast. Diagnosis: Paget's disease. Malignant tumor in breast.

230 *Cytology.* On thin-needle biopsy no typical Paget's cells. Numerous tumor cells of ductal origin with moderately polymorphous nuclei. Cell coherence absent. Mitoses (center of figure). Identical findings in axillary lymph nodes. Histology: Paget's disease of nipple. Partially intraductal, partially solid carcinoma of breast with axillary lymph node metastasis.

231 *Mammogram* (medio-lateral). Homogeneous thickening of breast with marked thickening of skin especially in mammillary area (lymphatic obstruction).

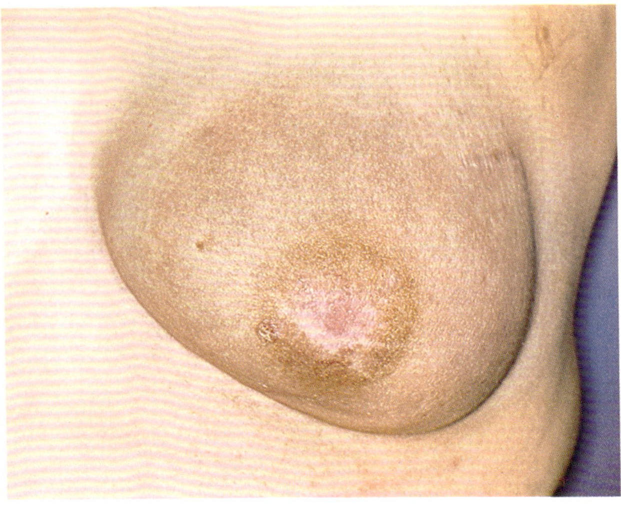

232 42-year-old female, radiation therapy 1 year earlier because of Paget's disease of left nipple. At that time normal palpation. Now routine follow-up examination. Painful induration of inner upper quadrant. Scarring of nipple and areola. No tumor cells on cytology.

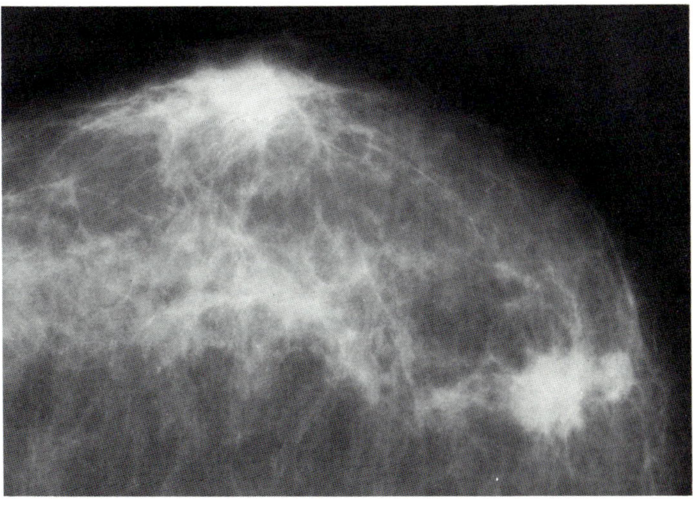

233 *Mammogram* (cranio-caudal). Increased retroareolar density of breast (radiation fibrosis). Near chest wall malignant tumor density with unsharp contour. Some microcalcifications.

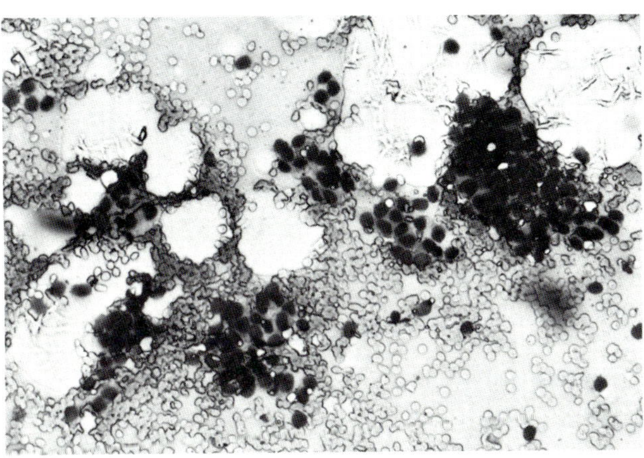

234 a

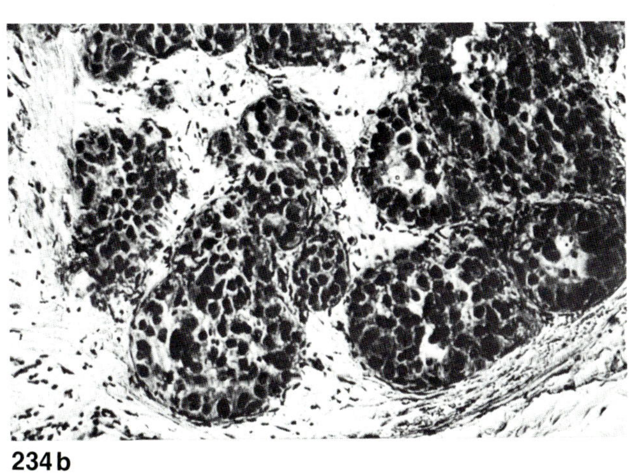

234 b

234 a, b. *Cytology and histology,* magnif 110×.

a) Cytology. After thin-needle biopsy multiple tumor cells arranged in small clusters but also dissociated. Slightly polymorphous nuclei. Moderate hyperchromasia. Erythrocytes.

b) Histology. Infiltrating lobular carcinoma. Tumorous infiltration of terminal ducts. Infiltration of surrounding stroma (not shown).

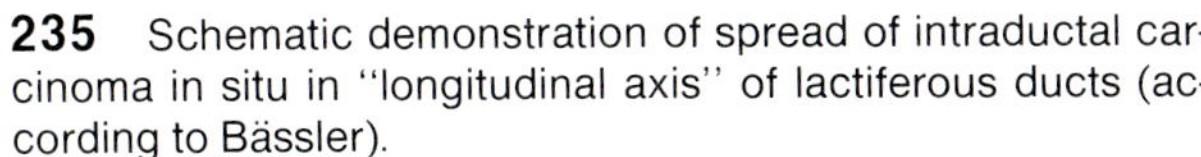

235 Schematic demonstration of spread of intraductal carcinoma in situ in "longitudinal axis" of lactiferous ducts (according to Bässler).

1. Intraductal tumor tissue grows into nipple: Paget's disease.
2. Spreading within the boundaries of ducts: ductal carcinoma in situ.
3. Invasion of tumor into terminal ducts of lobules: secondary lobular carcinoma in situ (prestage of infiltrating lobular carcinoma).

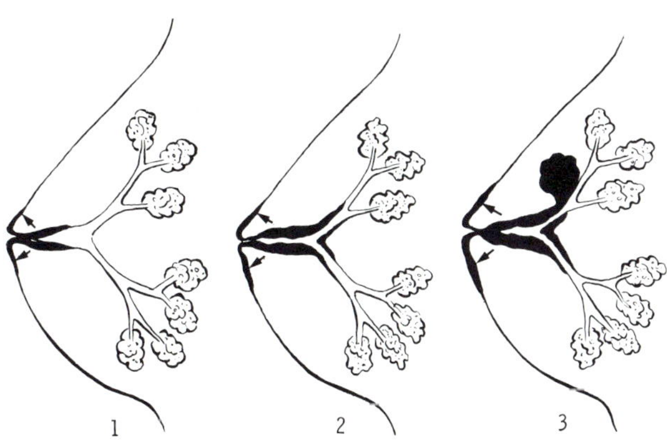

235

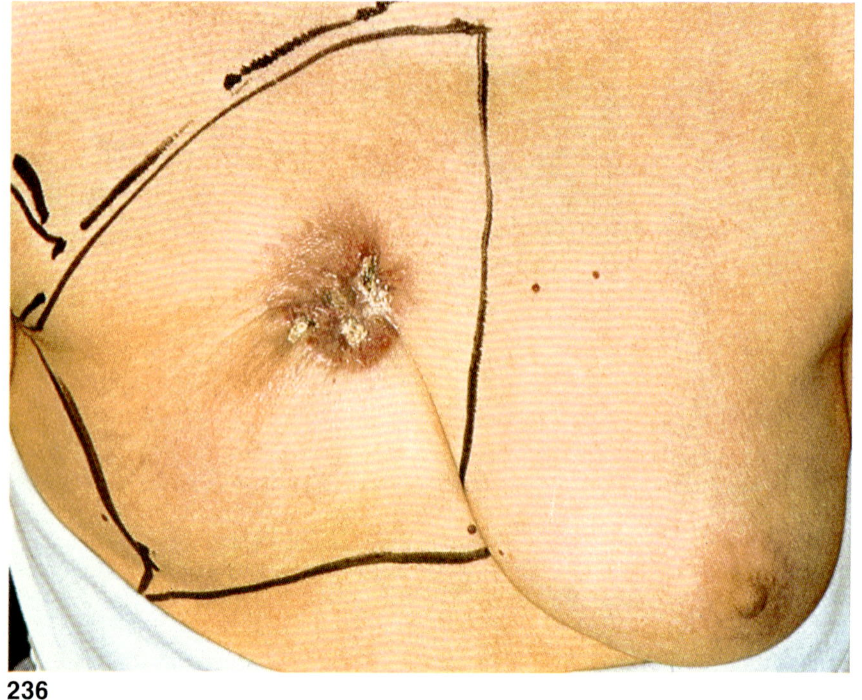

237

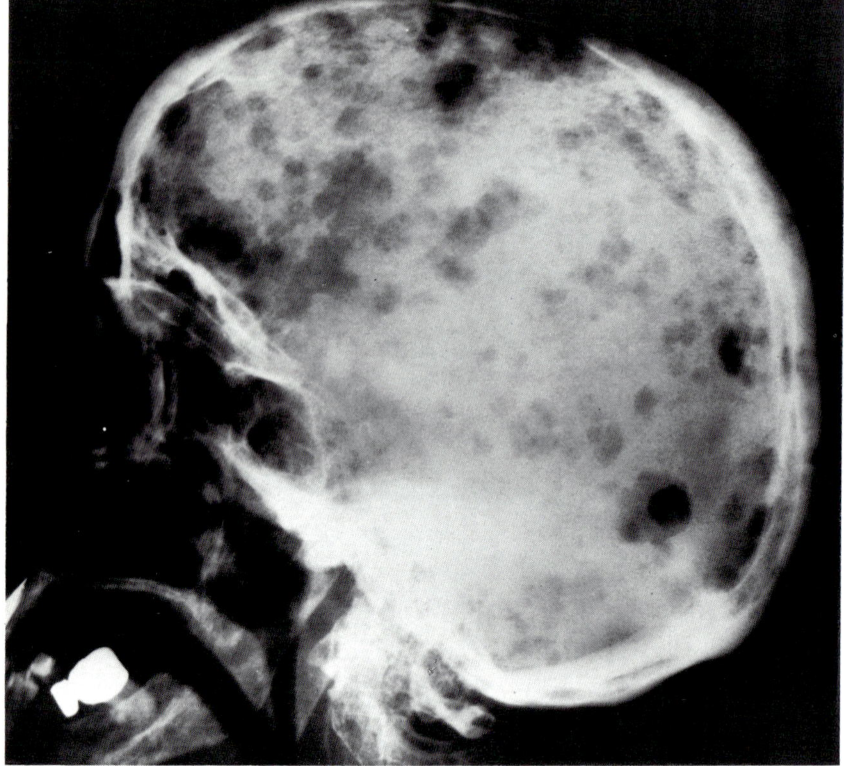

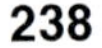

236 64-year-old nurse (nun). For 10 years Paget's disease of right breast (no therapy). Because of marked generalized skeletal pain consultation with physician. Right breast completely shrunken away and destroyed by tumor. Tumor surface palm-sized, red and covered with a whitish scab. Radiation port shown by markings (palliative radiation therapy).

237 Thoracic spine (lateral). Large and small osteoblastic metastases in bodies of several vertebrae at site of maximal kyphosis and inferiorly.

238 *Roentgenograph* (lateral) of skull. Multiple osteolytic metastases of entire calvarium.

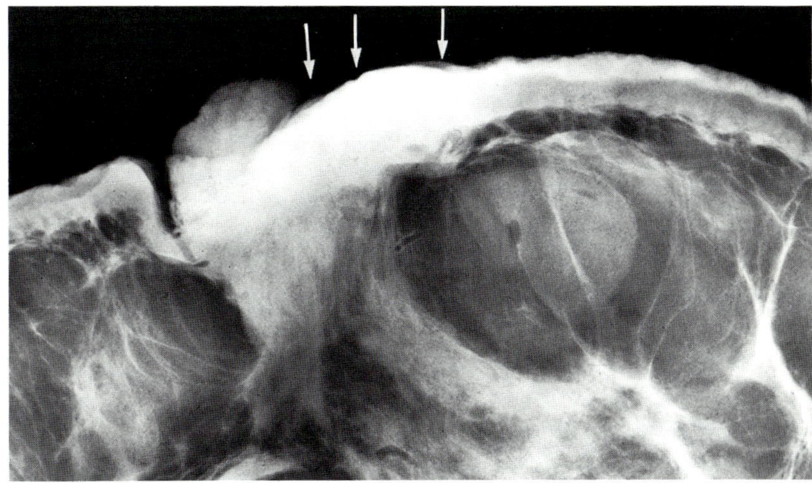

239

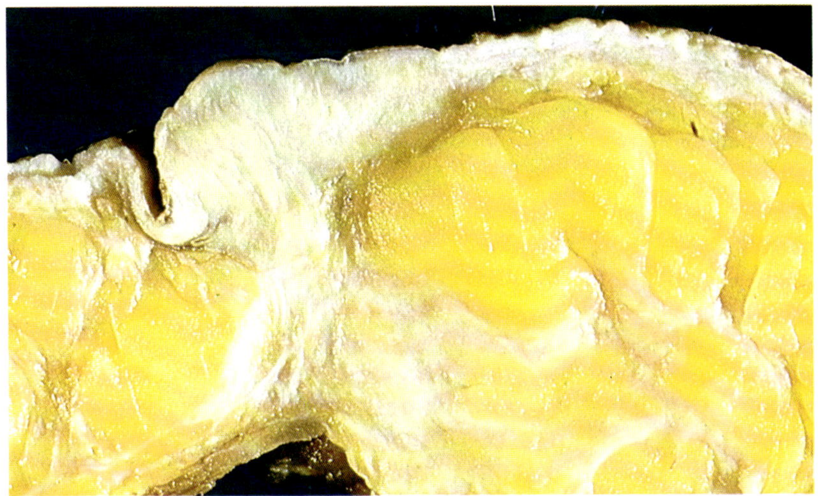

240

239 *Specimen radiograph* of right breast. Broadening of lateral portion of areola due to tumor (arrows). Thickening of the retroareolar space. Retraction of portion of areola opposite tumor. (Same case as in Fig 223.)

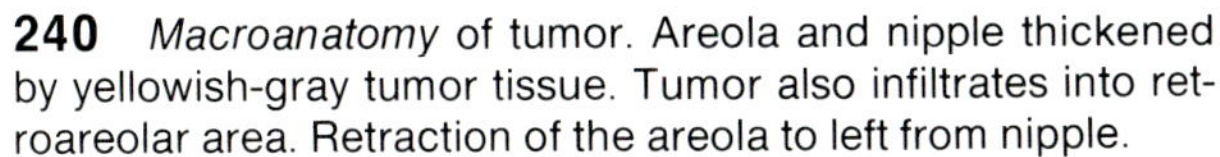

240 *Macroanatomy* of tumor. Areola and nipple thickened by yellowish-gray tumor tissue. Tumor also infiltrates into retroareolar area. Retraction of the areola to left from nipple.

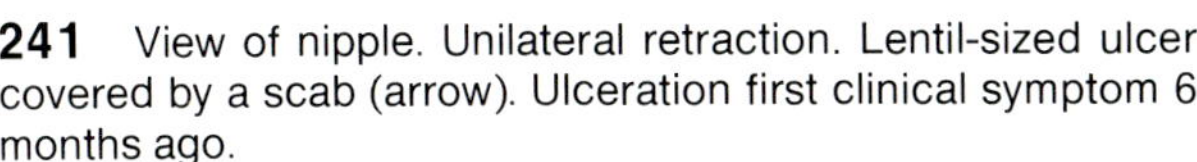

241 View of nipple. Unilateral retraction. Lentil-sized ulcer covered by a scab (arrow). Ulceration first clinical symptom 6 months ago.

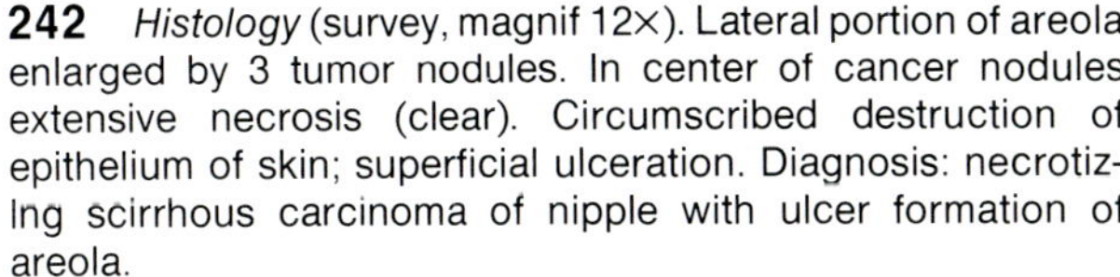

242 *Histology* (survey, magnif 12×). Lateral portion of areola enlarged by 3 tumor nodules. In center of cancer nodules extensive necrosis (clear). Circumscribed destruction of epithelium of skin; superficial ulceration. Diagnosis: necrotizing scirrhous carcinoma of nipple with ulcer formation of areola.

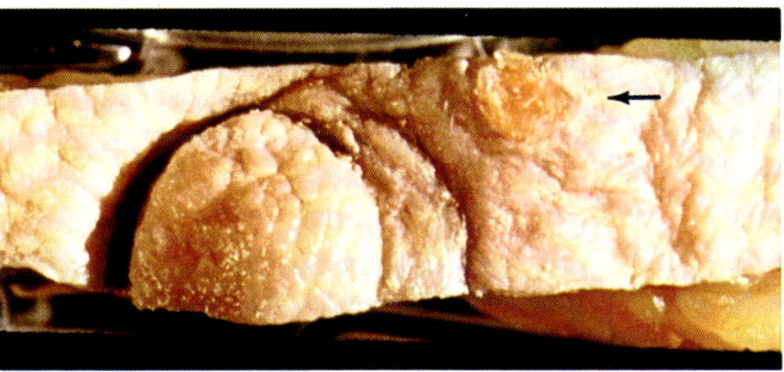

241

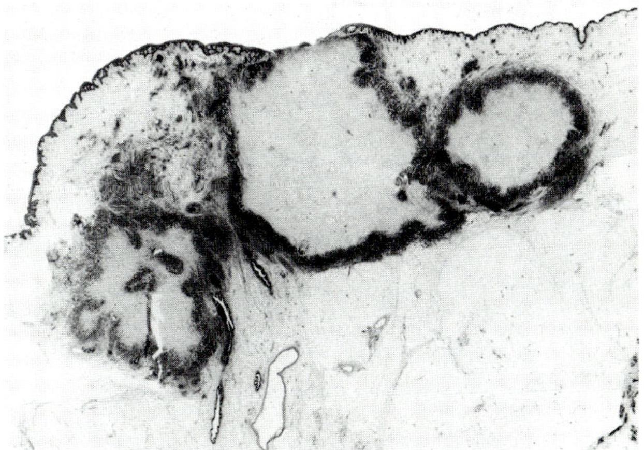

242

Differential diagnosis; difficult findings

The many morphological variants of breast carcinoma make all attempts at classification particularly of transitional and border-line cases, very difficult, especially for mammographic differential diagnosis. Most of the time errors in radiographic diagnosis are made in *postoperative* and *scarred* breasts. In our own material five cases of scarring were misinterpreted and carcinomas overlooked (Fig **243**). The mammogram does not differentiate carcinomas arising in scars from nonspecific scars (Fig **118**). The scar and the carcinoma in it appear radiographically as an oblong radiating density with projections to the skin. Coarse calcifications may be noted within these densities. Microcalcifications always suggest malignancy. In strands of scar tissue are histologically small nests of tumor epithelium which may not change overall scar structure radiographically.
In the *thermogram* scars normally are cold. Hyperthermia (after cooling of the surrounding area) suggests malignancy. There were, however, three carcinomas in thermographically absolutely normal scars. Whenever a carcinoma in a scar is suspected, thin-needle biopsy should be done to remove cells for cytological examination.
Small, up to lentil-sized, easily movable, subcutaneous nodules usually are thought to be cysts in older patients and fibroadenomas in younger patients; mostly correctly so. Nevertheless these areas should be aspirated, particularly if a circumscribed opacity cannot be confirmed in the mammogram. Subcutaneous nodules should not be missed with thin-needle biopsy. Thin-needle biopsy therefore will differentiate fibroadenomas, lipomas and malignancies (Fig **198**).
A very rare disease is so-called "chylous effusion" (passage of lymph into the interstitium).

The interpretation of the mammogram of a 61-year-old patient was very difficult in this context. The patient had reddish-blue, discolored, doughy skin in the right upper abdomen and inframammary region. Clinical impression was carcinomatous lymphangitis extending into the right breast. Mammogram of the right breast showed a nonhomogeneous band-like density suggesting carcinoma.
Chest radiograph showed bilateral pleural effusions so that at first a diagnosis of "carcinoma right breast with carcinomatous lymphangitis and pleural metastases" was made.
Thermographically the discolored skin of the abdomen was 1 °C warmer than the normal skin. Histological examination of the skin of the abdomen, however, did not confirm carcinomatous lymphangitis. Thin-needle biopsy of the right breast showed multiple, normal epithelial layers in the cytological smear. Comparison with a mammogram done 4 years earlier (at another institution) showed the densities of the right breast already there. Breast cancer, therefore, seemed unlikely.
The patient was studied in the United States two years ago because of the skin changes and pleural effusions. At that time "chylous effusion" was diagnosed since chyle was found in the pleural effusion.
The skin changes developed over the past eight years. They may be secondary to a disease of the lymph vessels with passage of lymph into the interstitium and pleural spaces. The etiology of this disease is unknown (Figs **262**–**267**).

62-year-old female. Tissue biopsy of right breast 3 years ago. Scar in upper outer quadrant. Patient thought she palpated small nodule in scar. Palpation of right breast was negative. There was minimal serous secretion from left breast (Figs 243–244). ▷

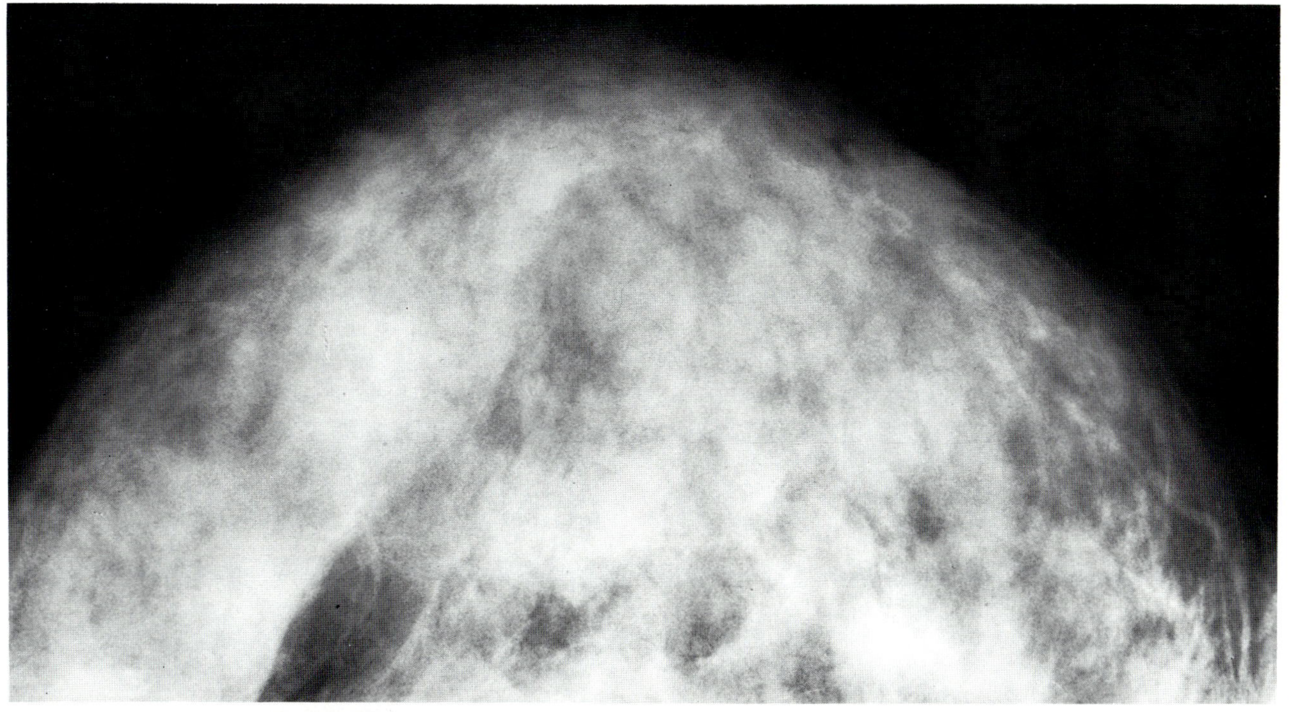

a

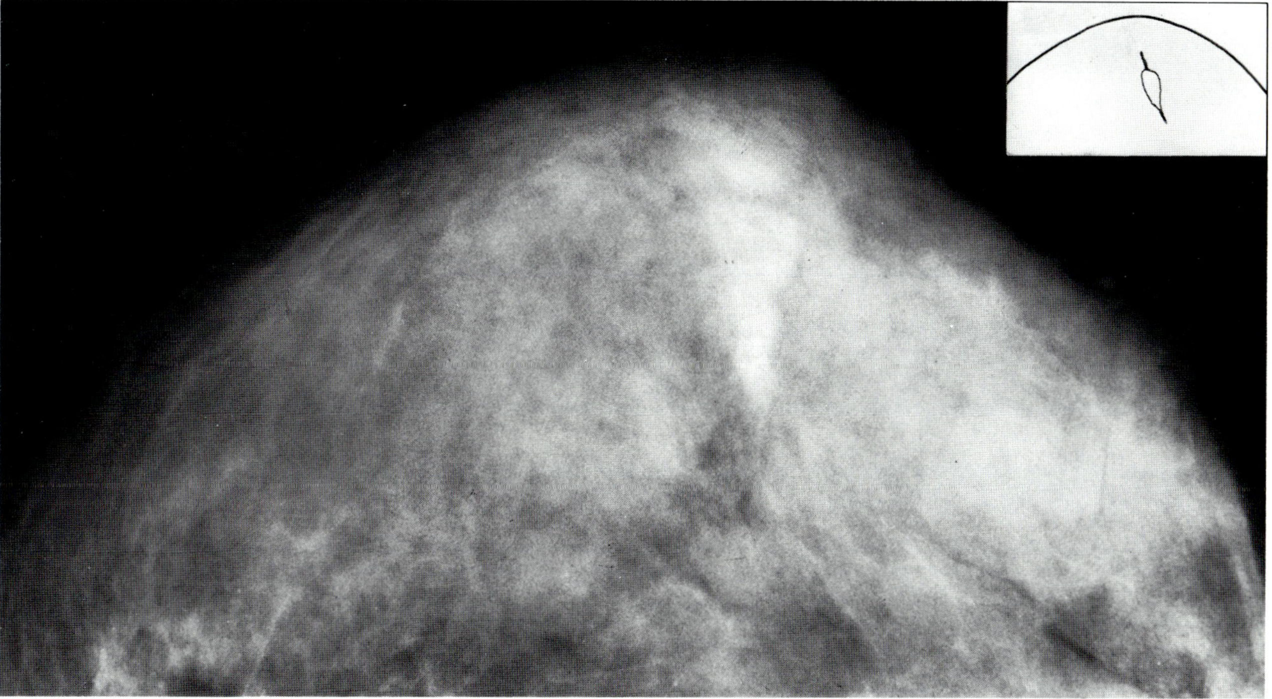

b

△

243 a, b. *Mammogram* (cranio-caudal).
a) Left breast.
b) Right breast.
Bilateral fibrocystic mastopathy. Multiple tiny opacities along the course of the ducts. Slightly thickened scar on right following biopsy.

244 *Thermography.* Bilateral symmetrical vascularization. No evidence of malignancy. Biopsy scar of right breast cold. No thin-needle biopsy. In spite of negative findings, surgical revision of scar was done to reassure patient. Histology, small, partially solid, partially scirrhous carcinoma growing in the scar.

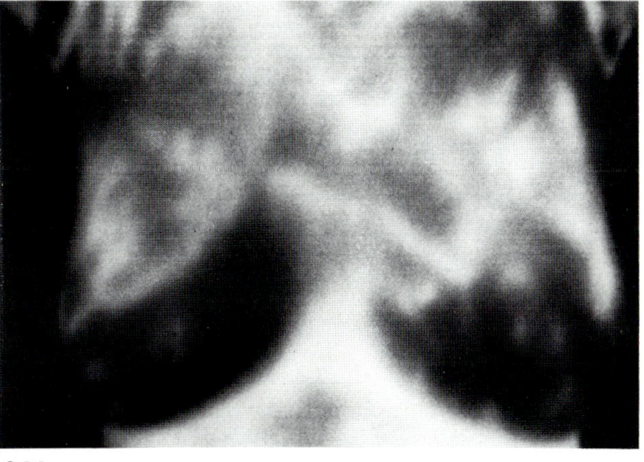

244

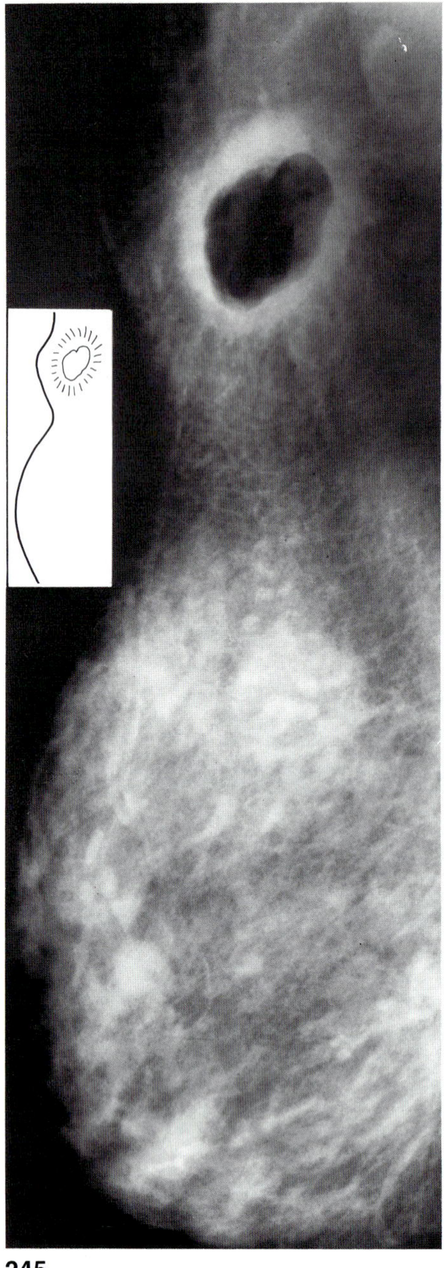

245

246

64-year-old female, right breast. Firm, movable tumor in axilla. Aspiration yields 5 ml of hemorrhagic fluid. Breast normal on palpation (Figs 245–247).

245 *Pneumocystogram of right axilla* (medio-lateral). Tumor seen following aspiration and filling with air. Irregular cavity with thick wall. Ill-defined delineation from fatty tissue of axilla. Suspicion of cystic necrotic tumor.

246 *Surgical specimen.* Cystic tumor opened. Irregular inner wall with punctate hemorrhages. Histology: metastasis of an adenocarcinoma.

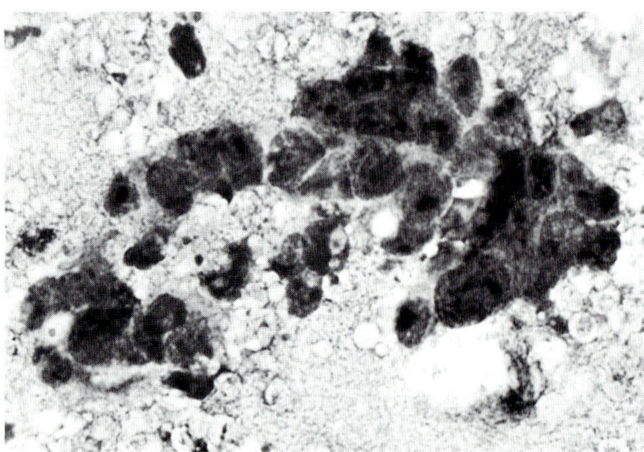

247

247 *Cytology,* magnif 180×. Sheets of tumor cells. Individual, dissociated epithelial cells. Polymorphous nuclei. Confluence and enlargement of nucleoli. Vacuole formation in cytoplasm. Suspicious for adenocarcinoma. Primary tumor at this date still unknown. (Aberrant breast with malignant degeneration possible.) Distant metastases after 4 years (lung, bone).

Diffuse Scirrhous Carcinoma, Clinical Course

59-year-old female. For 2½ years mammographic examinations because of fibrous mastopathy (Figs 248–256).
Bilateral, dense, coarsely nodular breasts. Last mammogram one year ago with thin-needle biopsy and galactography left: no evidence of malignancy. Only thermography showed hyperthermia of 1.5 °C surrounding right nipple.
Current follow-up examination. Clinically unequivocal carcinoma right. Markedly shrunken firm breast. Inspection of left breast, normal size. In upper outer quadrant dense plaque-like area. Slight secretion. Mammographically no change of architecture of breast when compared with previous examinations. Corresponding to clinical appearance, the right breast has become smaller and denser. No microcalcifications.

Thermography. Increased vascularization around right nipple. No thermographic change.

Bilateral thin-needle biopsy. Suspicion of small cell carcinoma bilaterally.

Histology (bilaterally). Diffusely growing small cell scirrhous carcinoma bilaterally. Changes in right breast more extensive than in left. Bilateral mastectomies followed by radiation therapy using fast electron beams. Extensive osteolytic metastases found radiographically in skull, entire spine and pelvis 8 weeks postoperatively. Patient's general condition is still good despite this.
This case indicates that in dense breasts early diagnosis of very rapidly growing tumors fails. Breast structures do not change significantly in mammogram with diffusely growing tumors. The only sign is gradual decrease in size of breast which becomes denser and finally stone-hard.

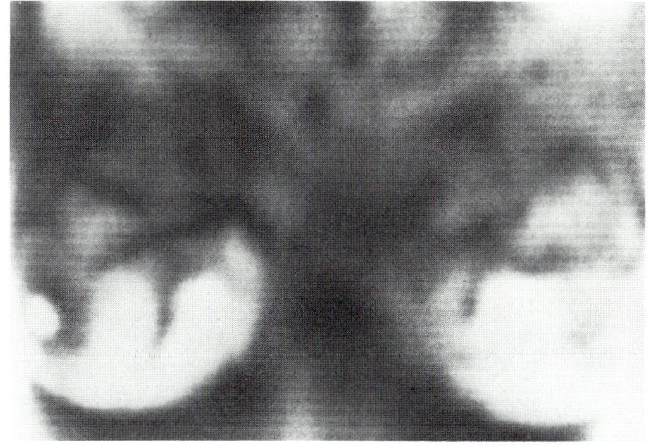

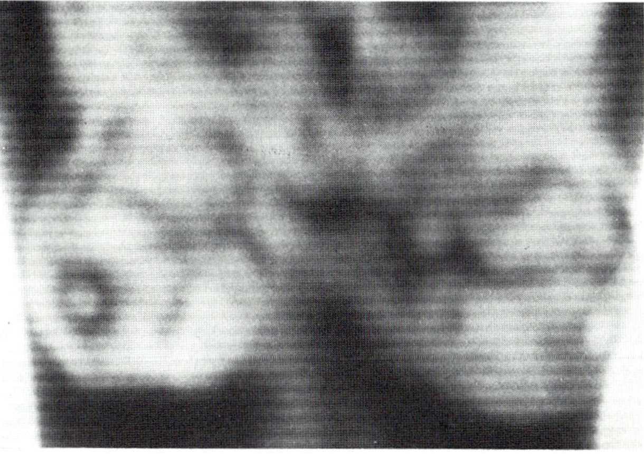

248 a, b. *Electronic thermovision.*
a) Left and right breast 1 year ago. Right: increased vascularization of inner upper quadrant. Hyperthermia of areola. Temperature difference 1 °C greater than left. Left: normal vascularization. Cold nipple. Cold areola.

b) Follow-up examination. Right breast smaller. No change in vascularization. On the left slight hyperthermia of vascular channel in inner upper quadrant.

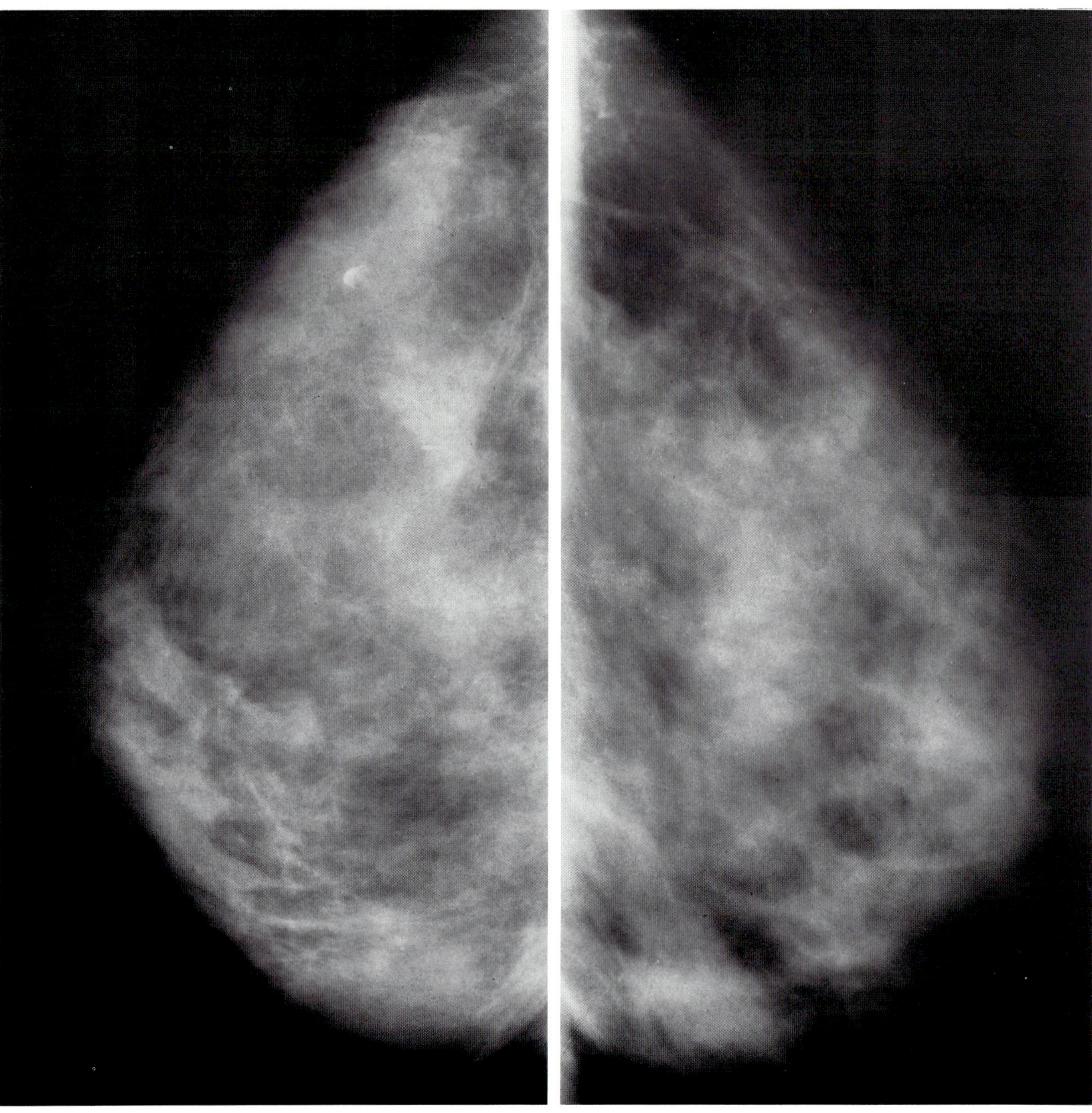

249 a, b. *Mammogram* (medio-lateral). Findings 2½ years ago.
a) Left breast.
b) Right breast.
Bilateral small and coarse opacities consistent with fibrocystic mastopathy. In center of right breast a somewhat more circumscribed nodular opacity. No suspicion of malignancy.

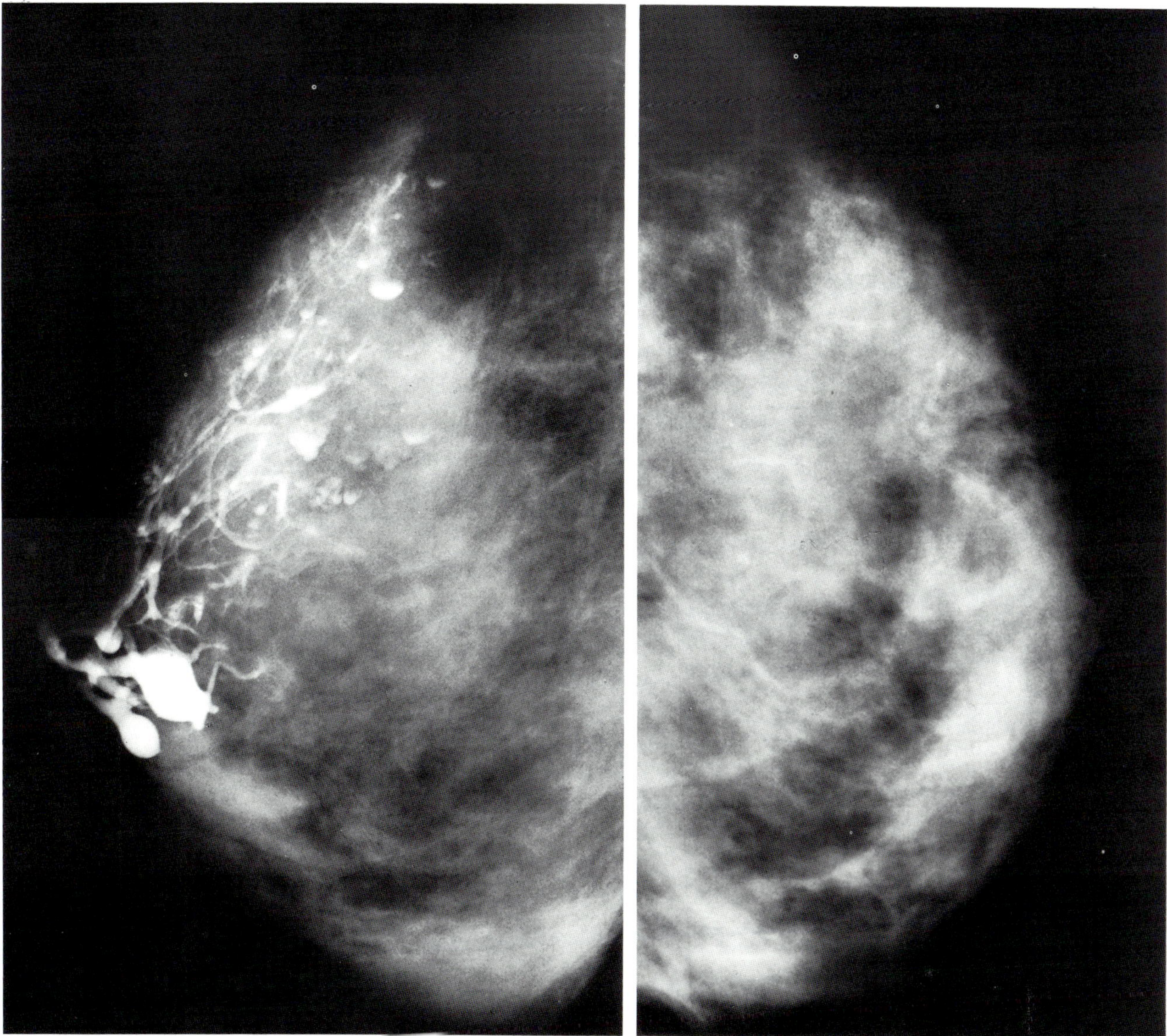

250 a, b. *Radiographic examination* 1 year ago.
a) Galactography left. Fibrocystic mastopathy with multiple contrast-filled cysts. Retroareolar ductal ectasia with obstructed ducts in lower quadrant.

b) *Mammogram* right (medio-lateral). No change (compare Fig. 249b). No suspicion of malignancy.

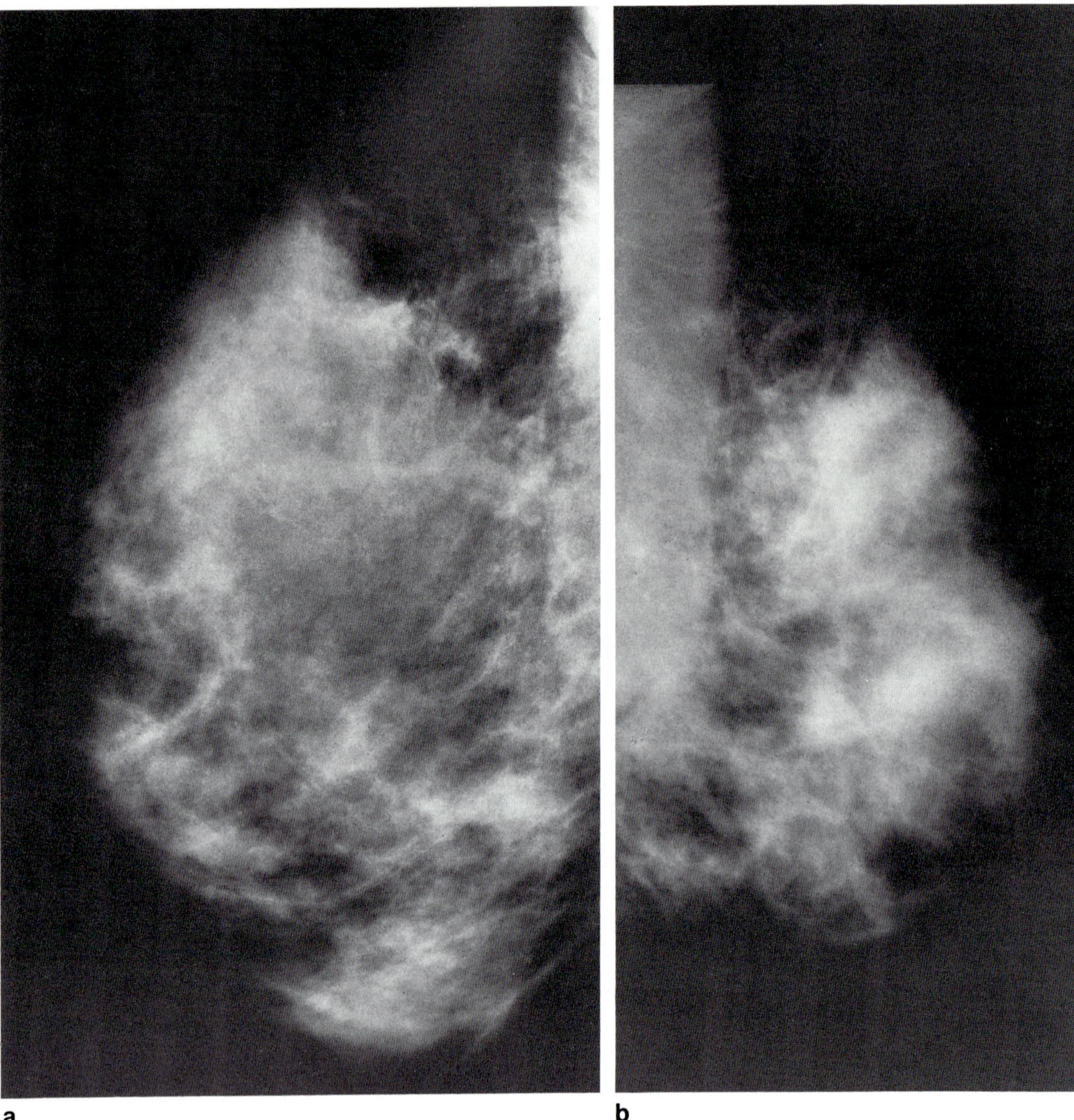

a b

251 a, b. *Current mammogram* (medio-lateral).

a) Left breast. No change since previous examinations (Figs 249a, 250a). Histology: diffusely growing small cell scirrhous carcinoma.

b) Right breast. Marked shrinkage of right breast. No circumscribed tumor density recognizable. Breast structures denser than on previous examinations. Clinically and histologically diffusely growing scirrhous carcinoma with marked shrinkage of breast.

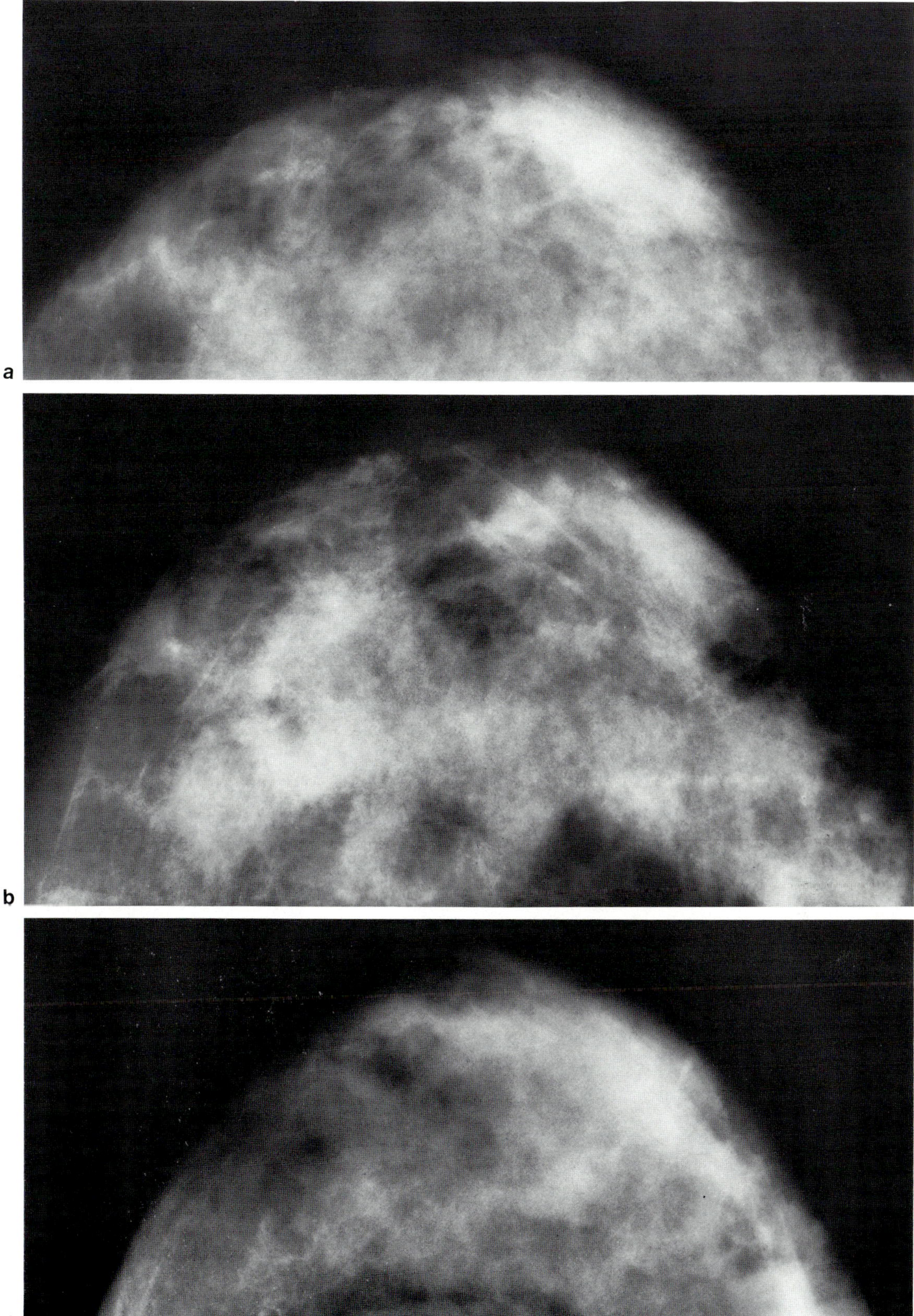

252 a–c. *Mammographic follow-up* right, second radiographic plane (cranio-caudal).
a) Findings 2½ years ago. Fibrocystic mastopathy. No evidence of malignancy.
b) Findings 1 year ago. No change.
c) Present findings. Shrinkage of breast. Increased density of breast. No localized tumor.

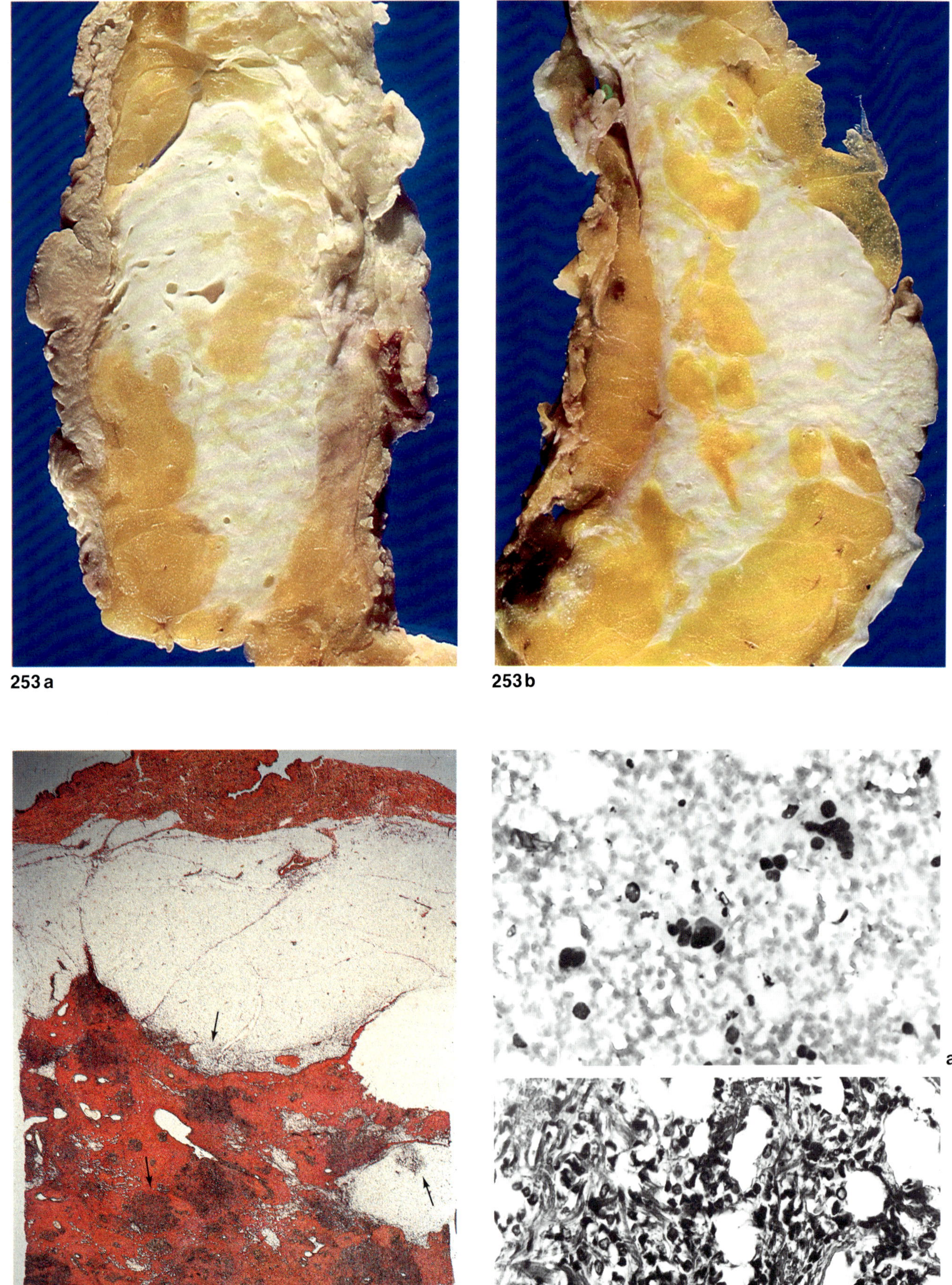

253 a

253 b

254

255 a

b

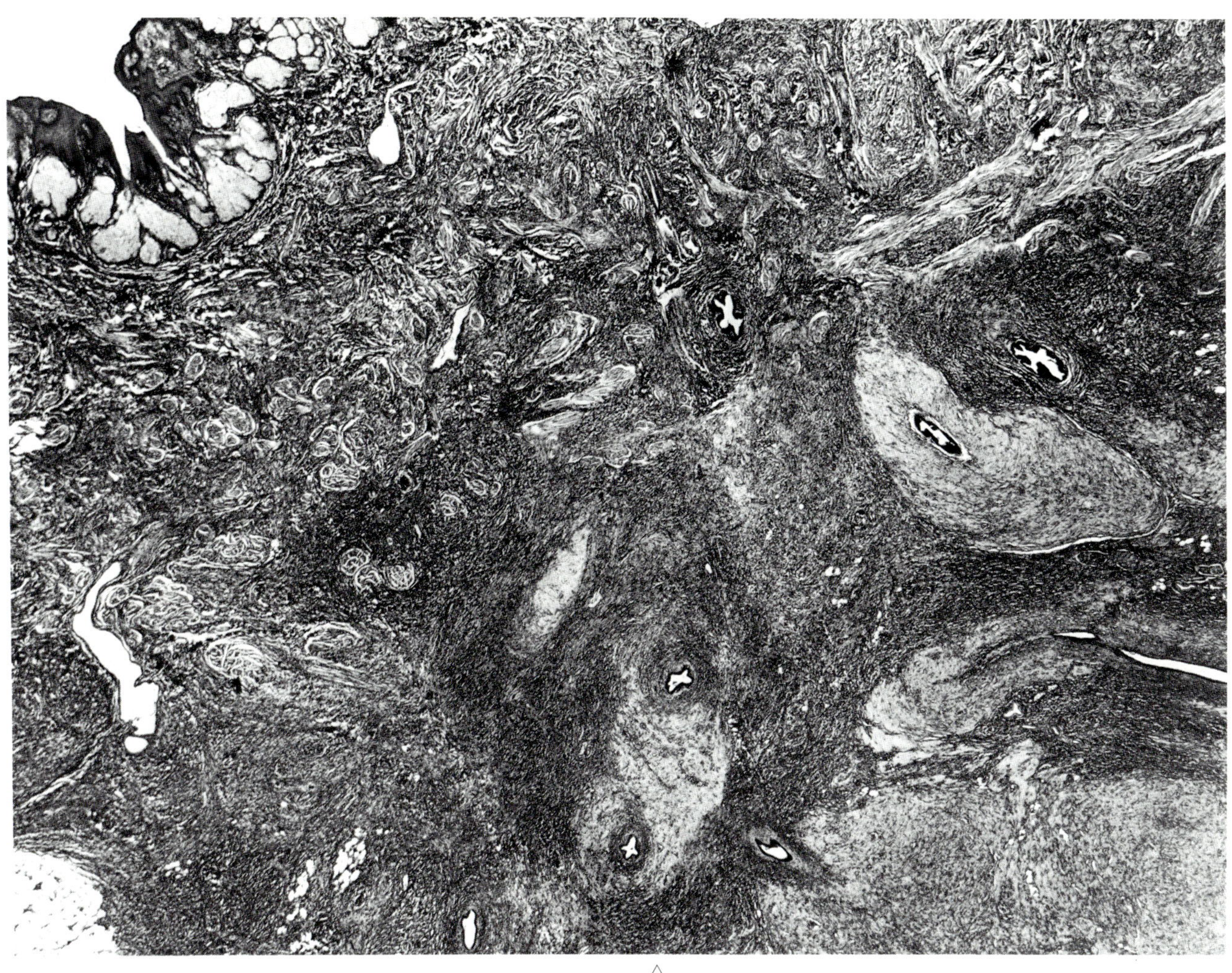

◁ **253** a, b. *Macroanatomy* of left and right breast.
a) Left breast. Breast gray-white, surrounded by yellow fat. Retroareolar dilated duct. No circumscribed tumor nodule. No retraction of skin or nipple.
b) Right breast. Gray-white breast shrunken by tumor, denser and without recognizable ducts. Slight retraction of nipple and areola. No tumor projections into surrounding fat.

◁ **254** *Histological picture* of section of Fig 253a (van Giesen stain, connective tissue red-brown, magnif 10×). Periductular fibrosis, diffuse penetration of the breast structures by small cell scirrhous carcinoma (arrows). Compare also with Fig 255b.

◁ **255** a, b. *Cytology and histology,* magnif 240×.
a) Cytology. Thin-needle biopsy shows small groups of tumor cells with small and moderately polymorphous nuclei. Cytologic appearance left and right identical. Suspicion of small cell carcinoma.
b) Histology (section of Fig 254). Small-cell, scirrhous carcinoma. Infiltration of fat. Marked formation of new connective tissue.

△
256 *Histological* structure of right breast, magnif 20×. Epidermis with sebaceous glands (above right). Marked periductular fibrosis. Smooth musculature. Diffuse infiltration of skin and perilobular connective tissue of breast by tumor cells (dark areas in center). Periductular intralobular connective tissue partially markedly thickened, fibroses, free of tumor.

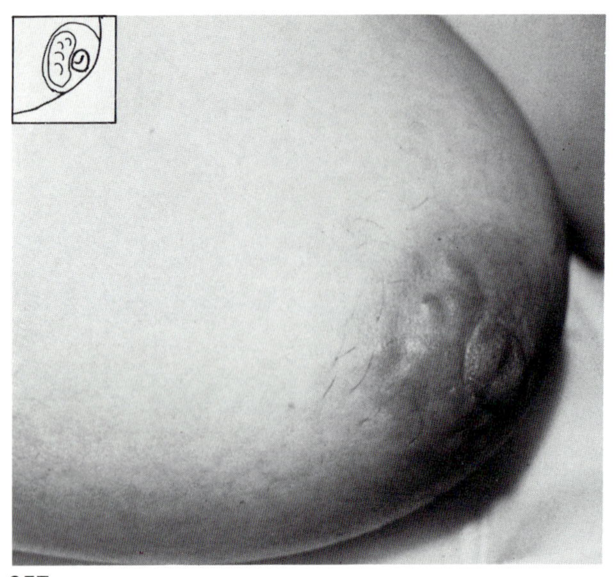

257

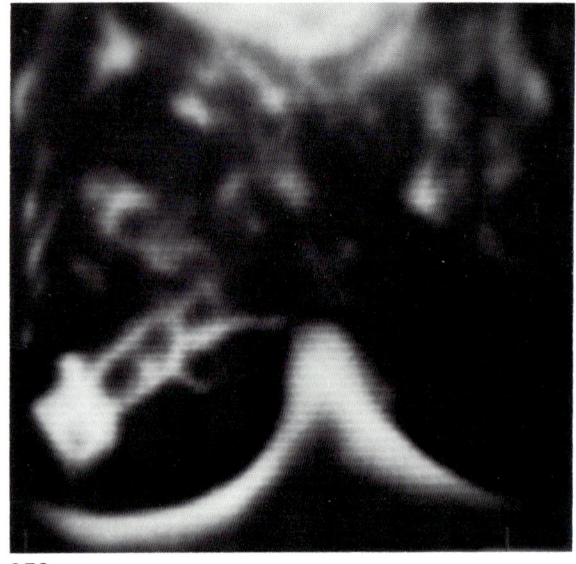

258

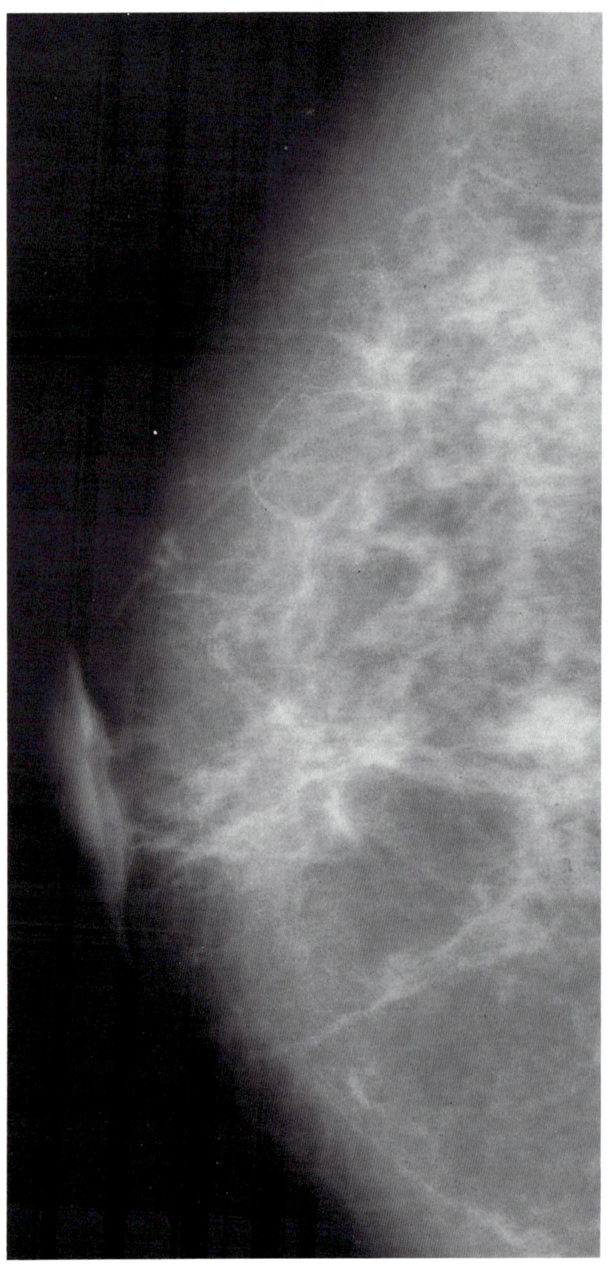

259 a

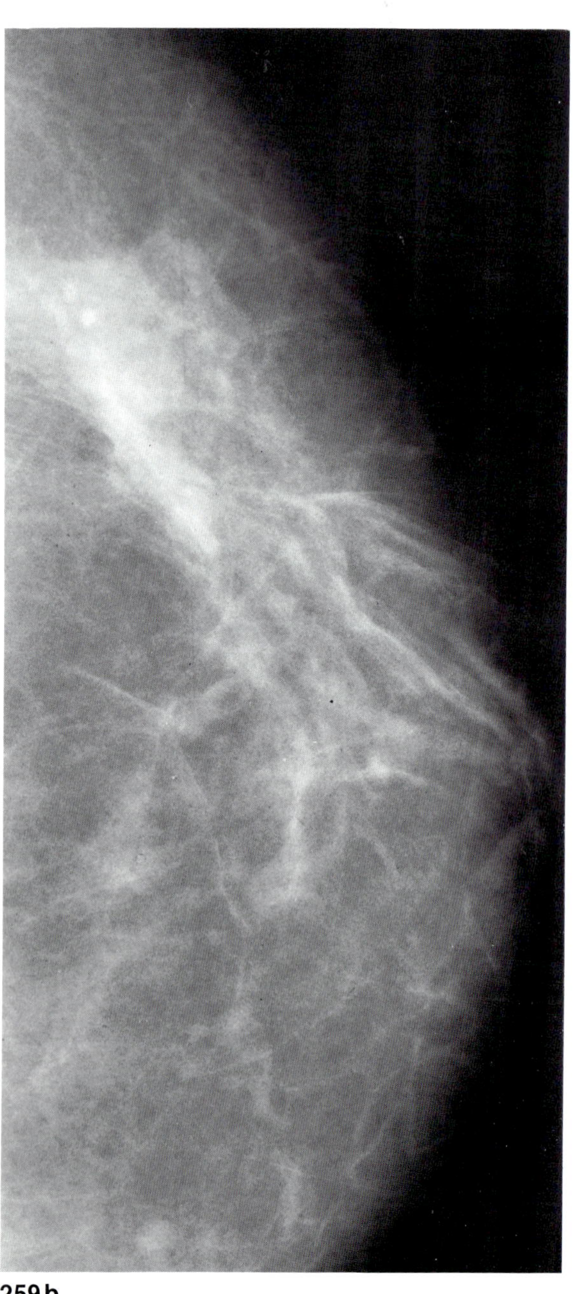

259 b

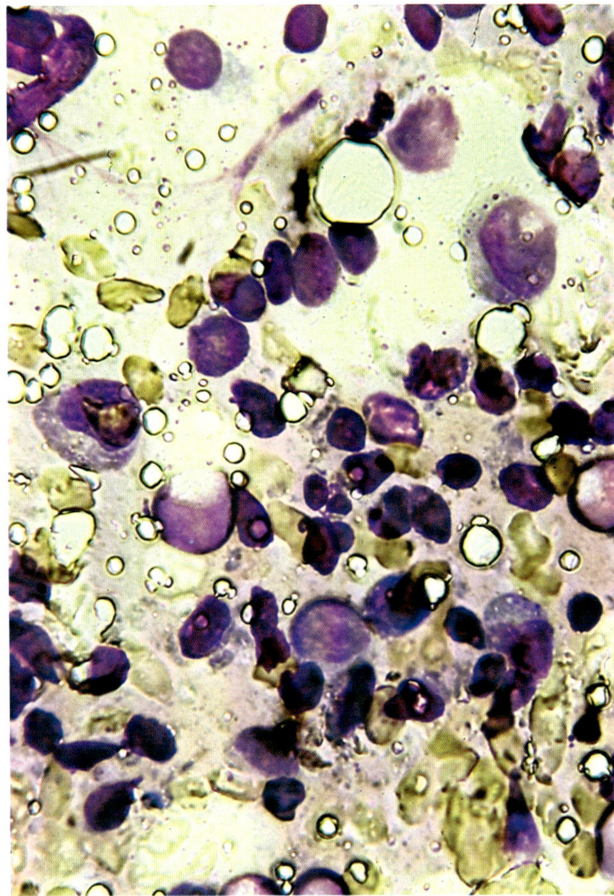

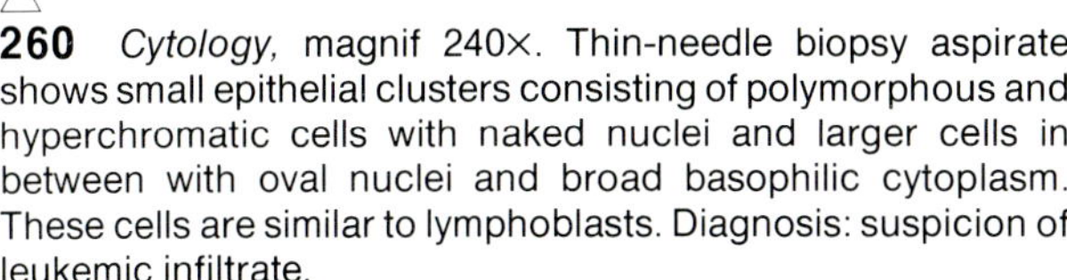

△

260 *Cytology,* magnif 240×. Thin-needle biopsy aspirate shows small epithelial clusters consisting of polymorphous and hyperchromatic cells with naked nuclei and larger cells in between with oval nuclei and broad basophilic cytoplasm. These cells are similar to lymphoblasts. Diagnosis: suspicion of leukemic infiltrate.

261 a–c. *Histology.*
a) Survey, magnif 40×. Epidermis normal. Subcutaneous, scattered, round-cell infiltration.
b) Magnif 105×. Irregular clusters of round cells lie between strands of smooth muscle.
c) Magnif 180×. Atypical naked nuclei. Lymphocytic cells with moderately polymorphous nuclei. Diagnosis: lymphosarcoma of lymphocytic type. Further studies negative for additional involvement of other organs by the lymphosarcoma.

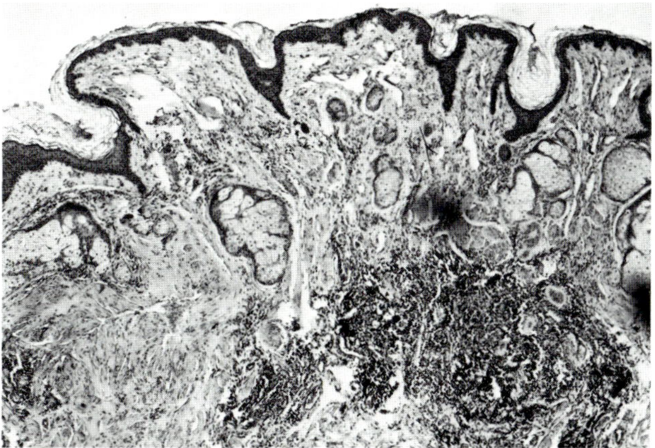

261 a

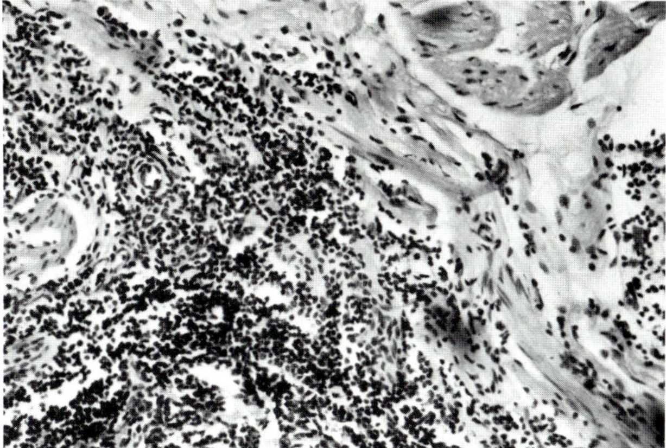

261 b

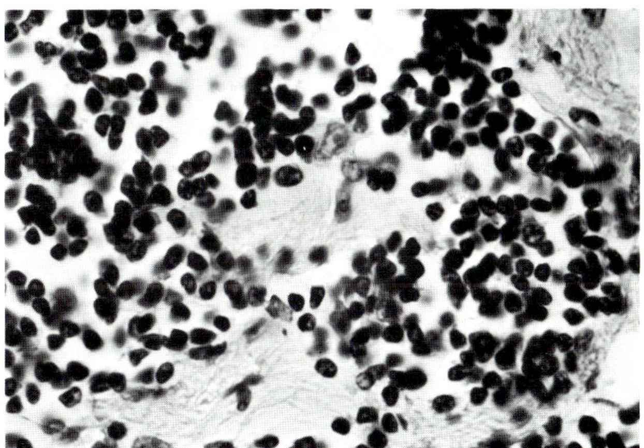

261 c

◁ **257** 52-year-old female. Cylindrical thickening of areola of right breast began 4 weeks ago. No pain, eczema, itching; no secretions. Palpation of breast normal. No swelling of regional lymph nodes. No hepatosplenomegaly.

258 *Electronic thermovision.* Hypervascularization and hyperthermia (2.8 °C) of right nipple. Increased vascular pattern of inner upper quadrant. Left breast thermographically cold.

259 a, b. *Mammogram,* medio-lateral.
a) Right breast. Thickening of areola. Small periductal opacities. No suspicion of tumor.
b) Left breast. Normal. No abnormal findings.

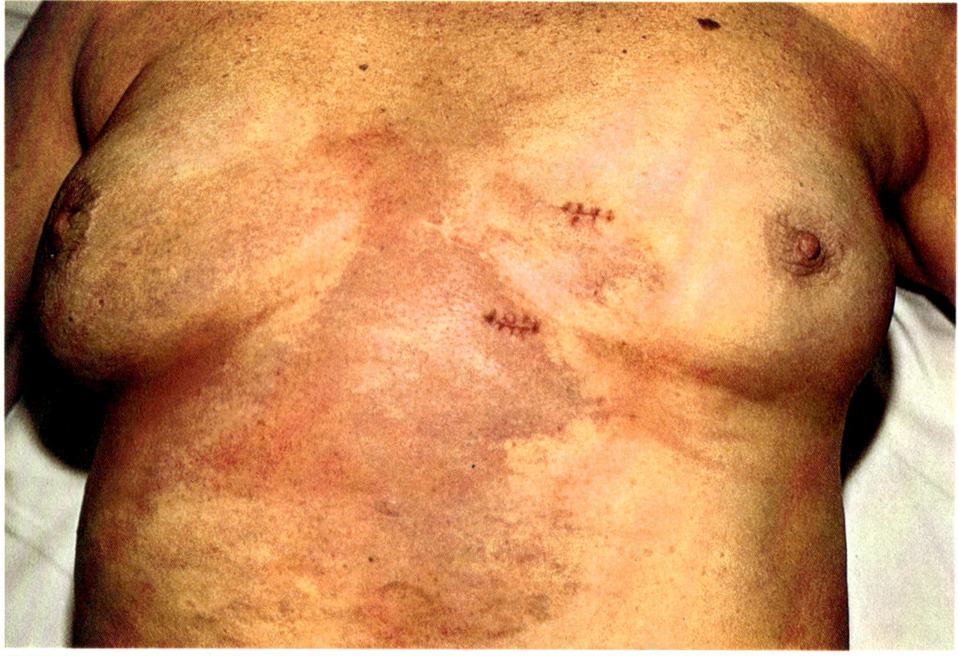

262

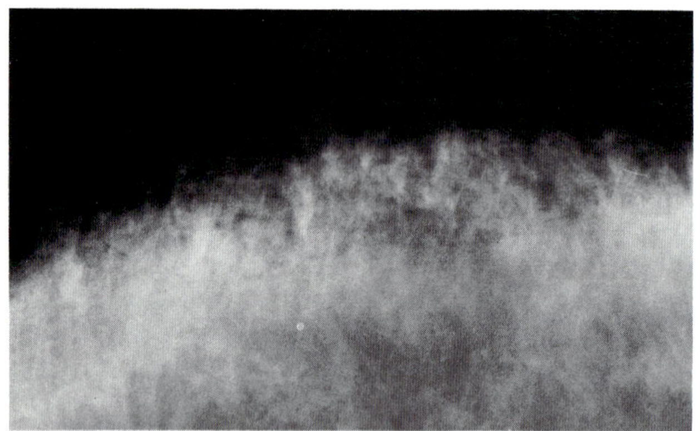

263

264

61-year-old female, right breast. For 3 years bluish-livid discoloration and edematous swelling of upper abdomen and undersurface of both breasts (right more than left). In mammogram 4 years ago vague thickening of structures of right breast. Tissue biopsy to exclude malignancy refused by patient at that time. Recurrent pleural effusion. Repeated thoracenteses always revealed chyle.
Changes of skin, right breast and pleura were interpreted in another country as passage of lymph into interstitium and pleural space: "chylous effusion." Tissue biopsy of skin of upper abdomen was histologically negative; in particular there was no evidence of carcinomatous lymphangitis of skin (Figs 262–267).

262 Changes in skin over both breasts and epigastrium. Extensive reddish-livid discoloration of skin extending to undersurface of right and to a lesser degree left breast. Two small scars secondary to previous skin biopsy.

263 *Soft-tissue radiographic examination* of discolored and thickened skin. Delicate, vertically directed, thickened lines of nonhomogeneous density. Suspicion of lymphangiectasia.

264 *Plate thermography* with measurement of temperature of skin over epigastrium. Diffuse superficial hyperthermia (1.5 °C) of epigastrium and of right inframammary skin fold (less extensive on left).

265 a, b. *Mammogram* (medio-lateral).
a) Right breast. Enlarged right breast. Irregular, band-like opacities (dilated lymph channels and interstitial edema?) decreasing from retroareolar space toward chest wall. Thin-needle biopsy: normal epithelium, no tumor cells.
b) Left breast. Normal. Retroareolar breast tissue without notable findings.

266 a, b. *Plate thermography* after cooling of both breasts.
a) Right breast. Diffuse hypervascularization with slight increase in temperature of nipple (Type II'). Significant finding is difference in vascularization between the two breasts.
b) Left breast. Normal vascularization with lateral vascular channel (Type I).

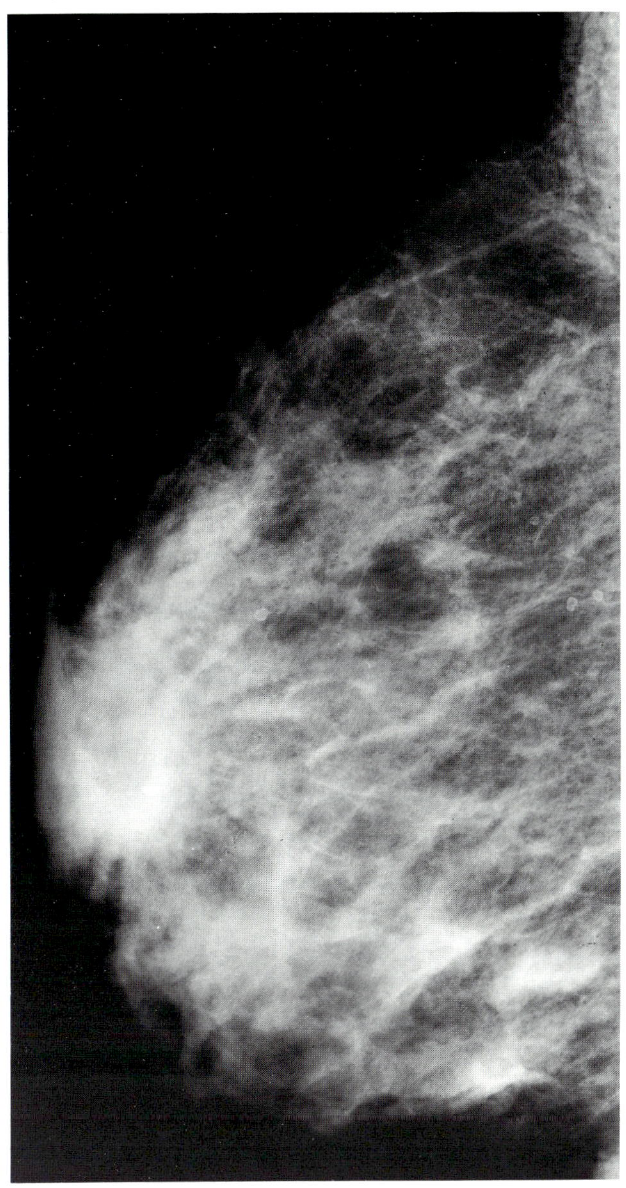
265 a

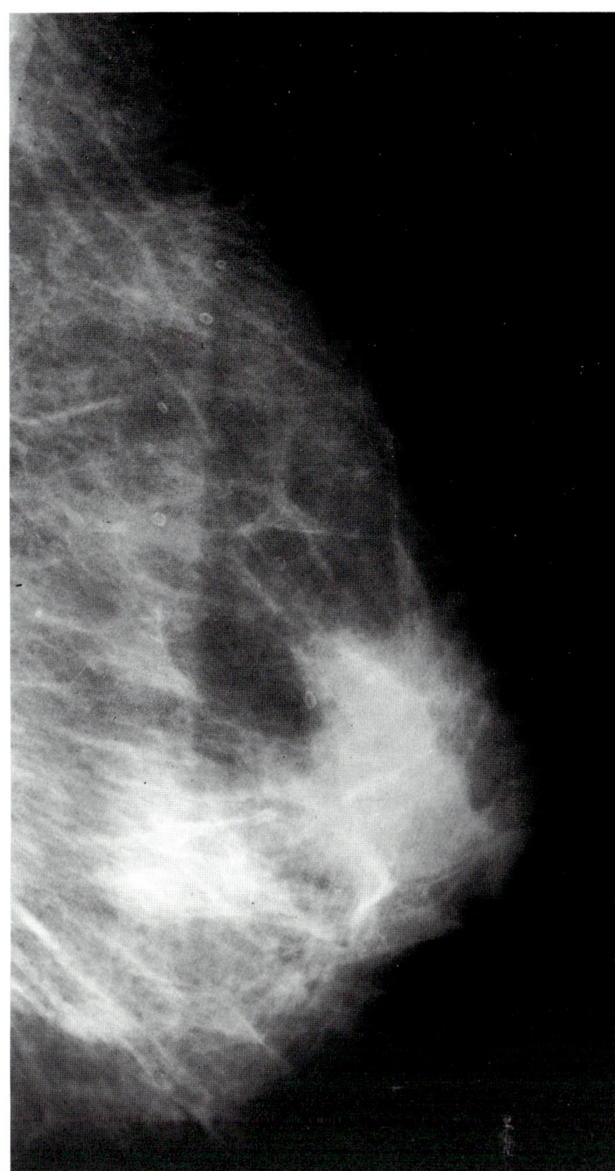
265 b

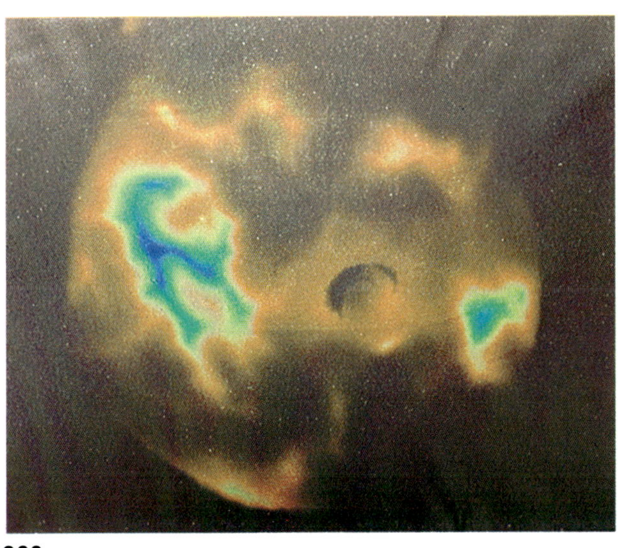
266 a

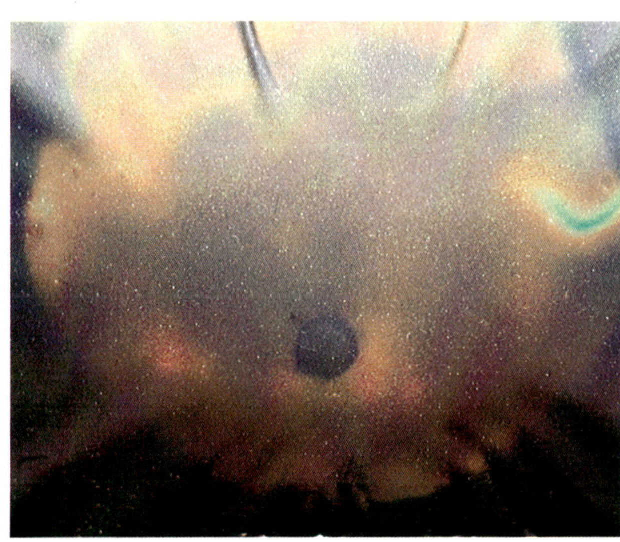
266 b

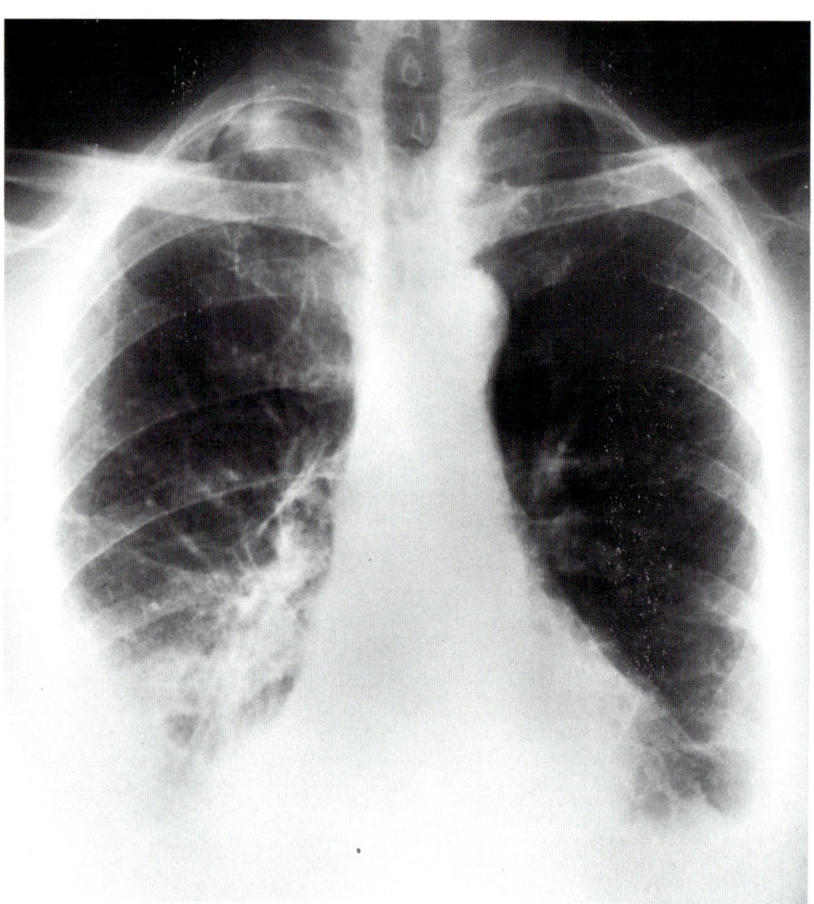

267 a

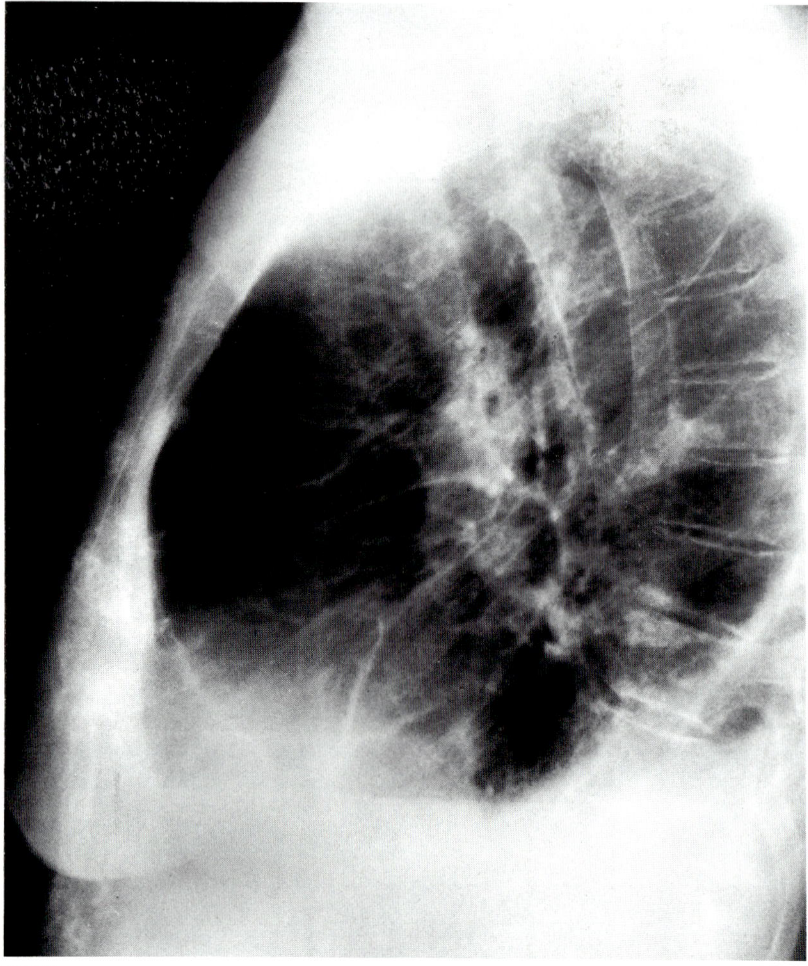

267 b

267 a, b. *Chest radiograph.*
a) Posterior-anterior.
b) Lateral.
Bilateral (right more than left) pleuritic reaction with loculated effusions. Heart and lungs otherwise normal for age. No pulmonary congestion radiographically or clinically.

Carcinoma of the male breast

Around the turn of the century, carcinoma of the male breast was a medical rarity. Although this disease is still rare, the number of malignant tumors of the male breast is increasing (GÜNTHER et al 1973). There is consensus in the literature that the prognosis in cancer of the male breast is poor. The major reason is that frequently the disease is thought of too late and the diagnosis is made when metastasis has already occurred. There is no histological difference between male and female breast cancer.

According to HAAGENSEN (1971) cancer of the male breast makes up 1% of all breast carcinomas. HOEFFKEN and LANYI (1977) found 1.2% of 1579 breast cancers to be in men. We found three among 259 malignancies in our patients (1.1%).

A summary of the incidence of male breast cancer in the world literature was reported by GÜNTHER et al (1973). *Clinically* there is a firm, retroareolar, often easily movable nodule. Occasionally there is secretion (Fig **268**). Paget's disease in the male breast is very rare.

A 56-year-old man with a lentil-sized, grayish-brown, slightly ulcerated erosion of the skin to the left of the areola showed, in mammogram, 10 stipple-like subcutaneous microcalcifications. Histologically Paget's disease was found.

According to HAAGENSEN (1971) the 10-year survival is up to 50%. Intramammary *metastases* from malignancies of other organs were found in three of our male patients. In two of them the metastasis was secondary to a malignant melanoma (Fig **271**); in the other it was secondary to a hypernephroma (Fig **183**).

Mammographic findings in male breast cancers are identical to those in women. Differentiation from gynecomastia may on occasion be difficult but is possible with thin-needle biopsy. According to HOEFFKEN and LANYI (1977) gynecomastia always lies behind the nipple while carcinoma is more eccentrically placed. Our own experience, however, contradicts this:

A 64-year-old man with recurrent bloody secretion from the right breast over a period of 5 years had a bean-sized palpable nodule *immediately* behind the nipple. Mammography showed a partially sharp, partially ill-defined opacity with retroareolar microcalcifications. Cytology and histology revealed a polymorphous comedocarcinoma (Fig **270**). On *thermography* the left nipple was 2°C warmer than the right.

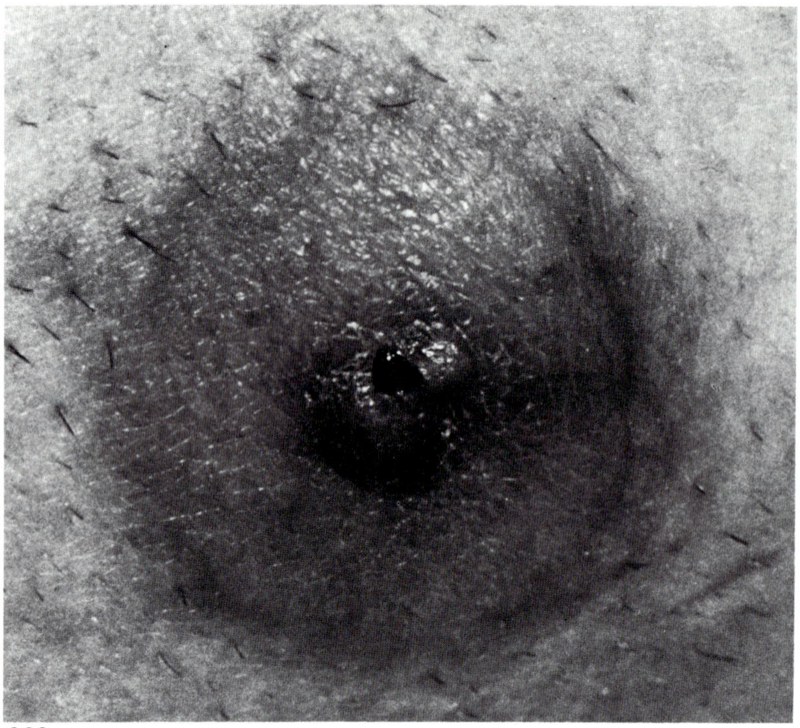

268

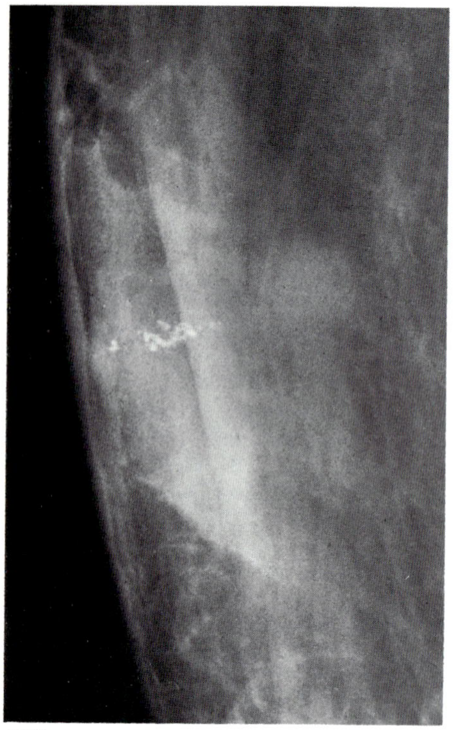

269

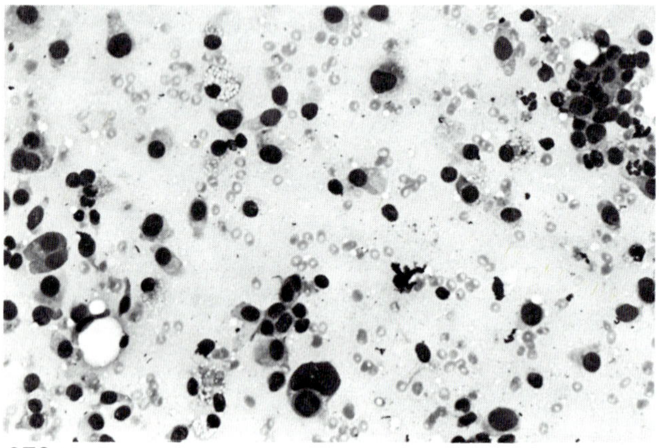

270 a

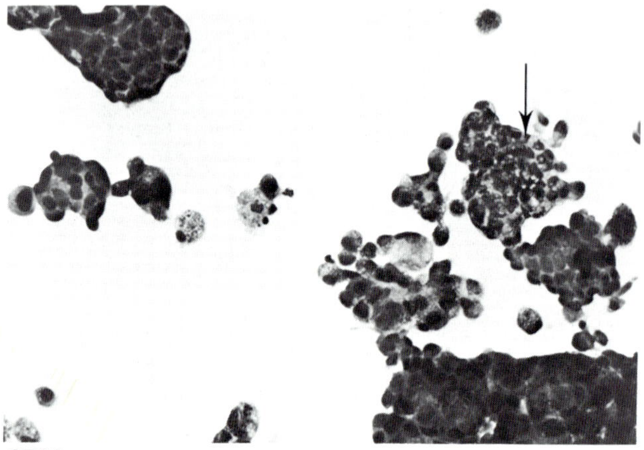

270 b

268 Right nipple and areola of 64-year-old male. For 5 years recurrent bleeding from right breast. Retroareolar, bean-sized, firm, nontender nodule palpable. Easily movable.

269 *Mammogram.* Ill-defined nonhomogeneous opacity with groups of microcalcifications. Suspicion of malignant tumor. (Courtesy, Dr. Mitrovics, Ludwigsburg, West Germany)

270 a, b. *Cytology.*
a) Secretion from nipple. Dissociated polymorphous tumor cells with hyperchromatic nuclei. Erythrocytes.
b) Thin-needle biopsy. Many clusters of tumor cells. Irregular size and shape of nuclei. Necrosis (arrow). Foam cells. Diagnosis: polymorphous breast carcinoma. Histology: comedocarcinoma with calcium deposits in ducts. Infiltrative growth. Axillary, lymph-node metastasis.

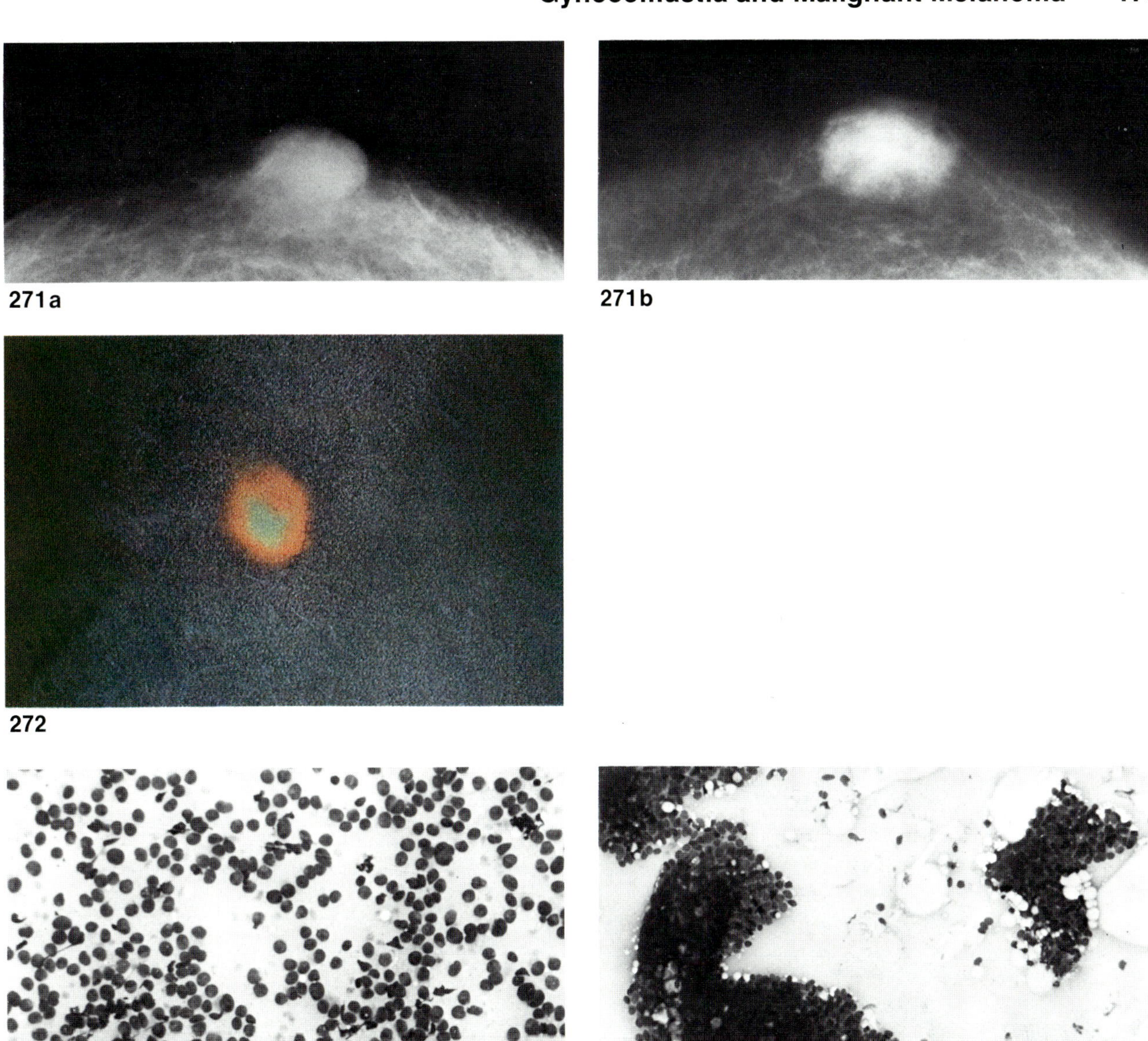

273a 273b

42-year-old male. Treatment for malignant melanoma on dorsum of foot 5 years ago. For 6 months formation of nodules in both breasts. Pain on left during past 4 weeks (Figs 271–273).

271 a, b. *Mammogram.*
a) Left breast (cranio-caudal). Nodular, retroareolar opacity, ill-defined at base; within it a smooth homogeneous nodule is identifiable, located medially at edge of breast. Suspicion of metastasis in view of his primary malignancy.
b) Right breast. Retroareolar nonhomogeneous opacity with partially smooth-, partially ill-defined contour. Diagnosis: gynecomastia.

272 *Plate thermography* left. Marked localized hyperthermia (3 °C) of left nipple and areola (Type IV^{II}): malignant. Right nipple thermographically cold.

273 a, b. *Cytological examinations,* magnif 60×.
a) Cytology left (obtained from surgical specimen). Numerous uniform small cells with predominantly naked nuclei. Absent cell coherence. No epithelial layers. Histology: amelanotic melanoma metastasis.
b) Cytology right. Normal large epithelial layers with small uniform nuclei. Single scattered bipolar cells with naked nuclei. Histology: gynecomastia.

The untreated and metastasizing carcinoma

Surgical treatment of breast carcinoma varies between extensive, radical and less extensive limited surgery. Each method can be combined with post-operative radiation therapy.
Problems of treatment have been discussed these past years on a world-wide basis in different ways. The older surgical and radiation-therapeutic concepts have been reevaluated.

Radiation therapy alone of carcinoma of the breast

Such treatment has been recommended and is used particularly in France (Gros 1963, Spitalier 1973). For several years we have observed ten patients treated exclusively with radiation therapy. The indication for radiotherapy only was either advanced age, increased surgical risk or advanced disease. The tumors were treated with a minimum of 6000 rad (tumor dose) with fast electrons using a 42 MeV-Betatron. The same radiation dose was delivered to axillary, supraclavicular and retrosternal lymph nodes.
Cellular tumors regressed more rapidly following radiation therapy than tumors rich in stroma.
Following tumor doses of 2000 to 3000 rad there is marked erythema of the skin, reaching its peak toward the end of the treatment. On occasion *epidermolysis* prevents further treatment. The epidermolysis changes to *scab formation*. The erythema will be healed 3 to 4 weeks following the completion of the radiation therapy treatment. Secondary to radiation, the *skin over the breast* often remains *hyperpigmented* for many years (Figs **232**, **283**).
Skin telangiectasia as seen with cobalt-60 teletherapy (Fig **279**), is less common after supervoltage therapy.
Complications of radiation therapy may be fibrosis of the breast, chest-wall muscles, soft tissues of the axilla, lungs and pleura. Fibrosis of chest wall and axilla may limit abduction of the arm. Contracting fibrosis of the axilla may cause edema of the arm and recurring thrombophlebitis of the upper arm.

Metastases

Breast carcinoma can be diagnosed when tumor diameter is 0.5 to 1 cm. As shown in Fig **274**, a breast carcinoma may metastasize when its diameter is only 0.06 cm—a very long time before it becomes clinically recognizable.
First each tumor develops subclinically. At present it is not known over what period of time this development occurs. It may be longer than generally assumed. The definitive diagnosis of a tumor occurs in the last third of the entire length of its growth period. According to Löhr et al (1972), in this period 10 to 20% of all patients already have distant metastases; 25 to 30% of all patients with breast carcinomas survive 10 years without recurrence. Late recurrences, even after 25 years, are not rare. There is a direct relation between the size of the primary tumor and the frequency of metastatic lymph nodes in the axilla. According to Bässler (1971) the frequency of axillary metastasis with a primary tumor 1.5 cm in diameter is 38%; over 5 cm 80%. According to Halama and Scherer (1964) and Halama (1966), in 50% of patients with metastatic breast carcinoma, metastases occur within 3 years after diagnosis. This is confirmed by our own experience.
Distribution of mestastases in the body is shown in Fig **275**. About 50% of distant metastases are in the skeleton; next come lung, liver, orbits, brain and skin. Metastatic involvement of bony structures and soft tissues of the orbits occurs in 8.9%, relatively commonly. Breast carcinoma metastases are found in either the skeleton or the soft tissues, but only rarely and in advanced disease are metastases found, both in soft tissues and skeleton.
Diagnosis of metastases on the body surface is not difficult because inspection, palpation and thin-needle biopsy permit early recognition. The most common form of surface metastasis is *local recurrence*. After mastectomy metastasis may occur in the area of the surgical scar, the operating field (the surrounding skin and tissue) and the pectoralis muscles. Axillary lymph nodes on the same side also belong to the group of local recurrences (Demarree 1951).
Frequency of local recurrence depends to a great degree on the technique of postoperative radiation therapy of the chest wall and the lymph nodes in the axillar, supraclavicular and retrosternal regions.
From 1966 to 1971 the *incidence of local recurrence* in 1000 patients treated for breast carcinoma with radiation therapy to the chest wall using the fast electron beam (electron-rotation-radiation therapy of thoracic wall and stationary radiation therapy to regional lymph nodes)

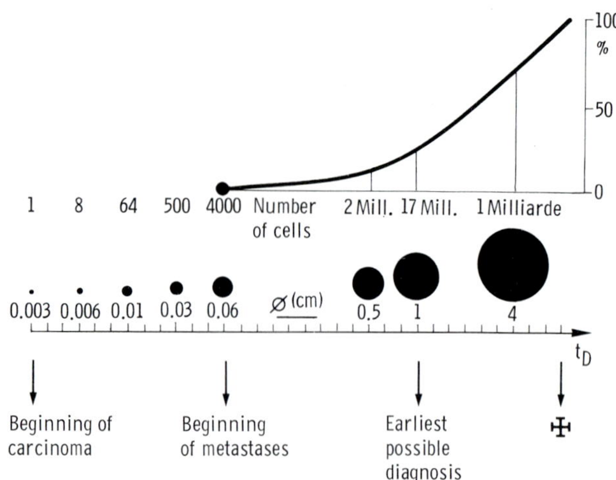

274 Local tumor growth (center) and frequency of metastases (above) in relation to doubling time of tumor (according to Krokowski).

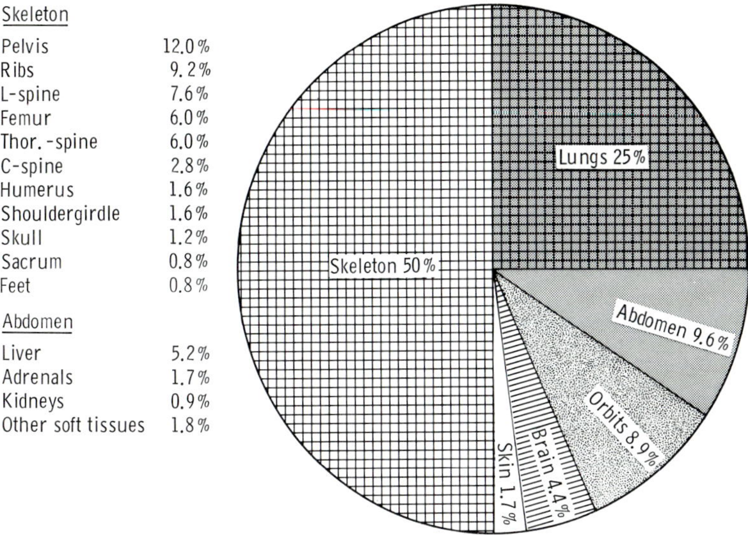

275 Organ involvement with distant metastases (according to Halama).

was 4.7%. However, in 6%, postradiation therapy necrosis of the ribs and ulcerations of the skin of the chest wall occurred.

Incidence of local recurrence with postoperative radiation of the chest wall using cobalt-60 teletherapy (tangential stationary ports) was 8.6%. *Without* primary postoperative radiation therapy of the operative field, the incidence of local recurrence was 25.6% (WÖLLGENS et al, 1973).

About $^2/_3$ to $^3/_4$ of all recurrences take place within the first 3 years; 90% in the first 5 years after primary therapy (VON FOURNIER et al 1972).

The early onset of carcinomatous lymphangitis often is misdiagnosed as an allergic reaction of the skin induced by the material of a breast prosthesis. This results in wasting time with antiinflammatory treatment before diagnosing and treating the metastasis (Fig **292**).

The diagnosis of *liver, brain and skeletal metastases* requires rather extensive instrumental and time-consuming efforts. *Bony metastases* are 85% *osteolytic* and 15% *osteoblastic* or mixed. Their high incidence on the one hand (often associated with prolonged debilitation) and the radio-therapeutic-success rate on the other demand earliest possible recognition of metastasis.

Commonly the pain caused by metastasis has equivalent radiographic skeletal findings, but patients may complain about diffuse or circumscribed skeletal pain without osteolytic or osteoblastic changes radiographically. It must be considered that bony morphologic changes can be shown radiographically only when calcium content of the metastasis has decreased 30% as compared with normal bone. On the other hand, radiographic signs of metastases in the skeleton may occasionally be found before the onset of symptoms.

Bone scintigraphy (isotope examination) will close the time gap between recognition of existing metastatic involvement and its clinical as well as radiographic manifestations in most cases. With this method skeletal changes were recognized 2 to 3 months prior to development of radiographic signs. For this reason, scintigraphy is being used as a screening method to determine the presence of metastases as early as possible in patients without symptoms. There are problems in its application; false positives are common because inflammatory arthritic changes may simulate metastases in the scintigram. False negatives, however, are rare.

Survival time

Survival time of untreated breast carcinoma is variable and depends on the degree of differentiation of the tumor and the immunity of the patient.

The average survival time according to HAAGENSEN (1971) is 2.7 years (Fig **276**). The longest survival time of an untreated carcinoma in our series of patients was found in a nun who had been hiding a Paget's disease for 10 years (Fig **236**). The patient confided her condition to her Mother Superior after skeletal pain (because of generalized metastasis) had become unbearable. After palliative therapy the patient has survived 2 years.

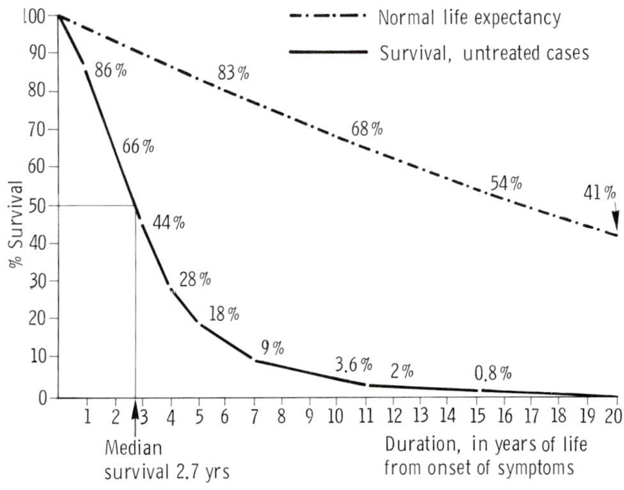

276 Average survival time of untreated breast carcinoma (according to Haagensen).

53-year-old female, right breast. Palpation negative. Mastectomy 4 weeks ago for scirrhous carcinoma, left. No tumor growth over a period of 12 months. The defense mechanism of the body apparently prevented local spread of the tumor. Danger of nonremoval of a nodule is related not as closely to its size as to the possibility of metastasis. In this case no distant metastasis after 2 years (Figs 277–278).

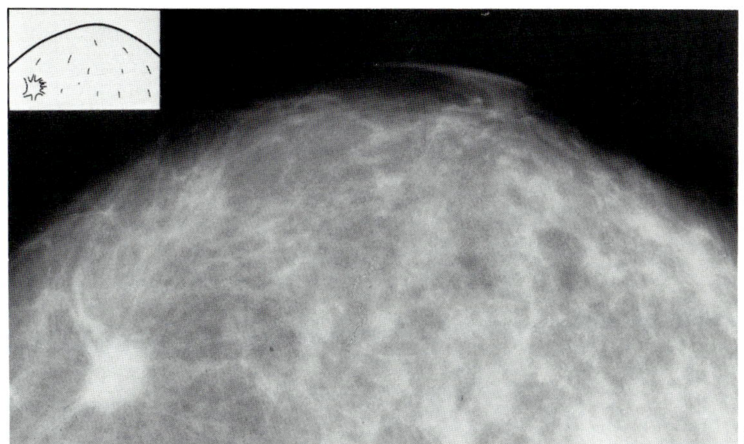

a

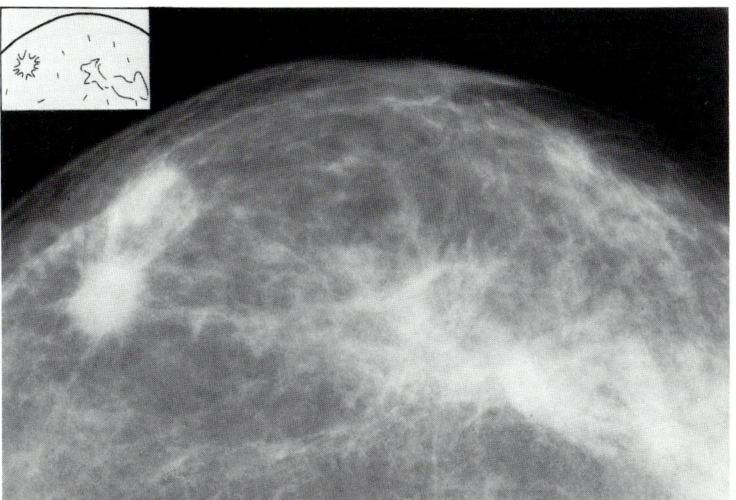

b

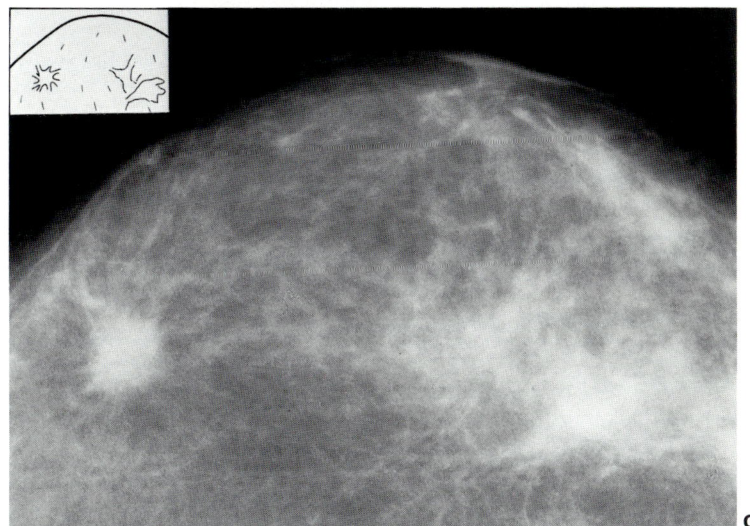

c

277 a–c. *Mammogram* right (follow-up examination, cranio-caudal).

a) First examination. In inner quadrant region homogeneous stellate tumor opacity: suspicion of carcinoma. Nodule not palpable; the surgeon, reading the radiographic report only hastily, made a biopsy of outer instead of inner quadrant. Histology: breast fibrosis.

b) Follow-up examination after 6 months. No tumor growth. No skin retraction. In region of biopsy nonhomogeneous, ill-defined opacity (scar formation). Attempt at tissue biopsy with a biopsy needle. Acute extensive bleeding secondary to injury of a vessel during introduction of needle into breast parenchyma. Histology of small tissue biopsy done under pressure of time—breast fibrosis. No therapy.

c) Follow-up examination after 12 months. No growth of carcinoma. Size unchanged. Thin-needle biopsy: numerous tumor cells.

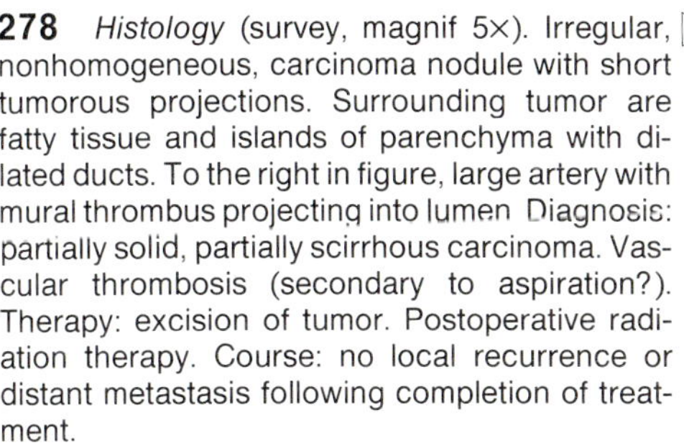

278 *Histology* (survey, magnif 5×). Irregular, ▷ nonhomogeneous, carcinoma nodule with short tumorous projections. Surrounding tumor are fatty tissue and islands of parenchyma with dilated ducts. To the right in figure, large artery with mural thrombus projecting into lumen. Diagnosis: partially solid, partially scirrhous carcinoma. Vascular thrombosis (secondary to aspiration?). Therapy: excision of tumor. Postoperative radiation therapy. Course: no local recurrence or distant metastasis following completion of treatment.

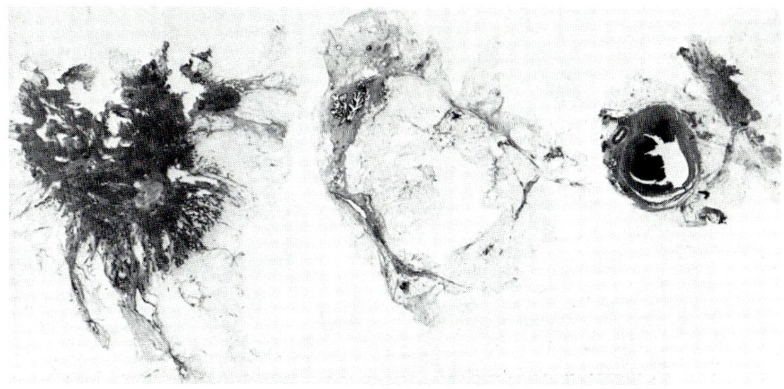

69-year-old female, right breast. Excision of tumor with postoperative radiation therapy (cobalt-60 teletherapy) 7 years ago because of adenocarcinoma. For 1 year ulcer in surgical scar with bark-like scab (Figs 279–281).

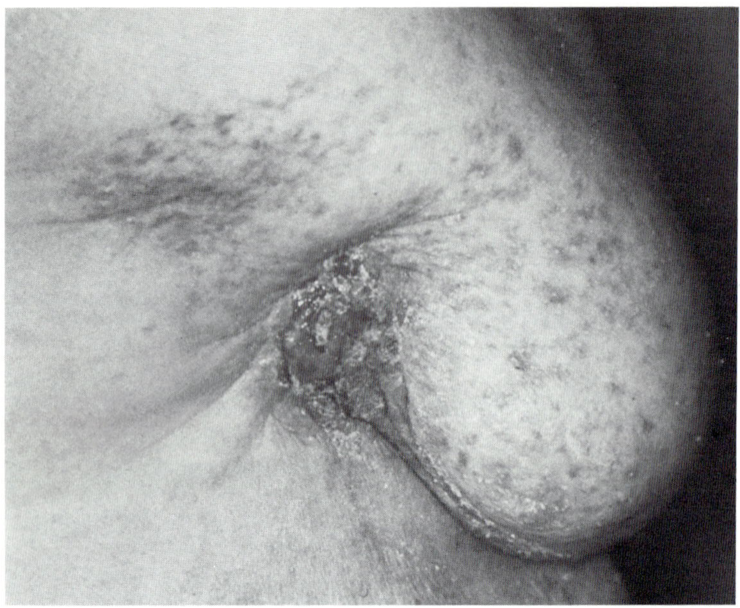

279

279 Right breast (lateral). Previous excision of tumor in right-outer quadrant region with decrease in size of breast. Multiple telangiectases of skin following radiation. In scar, 2 cm sunken ulcer with grayish-white-brown scab.

280 *Mammogram* (cranio-caudal). Circumscribed thickening of skin. Nonhomogeneous, diffuse, ill-defined opacity in region of previous tumor bed. Suspicion of local recurrence of tumor. Thin-needle biopsy.

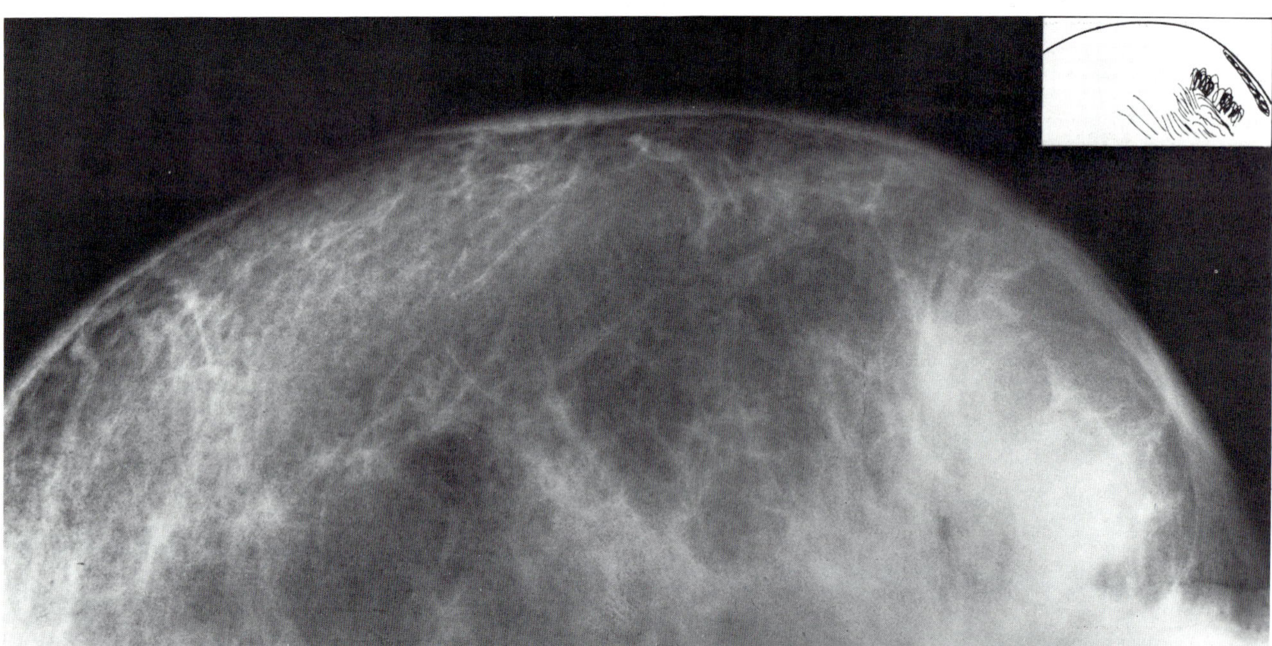

280

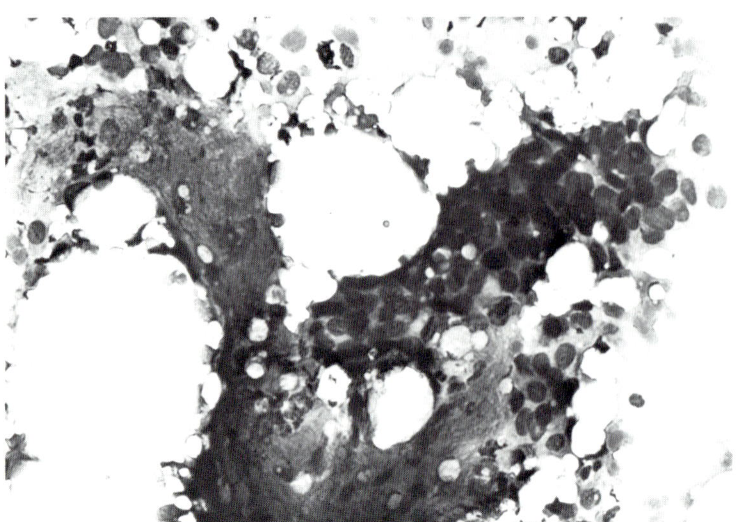

281

281 *Cytology.* Multiple, moderately polymorphous, dissociated carcinoma cells in two layers. Abundant mucus and debris. Therapy: mastectomy with removal of axillary lymph nodes (metastasis). Postoperative radiation therapy to chest wall with betatron (tumor dose 5000 rad). Course: generalized osteolytic skeletal metastases 1 year after completion of therapy. Death $1\frac{1}{2}$ years later.

63-year-old female, left breast. Previous local excision of a carcinoma in left upper outer quadrant. No postoperative radiation therapy. Local recurrence after 6 months. Again circumscribed excision of the tumor. No radiation therapy. Treatment with a mistletoe preparation. Mammography now after 1 year because of occurrence of another nodule and recurrent, spontaneous hematomas of left breast. On palpation multiple, easily movable nodules under scar. Walnut-sized lymph node in left axilla (Figs 282–289). Radiation therapy.

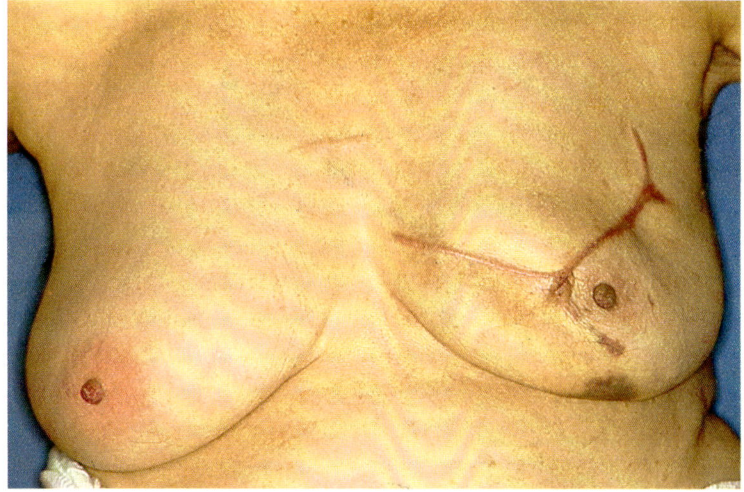

282

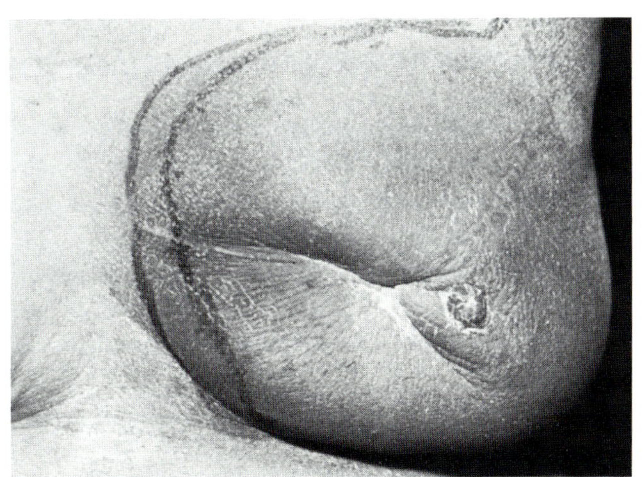

283 a

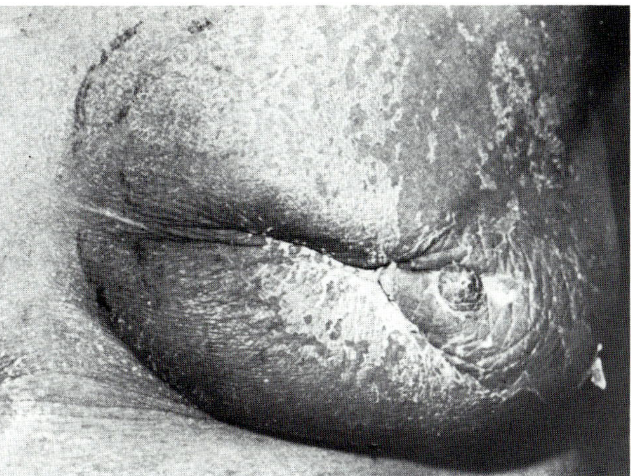

283 b

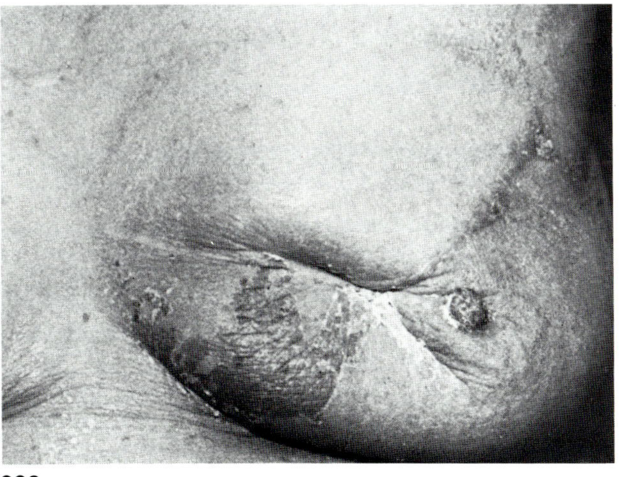

283 c

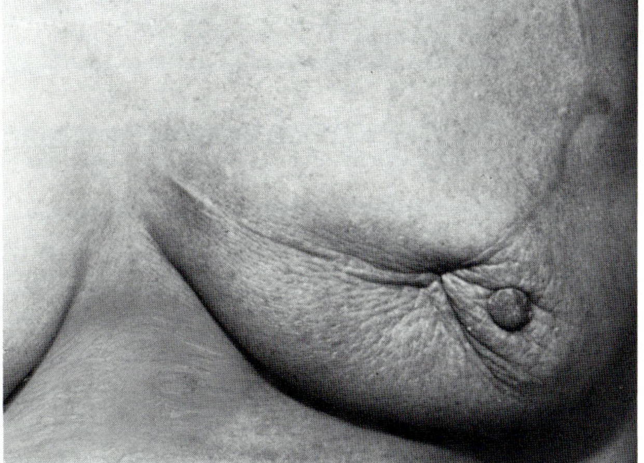

283 d

282 Two long scars in inner and outer quadrants. Hematoma at undersurface of breast. Right breast negative.

283 a–d. Changes in skin of breast during and after radiation therapy.

a) Three weeks after beginning radiation therapy (tumor dose 3500 rad). Marked erythema of skin. Slight swelling of breast.

b) At end of treatment after 5 weeks (tumor dose 6000 rad). Marked erythema with beginning epidermolysis.

c) Four weeks after completion of radiation therapy. Regression of erythema. Marked desquamation of skin.

d) Three months after completion of radiation therapy. Slight hyperpigmentation, otherwise no abnormal findings. At palpation increased consistency of fibrosed breast parenchyma.

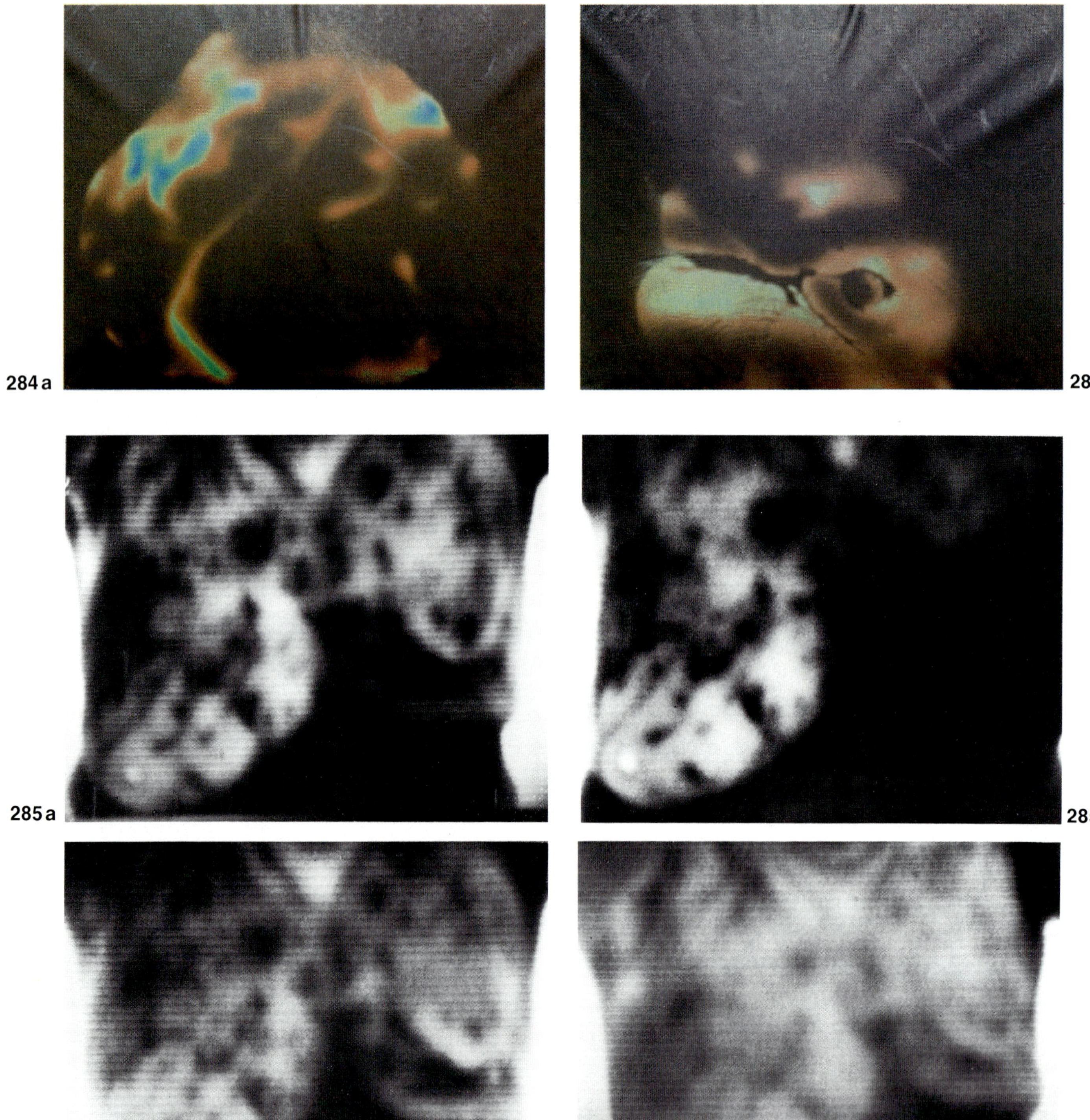

284 a, b. *Plate thermography* (first examination). Thermographic course.
a) Right breast. Inner and outer vessels show normal vascularity with anastomosing superficial vein.
b) Left breast. Scar, cold (retraction of skin with absent contact to plate). Under scar and periareolar area, marked hyperthermia of skin (2.5 °C): malignant.

285 a–d. *Electronic thermovision* (initial examination identical to plate thermographic picture).
a) Thermogram of skin following 1000-rad tumor dose. Band-like hyperthermia in area of scar on left. Right breast normal. Cold nipple.
b) Thermogram of skin after 3500-rad tumor dose. Very marked hyperthermia of entire left breast (dark). Right breast unchanged.
c) Thermogram 4 weeks after completion of radiation therapy. Regression of diffuse hyperthermia. Scar area still hyperthermic. Vascular pattern on right unchanged.
d) Thermogram of skin 3 years after completion of radiation therapy. Left breast markedly smaller. Scar still 0.5 °C warmer than surroundings. Right breast shows no change in vascularization.

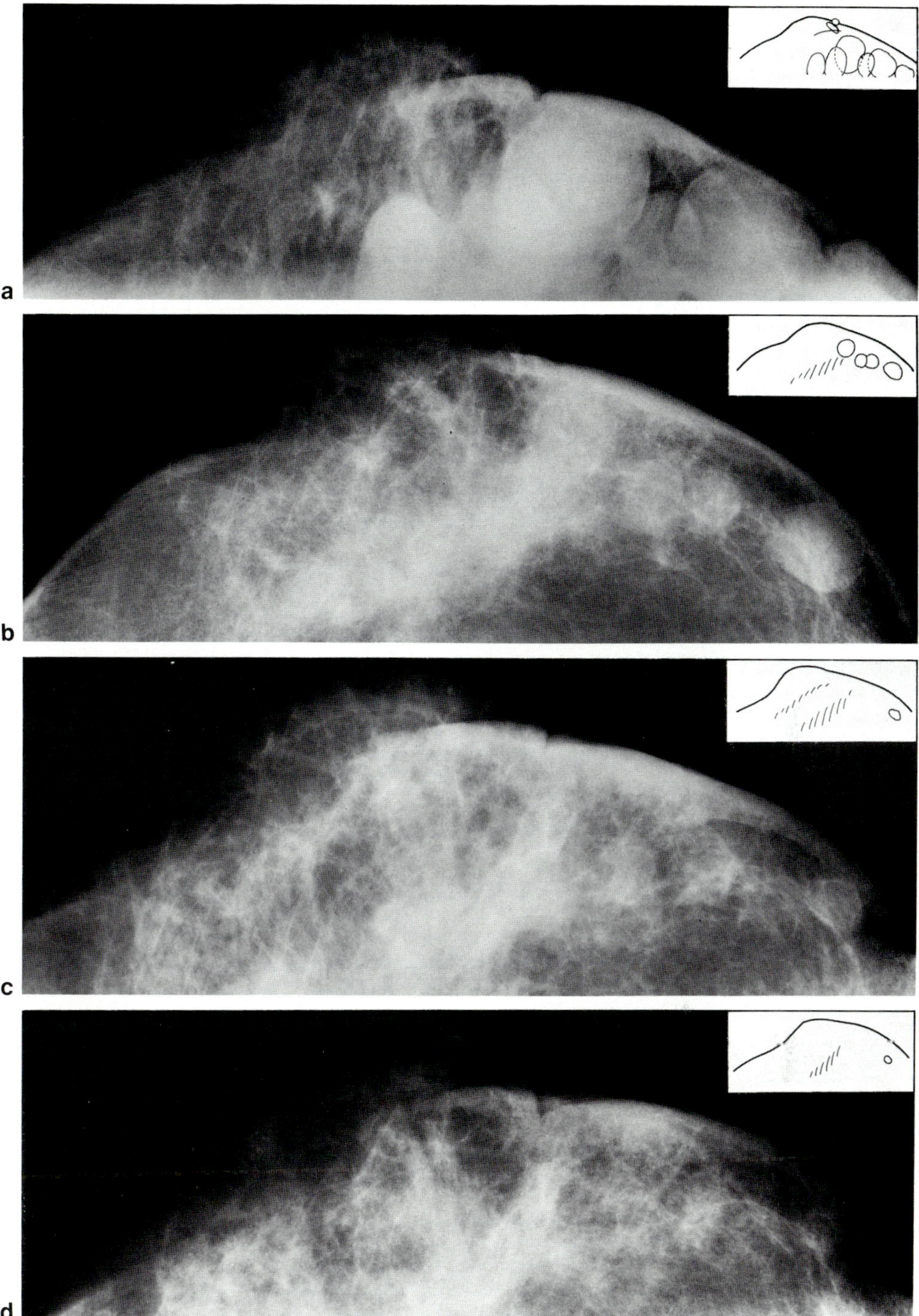

286 a–d. *Mammographic* changes in left breast.
a) Original examination. Previous excision of tumor with decrease in size of breast. Retraction of scar. Multiple, up to walnut-sized, homogeneous, smoothly defined opacities under scar in inner quadrant area.
b) Follow-up examination during radiation therapy (3500-rad tumor dose). Marked shrinkage of tumors. Nonhomogeneous thickening of breast (inflammatory reaction during radiation therapy). Thin-needle biopsy: markedly degenerated tumor epithelium (compare Fig 288b).
c) Follow-up examination 2 months after completion of radiation therapy. Increase of radio-opacity of breast (fibrosis). Small residual subcutaneous medial opacity. Thin-needle biopsy. In addition to degenerated tumor epithelium, active tumor cells without signs of degeneration (compare Fig 287c).
d) Follow-up examination after 9 months. Strand-like coarse fibrosis of breast. No nodules identifiable. Thin-needle biopsy: only connective tissue found in different areas of breast.

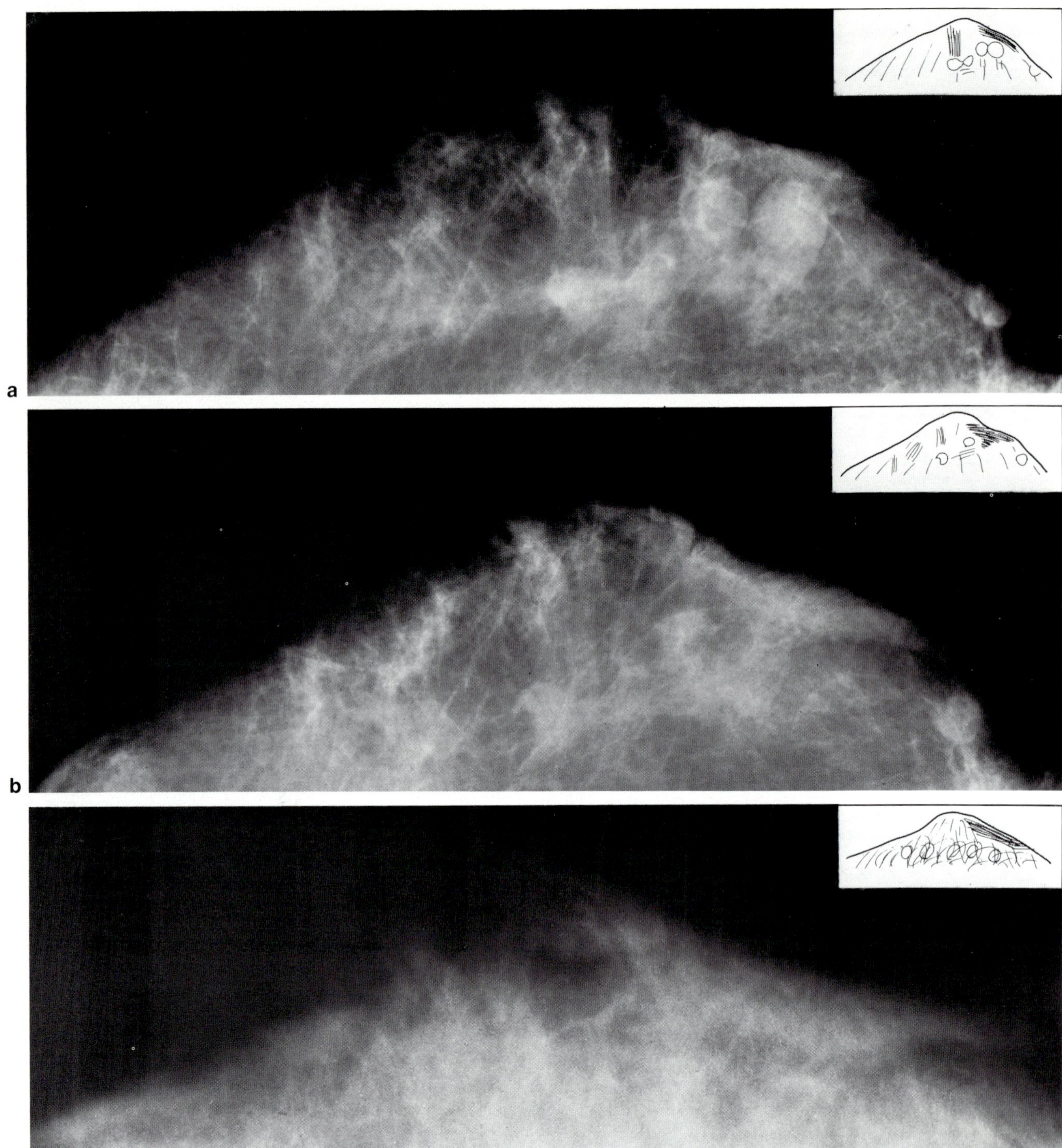

287 a–d. *Mammogram of left breast.*
a) Fifteen months after completion of radiation therapy. In interim 2 new nodules have grown: local recurrence. Thin-needle biopsy: on cytologic smear, tumor epithelium with marked lymphocytic reaction (compare Fig 288d). No therapy.
b) Follow-up examination 17 months after radiation therapy. Spontaneous regression of both nodules. Residual small nodule medially. Fibrosis of breast.
c) Follow-up examination 3 years after completion of radiation therapy. Recurrent tumor in the breast again 20 months after radiation therapy. Radiation therapy of recurrence with 3000-rad tumor dose (fast electron beam). After completion of first course of radiation therapy, complete regression of nodules without recurrence within 36 months. The radiation dose which totaled 9000 rad caused marked fibrosis of breast, chest wall and soft tissues of axilla, this resulting in marked limitation of abduction of the left arm.

In mammogram this fibrosis is recognizable by the dense structures and shrinkage of entire breast. The tumor nodules are destroyed.

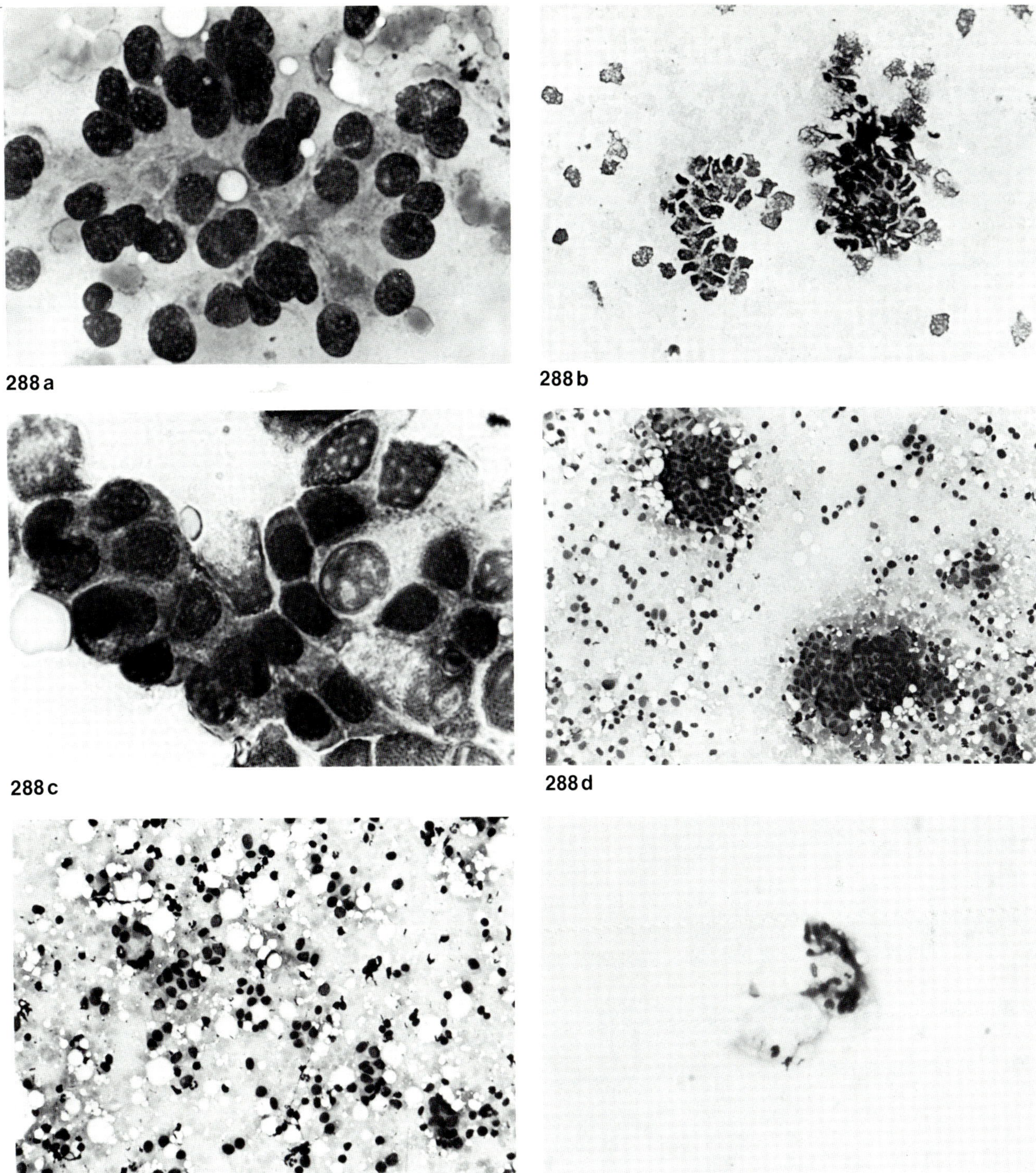

288 a–f. *Changes of cytology* during and after radiation therapy.

a) Original findings. Numerous tumor cells in loose clusters with slightly polymorphous nuclei. Magnif 240×.

b) Cytological appearance following tumor dose of 3500 rad. Two clusters of tumor cells. Marked degenerative changes of nuclei with finest, vacuole-like clear spots. Bizarre contours. Absent cytoplasm. Magnif 80×.

c) Cytological appearance 2 months after completion of radiation therapy. Next to markedly degenerated tumor cells hyperchromatic epithelium without signs of degeneration. Magnif 240×.

d) Follow-up cytology 15 months after radiation therapy. Multiple clusters of tumor cells with uniform nuclei. Between these clusters, very many lymphocytes. Magnif 80×.

e) Follow-up cytology 20 months after radiation therapy. Numerous lymphocytes next to small areas of tumor epithelium. Magnif 80×.

f) Follow-up cytology 36 months after radiation therapy. Some connective tissue and normal epithelium. Magnif 80×.

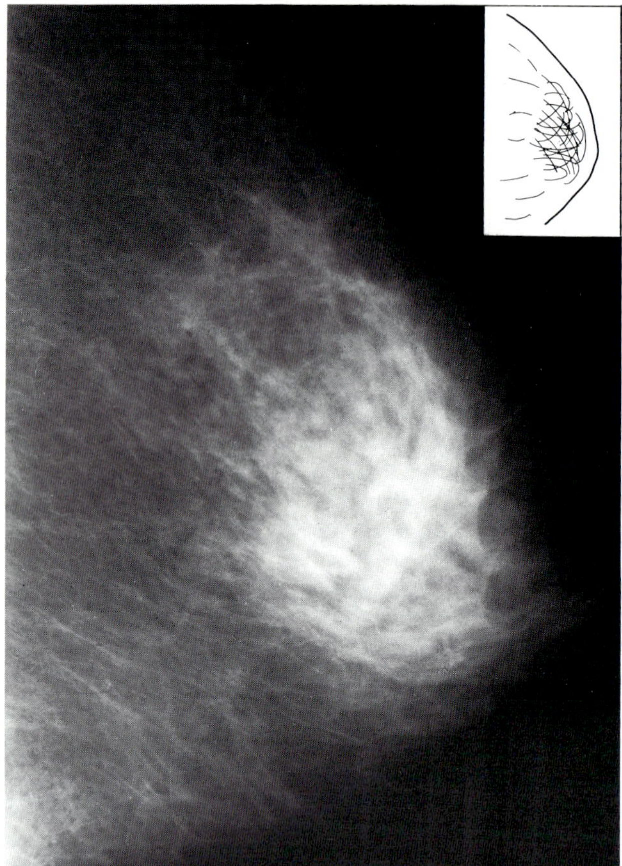

289 a

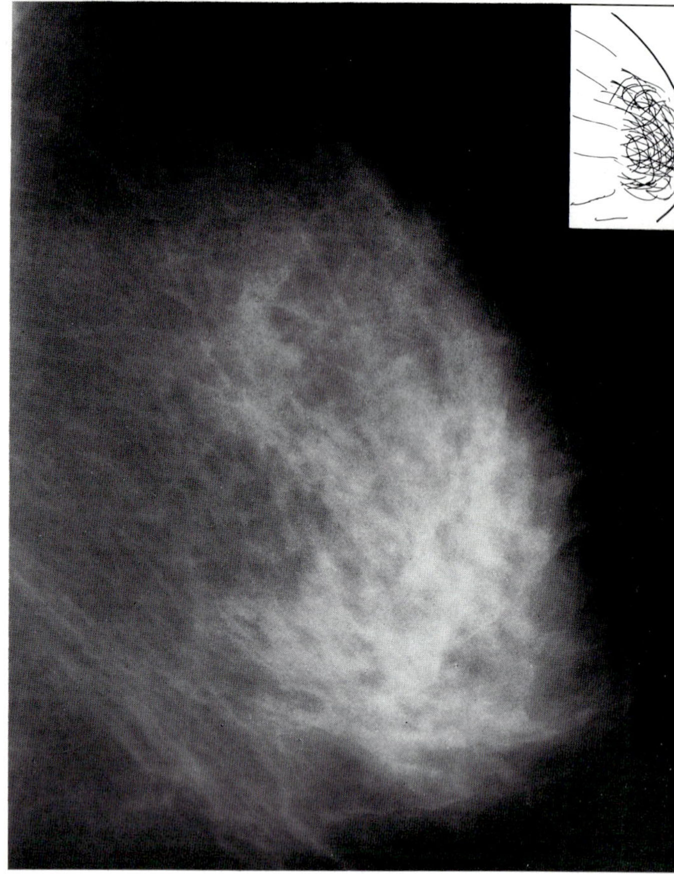

289 b

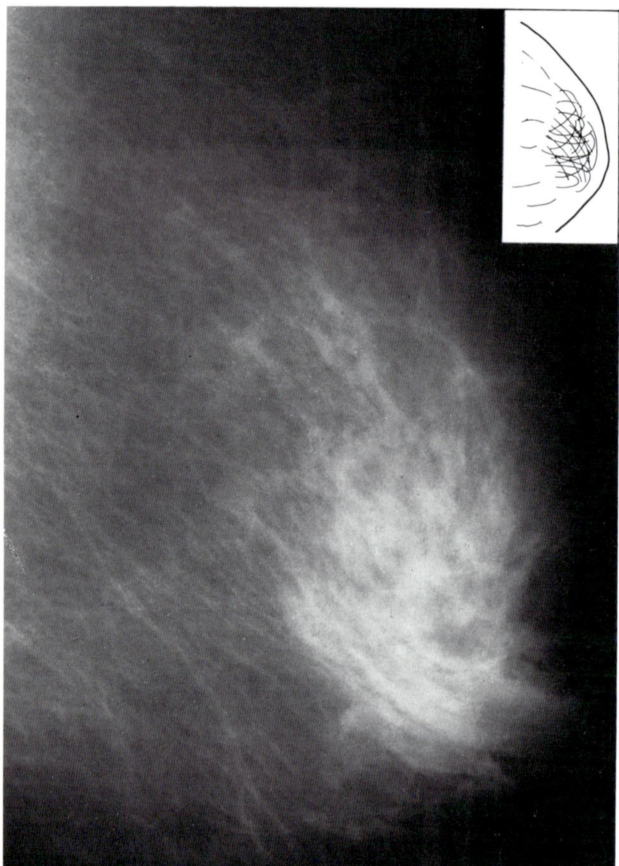

289 c

289 a–c. Changes of normal breast parenchyma following a single administration of hormone preparation of estrogen and gestagen because of local recurrence in left breast. *Mammogram* right (medio-lateral).

a) Original mammography. Normal structure of breast with small opacities along the ductules.

b) Mammogram 8 days after administration of hormones. Marked enlargement of breast with basic structure unchanged (proliferation of lobules and edema of perilobular connective tissue?). Clinically, marked feeling of pressure.

c) Follow-up examination 3 months after hormone administration. Breast now again completely normal. Normal glandular structures. Course: No distant metastases 4 years after first radiation therapy course began. General condition good. Limited range of motion of left arm because of radiation fibrosis.

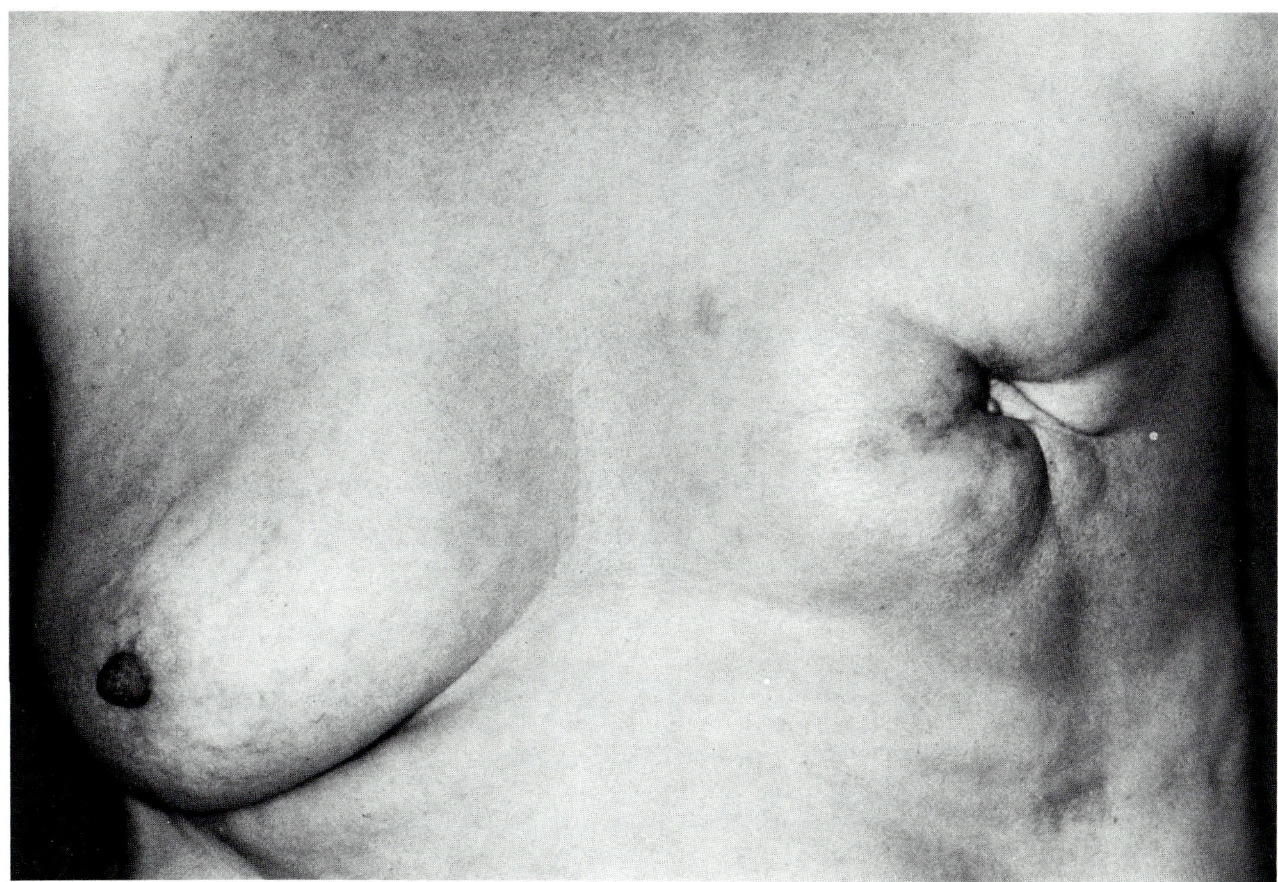

290

53-year-old female. Cherry-sized nodule in left breast 3 years ago. No therapy as patient wanted to wait for completion of her son's college education. Increasing shrinkage of breast (Figs 290–291).

290 Left breast markedly contracted after 3 years. Nipple and areola are drawn into breast by tumor and are no longer recognizable. Strand formation to axilla.

291 Appearance of tumor. Retracted and thickened nipple (above) with scirrhous retroareolar carcinoma. Tumor gray-white-yellow. The yellow, net-like strands in the tumor center are elastic fibers. Infiltration of pectoralis muscles (below in figure). Therapy: mastectomy with postoperative radiation therapy of chest wall and regional lymph nodes (metastasis in axillary lymph nodes). Course: Osteolytic metastases in pelvis and left femur 2 years after completion of treatment.

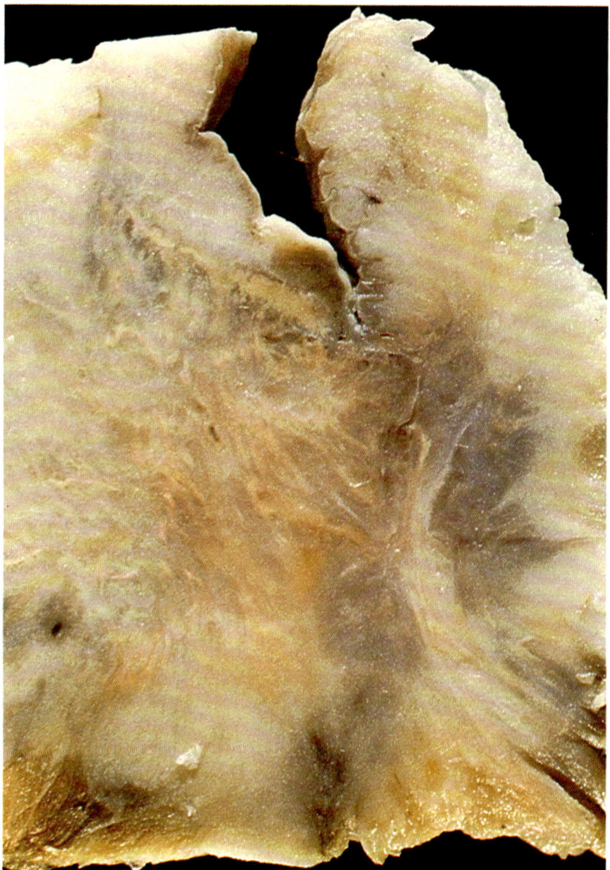

291

66-year-old female. Previous right mastectomy $3^1/_2$ years ago. For 6 months erythema and nodule formation of right chest wall associated with very marked itching (Figs 292–294).

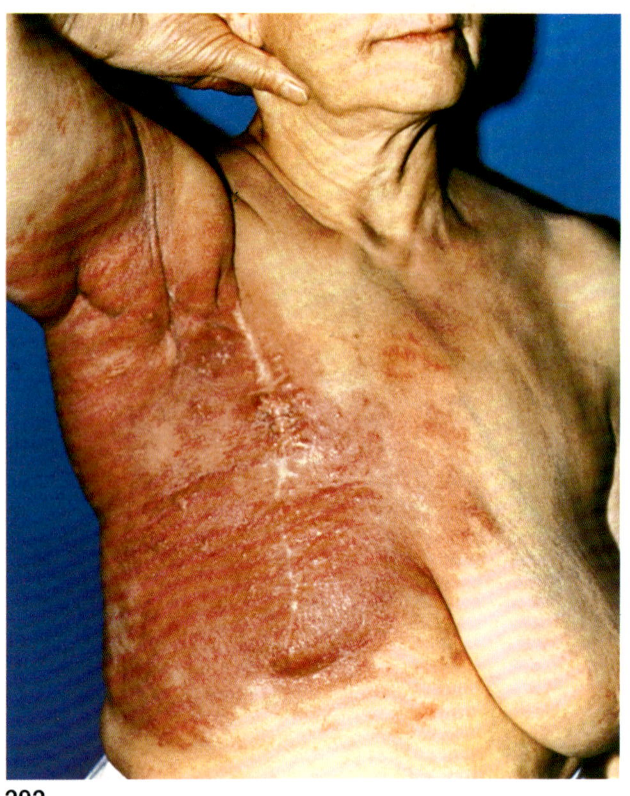

292

292 Marked erythema of skin surrounding scar and at lateral chest wall multiple small nodules. Suspicion of carcinomatous lymphangitis of skin with lenticular skin metastases. Thin-needle biopsy.

293 *Histology* of skin. Marked thickening of epidermis. Diffuse infiltration by lymphocytes and leukocytes. Extreme dilatation of epidermal lymph channels by tumor epithelium with marked formation of new connective tissue.

294 *Cytology.* Thin-needle biopsy from reddened skin reveals loosely arranged tumor epithelium. Round and oval nuclei. Coarse, spot-like chromatin structure. Increased and confluent nucleoli. Between tumor cells many leukocytes, lymphocytes and some debris.

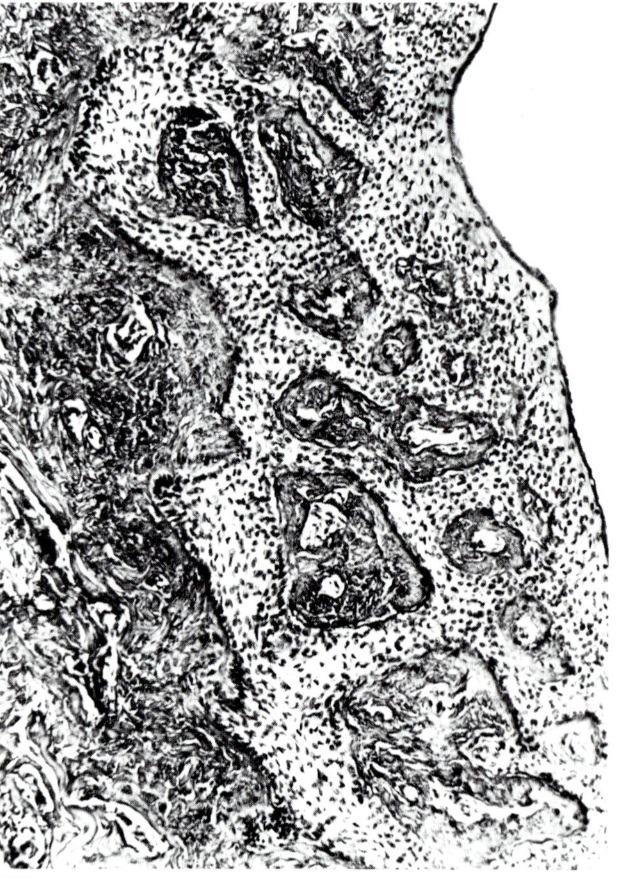

293

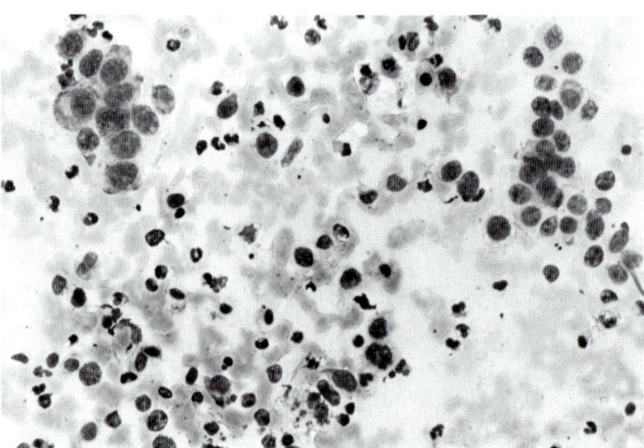

294

References

von Albertini, A.: Histologische Geschwulstdiagnostik, 2nd Ed. Thieme, Stuttgart 1974, 287

Ambrosi, C., Torresani, J., Saadjian, A., Jonve, A.: Méthode colorimétrique cutanée de thermométrie. Marseille Méd. 106 (1969) 689

Anastassiades, O.N., Pryce, D.M.: Fibrosis as an indication of time in infiltrating breast cancer and its importance in prognosis. Br. J. Cancer 29 (1974) 232

Arrata, W.S.M., Chatterton, R.T.: Human lactation: appropriate and inappropriate. Obstet. Gynecol. 3 (1974) 443

Bässler, R., Schulze, G., Schriever, D.: Histochemische Untersuchungen am Bindegewebe der hormonstimulierten Mamma. Beitr. Pathol. Anat. 140 (1970) 212

Bässler, R., Kreienberg, R., Scheidt, E.: Ergebnisse pathologischer und differentialdiagnostischer Untersuchungen an 4000 Probeexzisionen der Mamma. Arch. Gynaekol. 211 (1971) 48

Bässler, R.: Zur Definition und Dignität des Carcinoma in situ der Brustdrüse. Verh. Dtsch. Ges. Pathol. 59 (1975) 497

Bässler, R.: Pathologie der Brustdrüse. Springer, Berlin-Heidelberg-New York 1978

Baraldi, A.: Roentgen-mammo-mastia. Rev. Chir. 14 (1935) 321

Barth, V.: Mammographie und Zytologie in der Vorsorgediagnostik der Mamma. Röntgenber. 1 (1972) 22

Barth, V.: Die Feinstruktur der Brustdrüse im Röntgenbild. Thieme, Stuttgart 1979, in press

Barth, V., Deininger, H.K.: Informationswert der radiologischen Mammadiagnostik. Z. Allgemeinmed. 1 (1971) 1748

Barth, V., Deininger, H.K., von Babo, H., Kirchberger, R., Müller, G.: Vermeidbare diagnostische Irrtümer in Verbindung mit Röntgenuntersuchungen der weiblichen Brustdrüse. Dtsch. Med. Wochenschr. 98 (1973) 272

Barth, V., Kraus, B., Deininger, H.K.: Zur Diagnostik von Mammatumoren mit Hilfe von Gewebsstanzzylindern. Dtsch. Med. Wochenschr. 96 (1971) 2005

Barth, V., Kraus, B., Heuck, F., Ilbagian, K.: Kasuistischer Beitrag zum radiologisch-anatomischen Aspekt eines Mammakarzinoms neben einer proliferierenden Zyste. Fortschr. Geb. Roentgenstr. 117 (1972) 604

Barth, V., Müller, R., Deininger, H.K., Wöllgens, P.: Technische Fehlermöglichkeiten bei der erweiterten Mammadiagnostik. Dtsch. Med. Wochenschr. 98 (1973) 1724

Barth, V., Müller, R., Deininger, H.K., Wöllgens, P.: Klinik, Mammographie, Zytologie, Stanzbiopsie und Plattenthermographie in der erweiterten Mammadiagnostik. Vergleichende Untersuchungen. Dtsch. Med. Wochenschr. 99 (1974) 175

Barth, V., Müller, R., Mayle, M.: Die weibliche Brustdrüse im Galaktogramm. Dtsch. Med. Wochenschr. 100 (1975) 1213

Bauermeister, D.E., Hall, M.H.: Specimen radiography—a mandatory adjunct to mammography. Am. J. Clin. Pathol. 59 (1973) 782

Berndt, H., Landmann, R.: Zwei epidemiologische Typen des Mammakarzinoms. Arch. Geschwulstforsch. 33 (1969) 157

Berndt, H., Marwitz, S.: Mastopathie und Mammakarzinom. Arch. Geschwulstforsch. 32 (1968) 37

Black, J.W., Young, B.: A radiological and pathological study of the incidence of calcification in disease of the breast and neoplasms of other tissues. Br. J. Radiol. 38 (1965) 596

Black, M.M., Asire, A.J.: Palpable axillary lymph nodes in cancer of the breast. Cancer (Phila.) 23 (1969) 251

Black, M.M., Barclay, T.H.C., Cutler, S.J., Hankey, B.F., Asire, A.J.: Association of atypical characteristics of benign breast lesions with subsequent risk of breast cancer. Cancer (Phila.) 29 (1972) 338

Böhmig, R.: Mastopathia fibrosa cystica, ihre Epithelproliferationen und deren Beziehung zum Karzinom. Ergeb. Allg. Pathol. Anat. 45 (1964) 39

Bohatirchuk, F.P.: Erfahrungen der letzten 20 Jahre in der Anwendung der Mikroröntgenographie in der Medizinisachen Forschung. Fortschr. Geb. Roentgenstr. 87 (1957) 44

le Borgne, R.A.: The Breast in Roentgen Diagnosis. Impresora Uruguaya, South America, Montevideo 1953

Brandt, G., Bässler, R.: Die Wirkung der experimentellen Hypercalcaemie durch Dihydrotachysterin auf Drüsenfunktion und Verkalkungsmuster der Mamma. Licht-, elektronenmikroskopische und chemischanalytische Untersuchungen. Virchows Arch. A 356 (1972) 155

Brezina, K., Hernuss, P.: Das Röntgenbild der Parenchymstruktur der Mamma bei Uterus myomatosus. Radiol. Clin. Biol. 44 (1975) 24

Buchwald, W., Hylse, R.: Vermeidbare und nicht vermeidbare Fehlinterpretationen bei der Mammographie. Arch. Gynäk. 211 (1971) 42

Busch, W., Merker, H.J.: Elektronenmikroskopische Untersuchungen an menschlichen Mammakarzinomen. Virchows Arch. A 344 (1968) 356

Buttenberg, D., Werner, K.: Die Mammographie. Schattauer, Stuttgart 1962

Castano-Almendral, A., Gläntzner, H., Siedentopf, H.G.: Vergleichende mammographische und histologische Befunde. Arch. Gyn. 211 (1971) 43

Cowie, A.T., Folley, S.J.: The mammary gland and lactation, In: Young, W.C., Corner, G.W. (eds.): Sex and Internal Secretions, Vol. 2. Williams and Wilkins, Baltimore 1961

Cutler, S.J., Zippin, C., Asire, A.J.: The prognostic significance of palpable lymph nodes in cancer of the breast. Cancer (Phila.) 23 (1969) 243

Dabelow, A.: Der Entfaltungsmechanismus der Mamma. Gegenbaurs Morphol. Jahrb. 73 (1933) 69

Dauvillier, A.: Réalisation de la microradiographie intégrale. CR Acad. Sci. 190 (1930) 1287

Davies, J.D.: Pigmented periductal cells in normal and carcinomatous breasts. Arch. Pathol. 97 (1974) 369

Demarree, W.E.: Local recurrence following surgery for cancer of the breast. Ann. Surg. 134 (1951) 863

Dobrestsberger, W.: Die Fluidographie der weiblichen Brust. Elektromedica 4 (1967) 12

Doerr, W., Ule, G.: Spezielle Pathologische Anatomie III. Springer, Berlin 1970 (Heidelberger Taschenbücher 70 B)

Dominguez, C.M.: Estudio sistematizado del cancer del seno. Dol. Liga Urug. Cancer (Phila.) 4 (1929) 145

Douglas, J.G., Shivas, A.A.: The origins of elastica in breast carcinoma. J. Coll. Surg. Edinburgh 19 (1974) 89

Dubrauszcky, V., Cura, C.O.: Proliferative Vorgänge in der Brustdrüse und ihre Bedeutung bei der Geschwulstbildung. Gynaekol. Rundsch. 10 (1970) 241

Egan, R.L.: Experience with mammography in a tumor institute. Evaluation of 1000 studies. Radiology 75 (1960) 894

Egan, R.L.: Mammography: Report on 2000 studies. Surgery 53 (1963) 291

Egan, R.L.: Mammography, 2nd Ed. Thomas, Springfield 1972

Egan, R.L., Ellis, J.T., Powell, R.W.: Team approach to the study of disease of the breast. Cancer (Phila.) 23 (1969) 847

Evans, K.T., Gravelle, I.H.: Mammography, Thermography and Ultrasonography in Breast Disease. Butterworths, London 1973

Fergason, J.L.: Liquid crystals. Sci. Am. 211 (1964) 77

Finsterer, H., Prechtel, K.: Vergleichende cyto-histomorphologische Untersuchungen umschriebener krankhafter Brustdrüsenveränderungen. Arch. Gynaekol. 211 (1971) 57

Fleming cited from Vetter et al. 1974

von Fournier, D., Kubli, F., Kuttig, H., Curland, C., Hüter, J.:

Häufigkeitsverteilung der Malignitätszeichen bei der Mammographie. Med. Welt 26 (1975) 2211

von Fournier, D., Kuttig, H., Curland, St.: Zur Elektronen-Pendelbestrahlung der Thoraxwand. Strahlentherapie 144 (1972) 393

Franzen, S., Zajcek, Z.: Aspiration biopsy in diagnosis of palpable lesions of the breast. Acta Radiol. 7 (1968) 241

Friesen, H., Hwang, P.: Human prolactin. Annu. Rev. Med. 24 (1973) 251

Gallagher, H.S., Martin, J.E.: The study of mammary carcinoma by mammography and whole organ sectioning. Cancer (Phila.) 23 (1969) 855

Gallagher, H.S. (ed.): Early Breast Cancer, Diagnosis and Treatment. American College of Radiology, Wiley, New York 1975

Gershon-Cohen, J.: Breast roentgenology, historical review. Am. J. Roentgenol. 86 (1961) 879

Gershon-Cohen, J.: Atlas of Mammography. Springer, Berlin 1970

Gershon-Cohen, J., Colcher, A.E.: Evaluation of roentgen diagnosis of early carcinoma of the breast. J. Am. Med. Assoc. 108 (1937) 867

Gershon-Cohen, J., Berger, S.M., Curcio, M.: Breast cancer with microcalcifications. Diagnostic difficulties. Radiology 87 (1966) 613

Gershon-Cohen, J., Habermann, J.A.D., Brüschke, E.E.: Medical thermography: a summary of current status. Radiol. Clin. North Am. 3 (1965) 403

Gershon-Cohen, J., Hermell, M.B., Berger, S.M.: Detection of breast cancer by periodic x-ray examination; five year study. J. Am. Med. Assoc. 176 (1961) 1114

Gershon-Cohen, J., Strickler, A.: Roentgenologic examination of the normal breast: its evaluation in demonstration early neoplastic changes. Am. J. Roentgenol. 40 (1938) 189

Geschickter, C.F.: Diseases of the Breast, 2nd Ed. Lippincott, Philadelphia 1945

Goby, P.: Une application nouvelle des rayons X: La microradiographie. Compt. Rend. 156 (1913) 686

Gregl, A., Poppe, H.: Klinische und röntgenologische Symptomatik der sezernierenden Brust. J. Radiol. Electrol. 48 (1967) 723

Gros, Ch.M.: Les maladies du sein. Masson, Paris 1963

Gros, Ch.M., Bourjat, P., Gautherie, M.: Die Diagnose von Brustkarzinomen durch Infrarot-Thermographie. Fortschr. Geb. Roentgenstr. 116 (1972) 669

Gros, Ch.M., Walter, J.P., Girardie, H., Schmeltzer, A.: Ecoulements mammelonnaires lactoïdes et endostose. J. Radiol. Electrol. 46 (1965) 827

Grünberg, G., Rupp, N., Weiss, H.-D., Kramann, B.: Die Röntgensymptome der Milchgangserkrankungen in der Galaktographie und ihre Wertigkeit im Vergleich mit zytologischen und histologischen Befunden. Fortschr. Geb. Roentgenstr. 121 (1974) 335

Günther, D., Hennemann, H.M., Stoyanov, D.: Das männliche Mammakarzinom. Radiologe 13 (1973) 465

Gullino, P.M., Gromtham, F.H.: The influence of the host and the neoplastic cell population on the collagen content of a tumor mass. Cancer Res. 23 (1963) 648

Haagensen, C.D.: Diseases of the Breast, 2nd Ed. Saunders, Philadelphia 1971

Habermann, J.D.: The present status of mammary thermography. Cancer (Phila.) 18 (1968) 315

Halama, J.: Das metastasierende Mammakarzinom in strahlenklinischer Sicht, Radiologie 6 (1966) 27

Halama, J., Scherer, E.: Die Strahlenbehandlung der Orbitaltumoren. Münch. Med. Wochenschr. 106 (1964) 1976

Hall, P.: Gynecomastia. Monogr. Fed. Counc. Br. Med. Assoc. Aust. 2 (1959) 468

Hamlin, J.M.: Possible host resistence in carcinoma of the breast. A histological study. Br. J. Cancer 22 (1968) 383

Hamperl, H.: Zur Frage der pathologisch-anatomischen Grundlagen der Mammographie. Geburtshilfe Frauenheilk. 28 (1968) 901

Hamperl, H.: Sekretionserscheinungen in der mastopathischen Brust. Virchows Arch. B 18 (1975) 73

Hassler, O.: Microradiographic investigations of calcifications of the female breast. Cancer (Phila.) 23 (1969) 1103

Haupt, R.: Primärtumor und Metastase im histologischen Bild. Zentralbl. Allg. Pathol. Pathol. Anat. 113 (1970) 179

Heilmayer, L., Begemann, H.: Atlas der klinischen Hämatologie und Zytologie. Springer, Berlin 1955

Hellström, I., Hellström, K.E.: Some aspects of the immune defense against cancer. Cancer (Phila.) 28 (1971) 1269

Hess, F., Löhr, H.H.: Die Strahlentherapie des Mammakarzinoms. Radiologe 13 (1973) 457

Hoeffken, W., Lanyi, M.: Mammography. Saunders, Philadelphia 1977

Hofmann, W.D., Kern, G.: Die mikroskopische Untersuchung von Brustdrüsensekreten. Geburtshilfe Frauenheilk. 30 (1970) 525

Hüppe, J.R.: Die Optimierung der Mammographie aus klinisch-radiologischer Sicht. Radiologe 10 (1970) 128

Hutter, R.V.P., Kim, D.U.: The problem of multiple lesions of the breast. Cancer (Phila.) 28 (1971) 1591

Ingleby, H., Gershon-Cohen, J.: Comparative Anatomy, Pathology and Roentgenology of the Breast. Univ. Pennsylvania Press, Philadelphia 1960

Jackson, J.G., Orr, J.W.: The ducts of carcinomatous breasts with particular reference to connective-tissue changes. J. Pathol. Bacteriol. 74 (1957) 265

Jones, G.H.: Interpretation Problems in Thermography of the Female Breast. Karger, Basel 1969

Kleinschmidt, O.: In Zweifel-Payr: Klinik der bösartigen Geschwülste, Vol. 4. Hirzel, Leipzig 1927

Kley, H.K., Krüskemper, H.L.: Gynäkomastie. Dtsch. Med. Wochenschr. 100 (1975) 2612

Klose, H., Sebening, W.: Die Chirurgie der Brustdrüse. In: Kirschner, M., Nordmann, O. (eds.): Chirurgie, 2nd Ed., Vol. 5. Urban & Schwarzenberg, Berlin 1941

Koehl, R.H., Snyder, R.E., Hutter, R.V.P., Foote, F.W., Jr.: The incidence and significance of calcifications within operative breast specimens. Am. J. Clin. Pathol. 53 (1970) 3

Kramer, W.M., Rush, B.F.: Mammary duct proliferation in the elderly. A histologic study. Cancer (Phila.) 31 (1973) 130

Kraus, B.: Zur histologischen Klassifizierung des Mammakarzinoms. Z. Allgemeinmed. 34 (1973) 1675

Kraus, F.T., Neubecker, R.D.: The differential diagnosis of papillary tumors of the breast. Cancer (Phila.) 15 (1962) 444

Kreuzer, G., Boquoi, E., Meyer, R.D.: Die Diagnostik gut- und bösartiger Mammatumoren. Dtsch. Med. Wochenschr. 98 (1973) 691

Krokowski, E.: Betrachtung zur Dynamik des Geschwulstwachstums. In: Gottron, H.A. (eds.): Krebsforschung und Krebsbekämpfung, Vol. 5. Urban & Schwarzenberg, München 1964

Lamarque, P.: Microradiography. Radiology 27 (1936) 563

Lang, W.R., Renwick, S., Johnson, L., Wyse, E.: Benign mammary dysplasia. Med. J. Aust. 2 (1972) 147

Levitan, L.H., Witten, D.M., Harrison, E.G.: Calcifications in breast disease mammographic-pathologic correlation. Am. J. Roentgenol. 92 (1964) 29

Löhr, H., Hess, F., Karnahl, H.M., Wurche, K.D.: Postoperative Strahlenbehandlung des Mammakarzinoms. Chirurg 43 (1972) 119

Logan, W.W. (ed): Breast Carcinoma. The Radiologist's Expanded Role. American College of Radiology, Wiley, New York 1977

de Luca, J.T.: A statistical comparison study of patients undergoing breast biopsy at a community hospital over a 16-year period. Radiology 112 (1974) 315

Lundmark, D.: Breast cancer and elastosis. Cancer (Phila.) 30 (1972) 1195

McDivitt, R.W., Stewart, F.W., Berg, J.W.: Tumors of the Breast. Atlas of Tumor Pathology. 2nd Ser., Fasc. 2nd Armed Forces Institute of Pathology, Washington 1968

Macy, J.G.: Documenta Geigy, Wissenschaftliche Tabellen, Ciba-Geigy, Basel, and Thieme, Stuttgart 1975, 684–685

Menges, V., Troxler, A., Stadelmann, R., Wirth, W.: Galaktographie: Indikation und diagnostische Aussage. Fortschr. Geb. Roentgenstr. 120 (1974) 381

Minkowitz, S., Hedayati, H., Hiller, S., Gantner, B.: Klinisch-histopathologische Untersuchungen über die fibröse Mastopathie. Cancer (Phila.) 32 (1973) 913

Müller, K.-H.G., Barth, V.: Peau d'orange – kein sicherer Hinweis für diffus wachsendes Mammakarzinom. Fortschr. Geb. Roentgenstr. 120 (1974) 104

Müller, R., Barth, V., Heuck, F.: Plattenthermographie (Thermographie en plaque) der Mamma. Erste Erfahrungen mit einer neuen thermographischen Untersuchungsmethode. Dtsch. Med. Wochenschr. 99 (1974) 72

Müller, R., Barth, V., Spaich, I.: Kasuistischer Beitrag zum Krankheitsbild der Milchgangsfistel bei sezernierender Milchgangserkrankung. Fortschr. Geb. Roentgenstr. 119 (1973) 486

Murad, T.M., von Haam, F.: Die Ultrastruktur fibrozystischer Brusterkrankungen. Cancer (Phila.) 22 (1968) 587

Nizze, H.: Zum morphologischen Verhalten des Mantelbindegewebes bzw. Stromas in verschiedenen Brustdrüsenveränderungen. Arch. Geschwulstforsch. 40 (1972a) 320

Nizze, H.: Zur Biomorphose des Mantelbindegewebes der weiblichen Brustdrüse. Virchows Arch. A 356 (1972b) 259

Nunnerly, H.B., Field, S.: Mammary duct injection in patients with nipple discharge. Br. J. Radiol. 45 (1972) 717

Nyirjesy, J.: Galactorrhea without amenorrhea. Obstet. Gynecol. 32 (1968) 52

Olbricht, J.: Der Aussagewert der Plattenthermographie im Vergleich mit der klinischen und mammographischen Untersuchung. Diss. Marburg Univ. 1975

Ozzello, L.: Epithelial-stromal junction of normal and dysplastic mammary glands. Cancer (Phila.) 25 (1970) 586

Ozzello, L., Sanpitak, P.: Epithelial-stromal junction of intraductal carcinoma of the breast. Cancer (Phila.) 26 (1970) 1186

Picard, J.-D.: Le sein, the breast. Ann. Radiol. 17 (1974)

Pittner, J., Schmidt, G., Barth, V.: Die Hormontherapie des generalisierten Mammakarzinoms. Z. Allgemeinmed. 34 (1973) 1695

Prechtel, K.: Mastopathie und altersabhängige Brustdrüsenveränderungen. Fortschr. Med. 89 (1971) 1312

Prechtel, K.: Allgemeine Erläuterungen zur Histomorphologie von Brustdrüsenerkrankungen. Fortschr. Med. 92 (1974) 374

Quimet-Oliva, D., Hebert, G.: Galactography: a method of detection of unsuspected cancers. Am. J. Roentgenol. 120 (1974) 55

Rahn, J.: Das Mastion: I. Normale Anatomie, Physiologie und Biomorphose. Zentralbl. Allg. Pathol. Pathol. Anat. 115 (1972a) 326

Rahn, J.: Das Mastion: II. Zur pathologischen Anatomie unter besonderer Berücksichtigung des Mantelbindegewebes. Zentralbl. Allg. Pathol. Pathol. Anat. 116 (1972b) 22

Ries, E.: Diagnostic lipidol injection into milk ducts followed by abscess formation. Am. J. Obstet. Gynec. 20 (1930) 414

van Ronnen, J.F.: Het Roentgenonderzek van der Mamma Zonder Toepassing van Contrastmiddeln. Mouton, Utrecht 1956

Rummel, W., Kindermann, G., Weishaar, J.: Röntgenologische Milchgangsdarstellung (Galaktographie) bei pathologischer Sekretion aus der Mamille. Milchgangsexzision nach Urban und eine ihr angepaßte histologische Aufarbeitung. Geburtshilfe Frauenheilk. 29 (1969) 967

Sachs, H.: Erkrankungen der Brustdrüse der Frau. Chir. Prax. 15 (1971) 561

Salomon, A.: Beiträge zur Pathologie und Klinik der Mammakarzinome. Arch. Klin. Chir. 103 (1913) 573

Schremmer, C.N.: Myothelien und Mammakarzinom. Arch. Geschwulstforsch. 35 (1970) 114

Schwaiger, M., Herfarth, Ch.: Erkrankungen der Brustdrüse. In: Schwalm, H., Döderlein, G. (eds.): Klinik der Frauenheilkunde und Geburtshilfe, Vol. 7. Urban & Schwarzenberg, München 1967

Schwarz, S.R.: An improved method for the preparation of whole organ mounts for light microscopy. Localization of calcium salts and correlative radiolographic technics using whole breasts. Am. J. Clin. Pathol. 51 (1969) 511

Seifert, G.: Die Calciphylaxie der Langerhansschen Inseln beim Alloxan-Diabetes. Virchows Arch. 339 (1965) 29

Seifert, J.: Das Mammogramm und seine Deutung. Steinkopf, Darmstadt 1975

Selawry, O.S., Holland, J.F.: Cholesteric thermography for direct visualization of temperatures over tumors. Proc. Am. Assoc. Cancer Res. 7 (1966) 63

Shivas, A.A., Douglas, J.G.: The prognostic significance of elastosis in breast carcinoma. J. Coll. Surg. Edinburgh 17 (1972) 315

Sievert, R.: Two methods of roentgen microradio-photography. Acta Radiol. 17 (1936) 218

Silverberg, S.G., Chitale, A.R., Levitt, S.H.: Prognostic implications of fibrocystic dysplasia in breasts removed for mammary carcinoma. Cancer (Phila.) 29 (1972) 574

Snyder, R.E., Rosen, P.: Radiography of breast specimens. Cancer (Phila.) 28 (1971) 1806

Soost, H.J., Ries, P.: Die Zytologie der Brustdrüsensekrete und ihre Bedeutung für die Früherkennung des Mammakarzinoms. Geburtshilfe Frauenheilk. 28 (1968) 918

Spitalier, J.M., Pollet, J.F., Seigle, J., Robert, F., Amalric, R.: Cesium thérapie curative des cancers du sein à espérance conservatrice. Résultats. Excerpta Med. Sect. 16 Vol. 52 (1973) 301

Stegner, H.E.: Klinisch-histopathologische Korrelation beim Mammakarzinom. Arch. Gynaekol. 211 (1971) 46

Stegner, H.E., Pape, C.: Beitrag zur Feinstruktur der sog. Mikrokalzifikation in Mammatumoren. Zentralbl. Allg. Pathol. Pathol. Anat. 115 (1972) 106

Tabar, L., Kadas, J., Marton, Z., Nemeth, A., Kosaras, B.: The significance of mammography, galactography and pneumocystography in detection of occult carcinomas of the breast. Surg. Gynecol. Obst. 137 (1973) 965

Threatt, B., Appelman, H.D: Mammary duct injection. Radiology 108 (1973) 71

Tricoire, J., Mariel, L., Amiel, J.P., Poirot, G., Lacour, J., Fajbisowicz, S.: Thermographie en plaque. Press Méd. 78 (1970) 2483

Turkington, R.W.: Serum prolactin levels in patients with gynecomastia. J. Clin. Endocrinol. 34 (1972) 62

Underwood, J.C.: A morphometric analysis of human breast carcinoma. Br. J. Cancer 26 (1972) 234

Vaillant, W.K.Th.: Versuche zur Früherkennung des Mammakarzinoms durch Thermographie. Diss. München Univ. 1970

Vetter, L., Krauer, F., Wyss, H.: Galactorrhea. A report on 50 cases. Arch. Gynaekol. 216 (1974) 81

Vogel, W.: Die Röntgendarstellung von Mammatumoren. Arch. Klin. Chir. 171 (1932) 618

Walchshofer, E.: Über Rückbildungsvorgänge in der alternden Mamma. Dtsch. Z. Chir. 224 (1930) 137

Wallace, J.W., Champion, H.R.: Histological features of the primary tumour contributing to the prognosis in breast cancer. Br. J. Surg. 58 (1971) 862

Wallace, T.J.: Radiographic identification of calcifications in breast specimens. Cancer (Phila.) 21 (1971) 11

Walther, H.E.: Krebsmetastasen. Schwabe, Basel 1948

Warner, N.E.: Lobular carcinoma of the breast. Cancer (Phila.) 23 (1969) 840

Warren, L., Sr.: A roentgenologic study of the breast. Am. J. Roentgenol. 24 (1930) 113

Webster, G.V.: Gynecomastia in the navy. Mil. Surg. 95 (1944) 375

Webster, J.P.: Mastectomy for gynecomastia through a semicircular intra-areolar incision. Am. Surg. 124 (1946) 557

Weishaar, J., Rummel, W.-D., Kindermann, G.: Die Milchgangdarstellung mit wasserlöslichem Kontrastmittel bei sezernierender Mamma. Fortschr. Geb. Roentgenstr. 112 (1970) 1

Wellings, S.R., Jentoft, V.L.: Organ cultures of normal, dysplastic, hyperplastic and neoplastic human mammary tissues. J. Nat. Cancer Inst. 49 (1972) 329

Wellings, S.R., Wolfe, J.N.: Correlative studies of the histological and radiographic appearance of the breast parenchyma. Radiology 129 (1978) 299

Willemin, A.: Mammographic Appearances. Karger, Basel 1972

Witten, D.: The Breast. (American College of Radiology Atlas Series) Year Book, Chicago 1969

Wöllgens, P., Barth, V.: Die Therapie des Mammakarzinoms aus strahlentherapeutischer Sicht. Z. Allgemeinmed. 34 (1973) 1683

Wöllgens, P., Barth, V., Voss, A.Ch., Klöckner, D.: Das lokale Frührezidiv beim Mammakarzinom. Eine vergleichende Studie von 5 verschiedenen Bestrahlungstechniken bei 368 Patienten. Strahlentherapie 146 (1973) 1

Wolfe, J.N.: Mammography: errors in diagnosis. Radiology 87 (1966) 214

Wolfe, J.N.: Mammography: ducts as a sole indicator of breast carcinoma. Radiology 89 (1967) 206

Wolfe, J.: Xeroradiography of the Breast. Thomas, Springfield 1972

Zajdela, A., Ghossein, N.A., Pilleron, J.P., Ennuyer, A.: The value of aspiration cytology in the diagnosis of breast cancer. Experience at the Fondation Curie. Cancer (Phila.) 35 (1975) 499

Zajicek, J.: Monographs in Clinical Cytology. Aspiration Biopsy Cytology. Karger, Basel 1974. 136

Zinser, H.-K.: Mamma-Karzinom, Diagnose und Differentialdiagnose. Thieme, Stuttgart 1972

Zuckermann, H.C.: Mammography in the Diagnosis of Cancer of the Breast. In: Ariel, I.M. (ed.): Progress in Clinical Cancer, Vol. 1. Grune and Stratton, New York 1965. 185

Index

Numbers printed in normal print refer to page numbers.
Numbers printed in *italics* refer to figure numbers.

N

O

T

U

V

W

X